INTEGRATIVE FAMILY AND SYSTEMS TREATMENT (I-FAST)

INTEGRATIVE FAMILY AND SYSTEMS TREATMENT (I-FAST) | A STRENGTHS-BASED COMMON FACTORS APPROACH

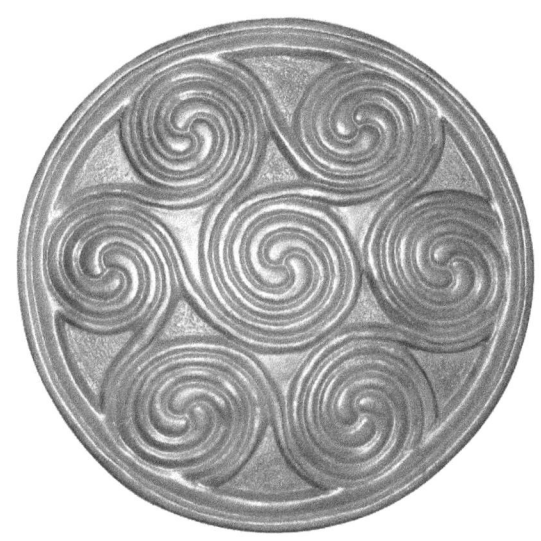

J. Scott Fraser, Ph.D., ABPP

David R. Grove, MSW, LISW-S

Mo Yee Lee, Ph.D.

Gilbert J. Greene, Ph.D., LISW-S

Andrew D. Solovey, MSW, LISW-S

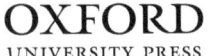

UNIVERSITY PRESS

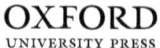

Oxford University Press is a department of the University of
Oxford. It furthers the University's objective of excellence in research,
scholarship, and education by publishing worldwide.

Oxford New York
Auckland Cape Town Dar es Salaam Hong Kong Karachi
Kuala Lumpur Madrid Melbourne Mexico City Nairobi
New Delhi Shanghai Taipei Toronto

With offices in
Argentina Austria Brazil Chile Czech Republic France Greece
Guatemala Hungary Italy Japan Poland Portugal Singapore
South Korea Switzerland Thailand Turkey Ukraine Vietnam

Oxford is a registered trademark of Oxford University Press
in the UK and certain other countries.

Published in the United States of America by
Oxford University Press
198 Madison Avenue, New York, NY 10016

© Oxford University Press 2014

All rights reserved. No part of this publication may be reproduced, stored in
a retrieval system, or transmitted, in any form or by any means, without the prior
permission in writing of Oxford University Press, or as expressly permitted by law,
by license, or under terms agreed with the appropriate reproduction rights organization.
Inquiries concerning reproduction outside the scope of the above should be sent to the
Rights Department, Oxford University Press, at the address above.

You must not circulate this work in any other form
and you must impose this same condition on any acquirer.

Library of Congress Cataloging-in-Publication Data
Integrative family and systems treatment (I-FAST) : a strengths-based common factors approach / J. Scott Fraser, Ph.D., ABPP [and 4 others].
pages cm
ISBN 978–0–19–936896–9 (paperback)
1. Family psychotherapy. 2. Family psychotherapy—Case studies. 3. Child mental health services. 4. Teenagers—Mental health services. 5. Evidence-based psychotherapy. 6. Integrated delivery of health care. I. Fraser, J. Scott.
RC488.5.I515 2014
616.89'156—dc23
2014000963

CONTENTS

Preface vii

PART ONE
I-FAST FOUNDATIONS

1	Integrative Family and Systems Treatment (I-FAST): A Meta-Model	3
2	I-FAST: Integrative Family and Systems Treatment	21

PART TWO
I-FAST PHASES, SKILLS, AND TECHNIQUES

3	Engaging	41
4	Tracking Interactions	61
5	Goal Development and Consensus	79
6	Frames, Framing, and Reframing	95
7	Initiating Change	109
8	Building Resilience and Terminating/Stepping Down	134
9	Some Final Thoughts on Practice	148

PART THREE
I-FAST SUPERVISION, AGENCY CONSIDERATIONS, AND SUSTAINABILITY

10	Teaching and Supervising I-FAST	159
11	Fitting I-FAST and Agency Together: Creating Sustainability	187

PART FOUR
RESEARCH ON I-FAST

12	Research on Integrative Family and Systems Treatment	205

REFERENCES	233
INDEX	243

PREFACE

This work has its foundations in collaboration and integration. We are deeply indebted to each other as well as to all of the therapists, administrators, families and agencies who worked with us over the course of developing this integrative approach. While each of us as co-authors have had long careers in doing, teaching and writing about family and systems therapy, we have each practiced from somewhat different approaches and models. As colleagues, we also realized that each of our approaches was effective and we respected each other's work. We have also all variously written and been passionate about psychotherapy integration, and so this project addressing integration across models of treatment with at-risk youth and families was a natural product of all of our values and interests. This integration has happened as a result of many hours of thoughtful dialogue, conversations and even through some heated arguments. Needless to say, we are all equal contributors to the development of *Integrative Family and Systems Treatment (I-FAST)* and we appreciate the learning that has emerged from among us as a team. This product has evolved over more than a decade.

As consultants and practitioners, we had also become aware of the growing pressures in the practitioner and agency communities to employ "evidence-based" approaches to treatment; and of the growing dissatisfaction of practitioners and agencies with trying to fit and sustain these pre-packaged approaches to their own unique styles, skills, agency designs and clients served. Practitioners were crying out, as it were, both in the literature and in practice, for evidence supported approaches that would better fit themselves, their practices, agencies and clients, and thus become more sustainable as well as affordable. There were and still are a number of excellent evidence-based models for working with at-risk youth and families, and yet each of them requires rather expensive training and ongoing supervision along with somewhat rigid guidelines of who to serve and exactly how to deliver each model. Practitioners longed for a more adaptable and flexible approach they could fit to their practice and manage on their own after initial introduction and training. They were feeling disempowered and longed for an empowerment model that would utilize their own strengths and build upon the strengths of their clients. This model and manual is a product of collaboration with a great number of agencies and practitioners, along with state mental health funding agencies over a great number of years to develop, refine and study the effectiveness of just such a flexible and effective treatment model. Our hope has been to develop a sustainable, evidence-supported family approach that allows families and practitioners alike to utilize and build upon their own strengths. This resulting model aims to be a meta-level treatment approach allowing practitioners to utilize their own perspectives and views while embracing broadly agreed upon components of all effective treatment across different approaches. It is designed to enable agencies and professionals to flexibly serve youth and families with diverse problems in diverse communities and cultures. It seeks to bridge the gap between approaches built on factors common to all effective treatment and those targeting more specific active ingredients. After long collaboration and development in the field of practice outside the university clinical research lab of more traditional approaches, we feel we have come close to those goals with this model we have chosen to call *Integrative Family and Systems Treatment or I-FAST*. For inquiries regarding I-FAST in general and information about I-FAST training please visit our web site at: IFASTmodel.org.

We have many people to thanks for this book; yet first our appreciation must go to Joan Bossert, Vice President and Publisher; Dana Bliss, Editor of Social Work;

and to all the other staff at The Oxford University Press. Their enthusiastic support for our work has made this book a reality.

Scott Fraser is deeply indebted to his family. To his mother, Frances Rose Preston Fraser, for her love and unflagging encouragement to "aim for the top of the tree!" And to his wife and lifelong partner, Beth, for being his rock; and to his children, Chris and Heather, as his pride and inspiration. Thank you is not enough.

Dave Grove is indebted to his mother, Miriam Brierley, who has offered unwavering support, his step father, Gerald Brierley who helped him develop a critical mind and encouraged him to participate in innovative research, and to his wife, Thazin Nu his closest companion.

Mo Yee Lee is especially thankful for her mother, Sho Yean Chan, who has given her the greatest gift of life; Kwok Kwan Tam for sharing his passion; and her two children, and daughter-in-law, Tze Hei, Hok Hei, and Brooke, for showing her how to be curious, creative, and playful about life.

Gilbert "Gil" Greene is thankful to his family-or-origin - late parents Grover and Julia and his brothers Don, Chris, Tony and Greg (deceased) – for teaching him about the rewards and challenges of family life. He is especially thankful to his daughter Gina, son-in-law Mark Hill, and grandson Dodge for their steady support and love while keeping him humble. And finally he wants to acknowledge the invaluable influence of some of his mentors: Drs. Palassana "Bal" Balgopal, Donald Brieland (deceased), Norman Denzin, Oakley Ray (deceased), Joseph Eades, and John Craft (deceased).

Andy Solovey is grateful to his wife Donna for her encouragement and support; and his three children Nick, Steven, and Anne who were willing to listen and engage in endless discussion about I-FAST. He would like to acknowledge his Mom, Olga, who passed away during the time this work was being written, and his Dad (Babe) who taught him to think outside the box.

In addition, a special thank-you goes out to Andy's colleagues and friends, and our collaborators at Scioto Paint Valley Mental Health Center. The clinic directors including Sue Peek, Ed Sipe, Mary Snyder, Kathleen Pallotta, and Vince Yaniga played a significant role in the initial implementation of I-FAST. Their hard work and dedication to the provision of excellent care to at-risk kids, and their families, is a tribute to what is possible in community mental health. Also to the staff of the Thompkins Child and Adolescent Services, especially Phil Washburn, Chuck Larrick, and Chris Gallagher for their collaboration. We are also indebted to the initial three-year funding support we received from the Ohio Department of Mental Health and the then director of the Office of Program Evaluation and Research, Dee Roth.

Lastly, we are deeply indebted to the clients and families we met, practitioners we have consulted with, and agencies we have worked with both in the US, Hong Kong, Germany and India. "To teach is to learn twice." (Joseph Joubert, 1754-1824) They have been our greatest teachers.

J. Scott Fraser
David R. Grove
Mo Yee Lee
Gilbert J. Greene
Andrew D. Solovey
January 20, 2014

I-FAST FOUNDATIONS

1

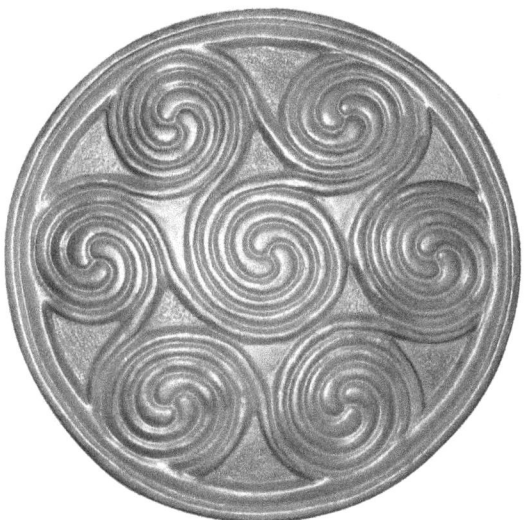

The Integrative Family and Systems Treatment, or I-FAST, is based on a set of flexible ideas and approaches common to most all effective treatments. It is essentially a systems approach that views all of us as functioning within multiple systems. This includes our clients as well as ourselves as interveners, the groups or agencies we work within, and the systems and agencies, communities, and cultures in which we are all imbedded. This also includes the idea that most all effective treatments have common golden threads that unite them. Problems and their resolutions are seen as spirals of interaction among all involved. Problems are seen as vicious cycles or spirals of problem engendering attempts to resolve a difficulty. Solutions or resolutions are viewed as virtuous cycles or again spirals of interaction that help all involved move on.

The ancient Celtic spiral design above and on the cover of this manual has been chosen on purpose. It presents a circle of concentric and interconnected spirals. This may be viewed as the multiple family members involved in each case seen, or the multiple systems involved with each family, or the multiple effective approaches to similar problems, and/or all of the above. The first set of chapters of this workbook lays the foundation for this view.

INTEGRATIVE FAMILY AND SYSTEMS TREATMENT (I-FAST)

A META-MODEL

INTRODUCTION

In recent years, there has been an increasing demand for practitioners that work with behavioral health concerns to use treatment approaches with a demonstrated record of effectiveness. This is particularly true for those working in social service, mental health, and criminal justice agencies dealing with youth who are engaged in disruptive, destructive, substance abusing, and other similar behaviors that put them at risk for placement outside the home. These youth and their families are classically involved with multiple agencies and systems such as schools, police, courts, child protective services, foster care, psychiatric hospitals, and juvenile detention centers, to name but a few. The costs of services to these youth and families are so high in terms of financial costs, time spent, and emotional pain and anguish to all involved that effective intervention approaches for this population have been vigorously pursued by policymakers, funders, researchers, and practitioners.

Although intensive treatment both in the home and in the office is widely used for treating families with a child or adolescent who is at risk for out-of-home placement, mental health and juvenile justice agencies are consistently challenged to develop and provide realistic family-centered treatment that meets local needs, can realistically fit within available budget and resource capabilities, and is effective in accomplishing common goals. These goals typically include preventing out-of-home placement or residential placement of the symptomatic child; empowering the families to develop competence and confidence in addressing emotional and/or behavioral problems of children; supporting the development and continuity of expertise in case managers and practitioners at the agency level; collaborating with institutions such as juvenile courts and children services that determine placement; and applying approaches that are cost effective in attaining these general goals. Meanwhile, funding sources are increasingly requiring mental health and court agencies to use evidence-based approaches when providing treatment for at-risk families.

Fortunately, several well-established evidence-based approaches to working effectively with these high-risk youth and their families have become available. These include such models as *Brief Strategic Family Treatment* (*BSFT*) (Horigan et al., 2005; Szapocznik et al., 2002), *Multisystemic Treatment* (*MST*) (Henggeler, Schoenwold, Rowland, & Cunningham, 2002; Schoenwald & Henggeler, 2005), *Multidimensional Family Treatment* (*MDFT*) (Hogue, Liddle, & Becker, 2002; Hogue, Liddle, Becker, & Johnson-Leckrone, 2002; Liddle, Rodriguez, Dakof, Kanzki, & Marvel, 2005), and *Functional Family Treatment* (*FFT*) (Alexander & Sexton, 2002; Sexton & Alexander, 2002). These approaches represent integrative models, meaning that numerous pure form family treatment approaches and strategies are woven into each respective format. Each model is, in fact, a product of integrating numerous pure form family treatment approaches and strategies into each respective format. Each of these approaches is also the result of admirable and sustained work by a number of dedicated clinical research teams. These approaches have shown such impressive results with youth involved in juvenile courts, with substance abuse, and with conduct disordered and other general mental health difficulties that they have come to be designated as evidence-based approaches.

That these approaches are considered to be evidence based is both good and bad news for agencies wanting to employ best practices. The good news is that there are several approaches available. The bad news is that they are all generally equally effective with the same kinds of client problems and populations. Thus, how does one choose among them? Further good news is that most of these approaches have become "franchised" in that agencies may purchase treatment and training packages and consultation to implement each of them. The bad news is that the programs may be rather expensive for agencies and may require a somewhat demanding adherence to an array of parameters, which the agencies may or may not be able to support easily. In addition to initial and ongoing training time and expense, there is the common demand for strict fidelity to the treatment model, usually provided by practitioners with advanced degrees in one of the mental health professions, along with regular linkages for consultation and data collection and reporting. Although there are excellent arguments in support of each of these requirements, they frequently pose hurdles for agencies in adopting and/or sustaining the implementation of these established approaches to treating at-risk youth and families.

Aside from these very real practical dilemmas, a broader question remains as to what common elements, if any, these evidence-based approaches share that support their effectiveness. If these factors could be in some way synthesized, might there be an integrated approach, which could be equally effective and offer greater flexibility and cost-effectiveness in adaptation? This question is in no way meant to diminish the outstanding work behind each of these current evidence-based approaches. The point is to see whether each approach needs to be adopted fully in the way it was developed in the "lab" of its clinical trials, or if a synthesis of common factors shared among these approaches might be equally effective.

Integrative Family and Systems Treatment (I-FAST) is a meta-model based on identified factors that established approaches to family treatment have in common. Figure 1-1 describes I-FAST as a meta-model at the levels of theoretical/philosophical constructs, evidence-based common factors, and specific practice techniques. At the theoretical level, the development of I-FAST is influenced by systems theory and social constructivism. Philosophically, I-FAST is strength based and emphasizes the abilities and resources of individuals and families to make their lives successful, worthwhile, and fulfilling. At the level of evidence-based common factors, we have drawn upon the work of Jerome Frank on the common factors in psychotherapy and healing (Frank, 1961; Frank & Frank, 1991) and the meta-analyses of psychotherapy conducted by Bruce Wampold (2001, 2010a, 2010b) to identify the following treatment components as central to positive treatment outcomes in families:

1. Therapeutic alliance with families that will facilitate the collaborative development of a common understanding of the problem, behaviorally specific treatment goals, and activities to achieve these goals with the family.

2. Collaboratively work with the family members to change interactional patterns that will result in solving presenting problems and achieving treatment goals through using rationales and procedures that are consistent with the family's frame/view of the problem.
3. Develop and maintain collaborative teamwork with community agencies that includes the development of a service packet addressing the organic needs of the family and the child (systems collaboration).

Based on theory and evidence-based common factors, I-FAST provides meta-frames on practice techniques at different phases in the treatment process. These three levels are illustrated in Figure 1-1.

LEVEL I

Theoretical and Philosophical Foundations

When considering what keeps problems going and what changes them, within I-FAST two major areas are investigated: how family members and helpers think about the problem and what they actually do about it. We refer to this as *viewing and doing*. The theory of *social constructivism* offers one way to understand how people view problems. *Systems theory* offers a way to understand how individuals within social systems act toward problems, that is, what everyone actually does in response to the problem. These are the two main theories that inform I-FAST.

SYSTEMS THEORY

Systems theory provides one way to conceptualize problems. A system is "[a] set of units or component parts that together make up a whole arrangement or organization"

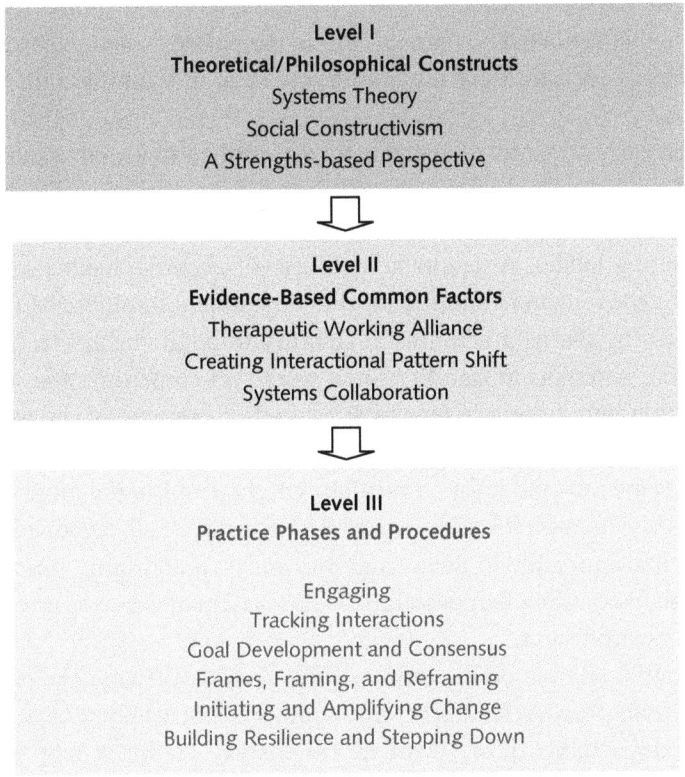

FIGURE 1-1
I-FAST as a meta-model.

(Goldenberg & Goldenberg, 2008, p. 472). For our purposes, the family and its members and the professionals involved with that family are the organization and units. Systems are goal directed, rule governed, and self-correcting. A primary goal of a system is to maintain itself as it interacts with its environment or to change itself as the environmental context of the system changes. These are referred to in systems theory as positive and negative feedback loops.

Negative feedback loops are *deviation reducing*. They are circular (nonlinear/recursive) processes of interaction among group members that seek to pull perceived differences from a desired norm or state back to the norm. If a child runs toward a busy street, parents call out warnings or act to stop her. If a youth stays out past his curfew, parents act to correct him, often instituting punishments to ensure that the violation doesn't happen again. In most instances, these negative feedback loops of interaction succeed in keeping the system or family well within its desired or normative patterns and rules.

Positive feedback loops are *deviation amplifying*. They are also circular interaction processes among group members, and yet the resulting interaction *increases* the differences from the initial starting points. A well-known mechanical example of this is the screech heard from holding a microphone too close to a speaker. A small noise from the speaker is picked up by the microphone, amplified by the system, put out in its louder form through the speaker, and then is picked up again by the microphone, only to repeat the cycle of amplification. This produces a deafening screech until the microphone is moved away, and the feedback loop is broken. The same happens in families when initial attempts at correction (or negative feedback) don't work. The youth may start arguing about having a too early time to be home. Parents may raise their voices, resulting in the same from the youth. Parents may then use harsher language and make harsher threats, met with the same from the youth. The youth may run from the home, followed by parents calling the police... and the escalating cycle evolves. Problems such as these are commonly seen in working with at-risk youth and families.

One of the early adapters of systems theory applied to social systems like families and the friends and agencies they are embedded within was Gregory Bateson (1972, 1979). Bateson described the evolution of interaction in human systems as a kind of alternating ladder. Attempts at stability (or negative feedback) at one level are followed by movement to another level of adjustment through positive feedback. This is followed by the next attempts at stability through negative feedback at that level, and so on. Attempts at stability often work, yet sometimes they create a trigger for escalation into a positive feedback cycle. For example, some attempts to get youths to come home on time work. Other times, the very attempt to correct the curfew violation is the kick point for an escalating fight, resulting in more curfew violations and a worse situation for all involved. Thus positive and negative feedbacks are linked. Sometimes attempts to create stability succeed and other times the attempt at stability is the very thing that destabilizes the system and moves it more and more away from its desired form.

There is one final note on the term *positive feedback*. Language can be confusing here. The term positive feedback says nothing about whether or not the escalating pattern is desired, good, or "positive." A positive feedback loop is simply one in which some deviation is amplified. The more of one thing that occurs is linked with the more of another thing happening. Positive feedback is escalation. We have noted the microphone-speaker screech and the curfew escalation between parents and youth, both of which have an implied negative value. We don't desire them. In this case, we would refer to these positive feedback loops as *vicious cycles*. The feedback escalated something *not desired*. However, there are as many or more examples of other positive feedback loops that increase desired results. A recent television commercial in the American market shows people observing kind deeds done by someone. Then the person who saw that kindness passes it on through another kind gesture for another. Someone else sees that kindness done and does another kind deed for another and so on. The message is to feed help and compassion forward, and then our culture will improve for it. The same happens when a child is commended for sharing or helping another child or an elder, for example. This may breed further reinforced helping, and so forth. Another example is asking someone how she could have possibly survived an overwhelming negative event. This implies a strength that that person must note, explain, and which may be built upon. In all of these examples, the positive feedback loop supports and amplifies *something desired, valued, or viewed as "positive."* We refer to the positive feedback loops in these instances as *virtuous cycles*. Whether a positive feedback cycle is labeled as a "vicious cycle" or a "virtuous cycle" is the result of a value judgment on what is being escalated. If what is being escalated or amplified is *not desirable*, we say it is a *vicious cycle*. If *desired* qualities or interactions are being amplified or escalated, we say that that is a *virtuous cycle*.

In most all effective treatment interventions, practitioners are noting, interrupting, and redirecting *vicious cycles*. At the same time, the goals of almost all effective interventions are to note, create, and then support *virtuous cycles*. This may seem easier said than done, and it often is. However, this process is at the heart of the I-FAST approach, as we will see.

For example: A Vicious Cycle Begins.

Parent yells and threatens child ⟶ Child acts out

Vicious Cycles

One primary implication of systems theory for I-FAST is the idea that problems are maintained by repeated interactions in response to the problem. As noted, we refer to these repeated interactions as *vicious cycles*, which are visually represented in Figure 1-2.

Once all members of a family and other involved systems determine that there is a problem, they all set about to solve it. In many instances, the usual solutions and resources that have been used by everyone involved *do* resolve the problem. On the other hand, if first attempts at the usual solutions do not work then more of the same solution is applied and actually intensified in frequency and intensity. A vicious cycle is under way. The initial difficulty has escalated into a true problem. In a manner of speaking, the vicious cycle may be referred to as an *interactional pattern* where all involved, including practitioners and other helpers, are drawn into the vortex of

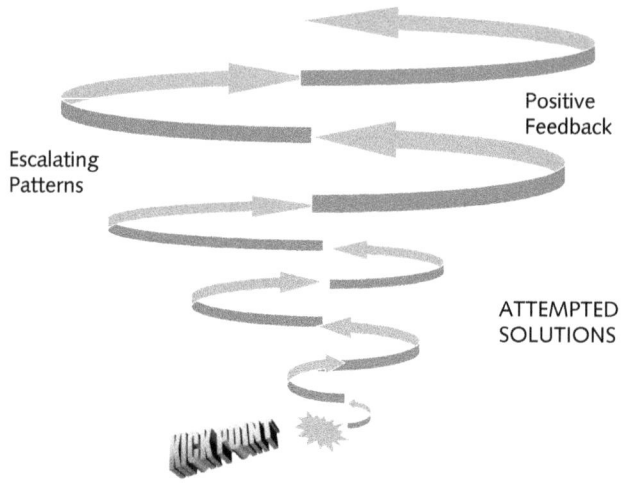

FIGURE 1-2
Vicious cycles.

repeated, rigid solutions that do nothing but escalate the cycle and make the problem worse. Further, none of this is done out of malice. Though everyone, including the identified clients, tends to become frustrated and often angry or depressed or anxious, we must assume that in most cases, they are all simply trying to solve the problem as defined by them in the very best way they can. A way of representing this solution-generated problem graphically appears in Figure 1-3. Both clients and natural helpers in their lives, as well as practitioners and other formal systems such as child protective services, schools, courts, and others get drawn into the same co-constructed definitions of the problem, drawing them into the same repeated patterns.

Changing Systems: Virtuous Cycles

Vicious cycles are positive feedback loops that keep the problem going and actually escalate it. The family and helpers are stuck in an interactional pattern that supports and increases the problem. However, just as some initial perceived difference or problem may have initiated this vicious cycle, another deviation, shift, or difference may similarly initiate a shift to a virtuous cycle. Such new or different responses can

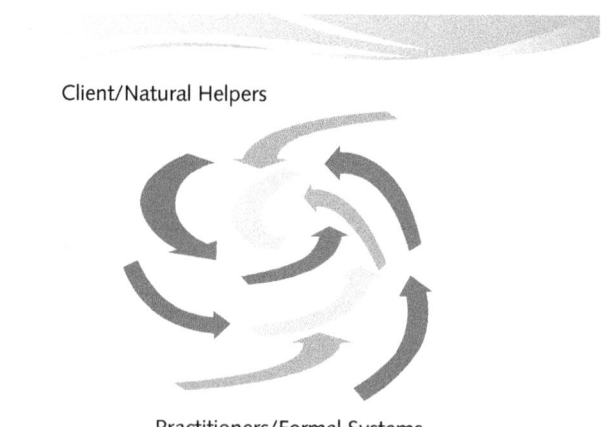

FIGURE 1-3
Problems as vicious cycles.

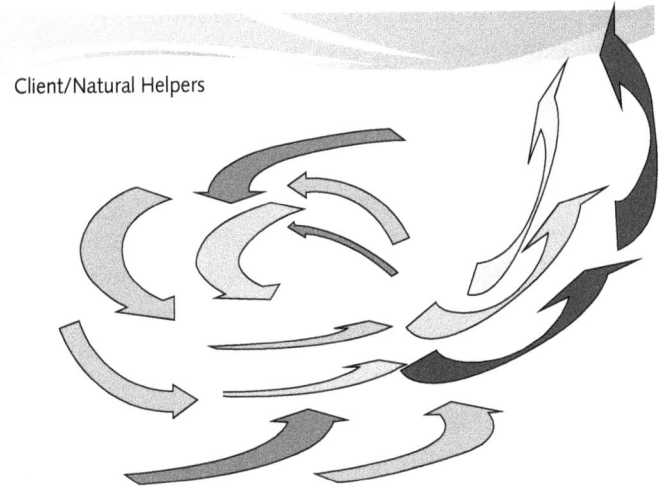

FIGURE 1-4
Intervention (clients/natural helpers).

change the system and create a domino effect throughout the organization. They are outside the box of what keeps the system going. For instance, systems theory suggests that change is constant in any system. As such, there must be times when the family is doing something different or interacts in different ways that do not keep the problem going. Identifying those *interactional exceptions* and setting a process going that utilizes them can change the system. This is called a *virtuous cycle*. Ultimately, a virtuous cycle will create enough change in the system that the system must reorganize and become a new system. Finding, amplifying, or creating responses to the problem that are outside the box of the vicious cycle that maintains it is the goal of intervention. A *virtuous cycle* is represented in Figure 1-4, showing the point when a vicious cycle is interrupted and redirected and a potential virtuous cycle is begun.

Practical Implications of Systems Theory

We have already discussed how interactional patterns, which support the problem, or vicious cycles, maintain and escalate problems. Commonly, such vicious problem cycles can begin when a family's interactions become incongruent with the life cycle and developmental tasks of that family (Haley, 1973). Families are not static systems. They must progress through developmental stages that require them to reorganize at each transition stage of development. This is a process of both assimilation and accommodation. It requires flexible adjustment and evolution of the family's ways of interacting. If cultural norms support greater independence and individuation of youth as they reach adolescence, then parents and other caretakers will need to gradually and often relatively quickly change from earlier correcting and guiding processes to support of more independent interaction with peers, clubs, school, and so on. If this shift is not made, then either the youth may be viewed as stuck in a "preadolescent dependence upon the family" or a vicious cycle of "rebellion" by the youth and escalating reactions from the family may start.

Interconnectedness and Wholeness

Systems theory also has major implications for how and with whom to intervene. Basic premises in systems theory include interconnectedness, wholeness, and interdependency. Systems theory assumes everything everyone does in a family interacts with everything everyone else in the family does. Although this may create very complex patterns, it often allows for very simple interventions. Because everything in a given family system interacts, a simple, unilateral intervention can change a complex family system. A so-called linear intervention may change a circular process. Interrupting a vicious cycle or identifying and amplifying ways it is already being interrupted can create a change that requires the entire family system to reorganize. In I-FAST, we may pick a particular person with a particular problem and assume that because everything is interconnected and interdependent, changing the interaction around that one problem will by necessity result in a multitude of additional changes. Systems theory allows for changing one person by changing another. An out-of-control teen can be helped by changing how his parents deal with him or her. Again, theoretically, the teen does not have to be seen directly by the practitioner. This assumption allows a practitioner to work primarily with whichever participants in a stuck pattern are the most motivated to change. In I-FAST one is not required to struggle to change a teen who is coming to treatment only to placate his or her parents. If the parents are the ones motivated to change, the practitioner can work with them to change their child's behavior. This principle allows us to encourage flexibility regarding whom to work with, allowing for working with individuals, whole families, or anyone in between.

Practically speaking, to change a family system, a change can be produced by one individual and that change must then be maintained until the rest of the group adjusts. This process suggests a treatment that involves three steps. In *step one*, a change is produced; in *step two* the family is helped to adjust to that change. In *step three*, the family is helped to own the change, build resilience, and welcomed back for another consult if they need it in the future. This requires three types of skills: how to get change going, how to keep it going after it is initiated, and how to help families own their successes and see the intervener or team as a helpful consultant they might use again if needed.

Change Is Constant

One basic assumption of systems theory is that change is constant. We are always interacting and changing within our environments and with ourselves. We are always adapting to new instances and to our own or others' growth and change physically, emotionally, and socially. As we discussed previously, we are always involved in the process of assimilating and accommodating to change. This is seen in what we have discussed about positive and negative feedback loops and vicious and virtuous cycles. Desired change may be seen as more and more of a good thing, as something we admire, support, and cheer for. Undesired change often serves as the trigger for corrective action that either works or results in escalating exactly the negative condition we hope to correct. As noted previously, these escalating negative changes are referred to as vicious cycles, or "the same damned thing over and over again." Our goal in the process of intervention is to observe the process of ongoing change in a system, whether it is an individual, a family, and/or larger systems. We need to note the defined problem patterns or changes going on in those systems. Then our task is to enter the process of ongoing change in that system and use that force of ongoing change to interrupt and redirect that changing process. We seek to initiate a new and desired virtuous cycle.

Once a vicious cycle is in full swing, most everything that happens among those caught within it is seen as negative. Those involved become frustrated, angry, and discouraged, and even start feeling hopeless. Vicious cycles tend to create world views, descriptions, and frames that are increasingly negative. A problem-saturated story is being shared by all involved, and everything that happens seems to be more of the same. Yet, within these ongoing and problematic patterns there are always exceptions to the rule: times when strengths are present, competencies are demonstrated, good deeds are done, and calm prevails. Negativity and weakness are rarely the rule in any ongoing patterned interaction, even if it is seen as dominated by a vicious cycle. There are always exceptions to the rules, and consequently every problem pattern includes these in one form or another (de Shazer, 1985). Such a view underlies a belief in the strengths and potentials of participants. Despite the multi-deficiencies and/or problems the families may perceive that they have, there are always times when they handle their life situations in a more satisfying way or in a different manner (Greene & Lee, 2011; Lee, Fraser, Greene, Solovey & Grove, 2003). These exceptions represent the family's "unnoticed" strengths and resources. By assisting people in noticing, identifying, amplifying, sustaining, and reinforcing these exceptions regardless of how small and/or infrequent they may be, people are already engaged in reinforcing the virtuous cycle for problem solving. Creating exceptions or redirections within vicious cycles and/or noting strengths in the face of adversity and times of differences from the problem pattern and then supporting, reinforcing, and amplifying them is another key process in the I-FAST model (Greene & Lee, 2011; Lee, Fraser, Greene, Solovey & Grove, 2003).

SOCIAL CONSTRUCTIVISM

Systems theory is closely related to the idea of social constructivism when we are working with human interaction. Simply speaking, the way we come to know and describe ourselves and others in our daily lives helps to define and channel how we then interact. If I have been brought up in the tradition that, for example, "children must be seen and not heard," or in the tradition of "spare the rod and spoil the child," my parenting will follow those rules or assumptions. If my parenting is guided alternatively, for example, by the idea that "you do your thing, and I'll do mine, and if we meet, it is likely to be beautiful," or "children are gifts from above and seeds to be watered, tended, and supported as they grow," then my parenting will likely follow a different path. Our way of viewing our world is shaped by and subsequently guides our doing within the world. Paying attention to the language and world view of all involved in any defined case, including attending to our own views, values, and language, offers a window into how systems define and direct their interaction. It also offers a window into how to facilitate change.

Constructivism posits that people come to "know" the world, to "know reality" by interacting with it—the people, the organizations, and the institutions within society. Thus, one's knowledge of reality is constructed through such social interactions (Berger & Luckman, 1967). The idea that a person's view of reality is socially constructed is not new. There are different "flavors" of constructivism but they all appear to have the following in common:

- There is not an objective social reality standing outside of individuals. Reality is not discovered but created by human observers.

- There is no such thing as an objective observer. The very act of observing changes that which is being observed.
- People are active participants in developing their knowledge of the world rather than passive recipients of stimulus–response interaction with their environment.
- Language and dialogue are integral to the social construction of reality.
- Our understanding of reality is co-constructed through social interaction.
- The cultural context affects how people interpret and co-construct reality.

Framing

Because communication can occur on more than one level at a time, *framing* helps explain how people communicate in ways that let others know at what level of abstraction a communication is to be taken and thus interpreted (Bateson, 1972). Lakoff (2008) explains that frames are smaller narratives that make up the more complex narrative of a person's life story. As in photography, the process of framing in social interaction involves focusing on one specific part of someone's reality and ignoring others (Fairhurst & Sarr, 1996):

> [j]ust like a photographer, when we select a frame for a subject, we choose which aspect or portion of the subject we will focus on and which we will exclude. When we choose to highlight some aspect of our subject over others, we make it more noticeable, more meaningful, and more memorable to others. Our framing adds color or accentuates the subject in unique ways. For this reason, frames determine whether people notice problems, how they understand and remember problems, and how they evaluate and act upon them. . . frames exert their power not only through what they highlight but also through what they leave out. (p. 4)

The framing process can be facilitated in a number of ways, such as:

- Showing special interest in what the other person is saying that is consistent with the desired frame
- Shifting the conversation to the desired frame by asking leading questions
- Telling stories and anecdotes consistent with the desired frame
- Connecting seemingly different ideas in conversation that are consistent with the desired frame

For a frame to be acceptable to the other person it must make sense to him or her; it needs to be consistent with his or her mental model (assumptions) of the world. At the beginning of treatment families often feel stuck, defeated, deficient, disempowered, and hopeless, with a low sense of personal agency, a negative view of self, and little if any confidence that positive change is possible. For practitioners to conjointly create positive change they need first to learn the family's frame for their presenting problem and then in conversation prime ideas that can become associated with the client's existing frame, which then can used in expanding it.

Social constructivism is the meta-construct that guides practitioners' ways of understanding the world view and language of their clients and the larger systems with which they are involved. Practitioners in I-FAST must come to terms with the idea that there is no one true reality. There can be multiple useful versions of reality, each of which will have been co-created by the individuals and members of the systems with which the practitioner is working. The social constructivist perspective encourages practitioners to be flexible and open to multiple points of view. Each viewpoint may be seen as a meta-frame with a wide range of frames within it for understanding the world and the behaviors of self and others. Paying attention to the frames being used by clients and larger systems involved with each case allows the practitioner to understand and have compassion for the behaviors of all involved with the case. It also allows practitioners to engage in the gentle art of reframing, de-framing, and the like to initiate and support the process of change. We will have much to say about this process as we move forward into sections describing the details of practice itself.

Philosophical Foundation: A Strengths-Based Perspective

I-FAST is premised on a "strengths-based" view of clients and the systems with which the clients are involved. This is to say that problems are rarely viewed as a result of deep-seated pathology, malevolent motives, or predetermined by negative histories. All involved with each case are viewed as having a wide range of positive qualities, values, and skills. They are assumed to be acting with the best of motives to try simply to resolve the problems at hand. The task of the practitioner is always to seek out and build upon strengths and points of resiliency.

According to McQuaide and Ehrenrich (1997), strength involves "the capacity to cope with difficulties, to maintain functioning in the face of stress, to bounce back in the face of significant trauma, to use external challenges as a stimulus for growth, and to use social supports as a source of resilience" (p. 203). The following positions flow from this stance, and represent premises of the I-FAST approach:

- Each person has varying levels of physical and intellectual strengths, abilities, and possibilities unique to him or her.
- People with high levels of strengths have good coping abilities; positive self-esteem; and a sense of self-efficacy, empowerment, resilience, and so forth (Saleebey, 2002).
- All people have strengths, including those with severe and/or multiple problems.
- A basic tenet of human behavior is that change is occurring all the time, even for people with long-term serious problems. For most people, their problem does fluctuate in frequency, intensity, or severity (Breulin, 1989). In fact, there may be times when they are entirely free of their problem.
- Consequently, it is worthwhile to try to identify what is different at those times. What is the client doing to make his situation better? What is different in his significant relationships and/or his environment at the times when his problem is better or not present? Can we not, together with the client, identify the strengths (resources, competencies, and assets) that are present at those times and work with the client to amplify those solutions to make desired changes so the situation is no longer a problem?
- A growing body of knowledge indicates that the latter is not only possible but also preferred.

LEVEL II

Evidence-Based Common Factors

I-FAST is a meta-model based on identified factors that established approaches to family treatment have in common. In developing I-FAST we have drawn upon the work of Jerome Frank on the common factors in psychotherapy and healing (Frank, 1961; Frank & Frank, 1991) and the meta-analyses of psychotherapy outcome effectiveness conducted by Bruce Wampold (2001, 2010a, 2010b). In analyzing change processes in various forms of treatment, cults, and indigenous practices in non-industrialized countries, and the placebo response in medical and psychological treatments, Frank concluded that there are four common factors that actually account for people changing. As summarized by Wampold (2010a, pp. 36–37) these factors are:

- **Relationship.** In the context of a trusting, emotionally charged relationship, the practitioner/healer is given special status and perceived to have powers to heal. In family treatment, the practitioner is a credentialed professional that clients perceive to be effective and to work in their best interests.
- **Rationale.** A rationale or "myth" explains the problem and offers a direction for resolution. The actions of the practitioner have a rationale provided by a myth or theory that the client perceives to be cogent and powerful. The rationale does not need to be scientifically sound but what is important is that clients accept the healer's explanation for their distress and the solution to the presenting problem. For practitioners the rationale or myth is the theoretical approach they use in their work with clients.
- **Procedures.** A set of procedures that are consistent with the rationale of the theory/myth is put in place to achieve that resolution.
- **Supportive structure.** A supportive relationship reinforces the practice of those procedures and their new direction.

In his meta-analyses of psychotherapy outcome studies conducted over the course of several decades Wampold (2001, 2010a) concluded that:

- No bona fide coherent therapeutic approach is more effective than any other bona fide coherent therapeutic approach.
- Bona fide coherent evidence-based therapeutic approaches are no more effective than comparison control conditions that were structurally equivalent.
- Practitioners must have confidence and competence in their chosen therapeutic approach (practitioner allegiance).
- Clients must be accepting of (buy into) the practitioner's rationale and treatment approach (procedures and rituals).
- If the client is not responding to the chosen treatment approach (making progress) then the practitioner needs to make adjustments to the treatment.

Wampold referred to the common factors as the basis for a *contextual approach* to client change in contrast to a medical model of treatment. A contextual model suggests that all effective treatment is based on:

- A therapeutic working alliance
- A frame or rationale for shifting interactional patterns around the problem and/or focusing on interactional exceptions
- The support to implement and follow through with the procedures to achieve these shifts in interactional patterns

These three basic elements common to all effective treatment are well supported in the general treatment literature as well as for family treatment in particular (cf. Norcross, 2002; Sprenkle, Blow, & Dickey, 1999) and provide the foundation for core elements of I-FAST: the therapeutic alliance, interactional patterns, and general process of change and systems collaboration.

The Therapeutic Alliance

Sprenkle et al. (1999) state: "[i]f there could be said to be a 'gold standard' finding in the MFT [marital and family treatment] research literature, it would be that the quality of the client-practitioner relationship is the *sine qua non* of successful therapy" (pp. 334–335). The literature repeatedly emphasizes the important role of the therapeutic alliance in facilitating positive treatment outcomes in working with clients and families. Bordin (1979) theorized that the therapeutic alliance could be accounted for with three constructs: the development of positive affective bonds, mutual agreement on goals, and mutual agreement on tasks for achieving those goals. Building on Bordin's definition, in family treatment the therapeutic alliance has been defined to include (Friedlander, Escudero, & Heatherington, 2006):

- Engagement, which includes the family's agreeing with the practitioner on the goals and tasks of treatment
- The family having a positive emotional connection with the practitioner
- The family experiencing a sense of safety within the treatment context
- The family developing a shared sense of purpose for the treatment

As an example of these common factors, the therapeutic alliance alone has been supported as one of the major necessary yet not always sufficient conditions of effective treatment (Horvath & Bedi, 2002). So, if one follows the widely used definition of a therapeutic alliance of Bordin (1979), we would expect to find all of these elements present in the relationship of all of the evidence-based approaches to high-risk youth. These elements include:

- **Positive bonds** between clients and practitioners such as mutual trust, liking, respect, and caring
- **Consensus about and commitment to the goals** of treatment and to the means or tasks of treatment by which these goals may be attained

- **A partnership** in which all parties are actively committed to their roles in the process of treatment and belief that all others are also enthusiastically engaged in the same process

Interactional Patterns and General Process of Change

I-FAST is informed by *systems theory*. A family is a system, which is part of larger systems. Systems theory posits that the whole is greater than the sum of its parts. That is, to understand a system one must have knowledge not only of the individual system members but also of the nature of the interactions and relationships between and among the system members. These interactions become repetitive and patterned over time. For families, these repetitive patterns become the family rules (assumptions/premises) that organize how the family functions. Because family members live these rules day in and day out they take on a life of their own: family members tend not to question them and assume (take for granted) that this is the way the world works or at least should work.

A system is also goal oriented, with the primary goal being its continued existence and survival. Consequently, families develop and seek to maintain a certain patterned regularity and stability. To maintain its integrity, a system needs to be capable of processing feedback from its larger environmental context about the behavior of its members; its output becomes input to it from the environment. Within its rules, family members also give each other feedback about each other's behavior. Feedback processes are especially important in parents raising their children. When parents respond to their children's behavior it is often to reinforce desired behavior and/or to correct undesired behavior.

In family life there are difficulties and there are problems. Difficulties tend to be unpleasant situations that draw action to either change, assimilate, or accommodate. Families most often solve difficulties, and so this points to strength that is helpful for practitioners to acknowledge. Usually by the time a child's behavior has become problematic enough to seek professional mental health treatment services, the parents' attempts to solve the problem that perhaps worked in the past are no longer successful. Not knowing what else to do within its rules and assumptions, and feeling out of control of the child, parents usually end up trying even more of what has not worked in escalating spirals with their child to regain control. The parents and child are now in a *vicious cycle* and often a power struggle; where previously there was only a "difficulty" there is now a "problem." The parents and child are now in a *positive feedback loop* in that the more the child misbehaves the more the parents try more of what is not working to attempt to solve the child's problematic behavior, and the more the parents use these unsuccessful attempted solutions the more the child misbehaves.

Sprenkle, Davis, and Lebow (2009) state that "conceptualizing problems in relational terms is the one distinctive element common to all larger system therapies" (p. 35) and "relational therapies pay special attention to the interactional cycles among the various subsystems that constitute the larger system in which the problem is embedded" (p. 36). In families in treatment the most common interactional cycle (pattern) of interest involves parents and children. In fact, according to Diamond and Diamond (2002), "[i]mproving parenting practices may be the single most common and potent mechanism of change in family-based treatments" (p. 54).

Sexton has identified understanding problems of severely disturbed youth within the context of how adults habitually respond to the youth's problem behaviors. Interactional patterns that maintain the problem, what we are referring to here as vicious cycles, have been identified as a common factor. The interruption of these patterns, or the identification and amplification of existing exceptions to these patterns, has also been identified as a common factor (Fraser & Solovey, 2007); Fraser and Solovey have referred to this as the *general process of change*.

The process of change in social systems involves what has been called *first- and second-order change* (Fraser & Solovey, 2007; Watzlawick, Weakland, & Fisch, 1974).

- **First-order change**. In first-order change solutions that follow the current ideas and rules within a system are applied to perceived difficulties. These solutions may resolve the difficulty. Alternatively, they may either not resolve or even escalate the perceived difficulty, frequently resulting in reapplication of the same kind of solution. This often creates vicious cycles, or what are often called solution-generated problems.
- **Second-order change.** At these points, a distinctly different form of solution is required to break the vicious cycle. This solution is most often viewed as counterintuitive or paradoxical from the initial frame or rationale in that it frequently requires a reframing of the original viewpoint and/or a reversal or redirection of former solutions. This sort of change is what has been called *second-order change*, and it has been described as a common or "*golden thread*" that runs through most evidence-based practices (Fraser & Solovey, 2007).

The best way to explain the general process of change is that it is a point of view on how all change occurs in human interaction. It's a theory of change. It is built upon social constructivism and systems theory. Two aspects of this process have been called *first-order change* and *second-order change*. Simply speaking, first-order change is what we do as we act on our agreed on definitions of our realities. It does change things within that defined reality, and yet it also confirms that reality and often keeps things the same or escalates them if there is a dilemma to be solved. Second-order change essentially "steps outside the box" of our definitions of the way things are and opens a new set of ways to act or to solve a problem if there is a dilemma. Second-order change also often appears illogical, paradoxical, or counterintuitive when viewed from our original definitions of our situation and their resulting actions or solutions.

Systems Collaboration

A final set of assumptions is really a specific assumption that should be made explicit on its own. *All human interactions take place within multiple embedded systems* (Bronfenbrenner, 1979). This suggests that all problems, especially those of high-risk youth and families, are embedded within numerous social systems and are best treated through interactions with as many of those systems as are directly and indirectly involved. A corollary of this assumption is that these multiple systems (including those of the practitioner and agency treating the clients) operate on the same process of change principles outlined earlier. Thus, such systems are as likely to become drawn into the same sort of vicious cycles of solution-generated problems as are the identified clients and their families.

Many if not most at-risk families are involved with several different agencies and their representatives, that is, mental health, social services, juvenile court, and so on. The interactions families have with other systems outside the family, that is, schools and so forth over time also can become unquestioned rules that affect the family's organization. As within family patterns, the attempts of these systems to help at-risk families solve problems can often maintain the problem. Consequently, system collaboration is an integral part of I-FAST.

In addition to the coordination of community and natural resources/supports to meet the needs of children and families across multiple life domains, systems collaboration also constitutes a crucial component in changing interactional patterns involving at-risk families. Juvenile courts, child welfare agencies, and/or psychiatric hospitals are often involved with these families to "help" them when their problematic child is out of control by restraining the child using different venues such as removing the child and placing him or her in residential care, foster care, or a hospital. In those situations, the family's interactional pattern with their child was not changed for two reasons: (1) the goal of the intervention was safety, not change in how parents deal with the problems the child has; and (2) the child was settled down by outsiders, not by the family. If parents are to be helped to reassume control of their out-of-control child, or if they are to be empowered to help their child, the agencies that have power to remove their child or to dis-empower parents must be included in the treatment process because how these agencies intervene can either change family patterns or reinforce them. System collaboration, as such, is fundamental to successful outcomes in families both via providing resources and supports as well as working together to create a context for permanent (second-order) change in the interactional patterns.

Summary of Foundation Concepts

The essence of the basic foundation concepts of I-FAST can be summarized as follows. This may help the reader remember and stay clear on the foundations of the approach.

- **Systems theory**
  - Vicious cycles keep problems going.
  - Virtuous cycles reorganize the system in a helpful way.
- **Social constructivism**
  - Reality is relative.
  - Reality is co-created.
- **Socially constructed reality**
  - Co-created premises guide our viewing and doing . . . channeling our interactions.
  - This applies to ideas on the nature of problems and how to resolve them.
  - Applies equally to practitioners' theories and practices in treatment.
- **The Process of Change**
  - **First-order change**:
    - A change in intensity, frequency, location, duration, and so forth of interactions (solutions)
    - Variations of similar interactions within the accepted premises and patterns of a system

- Often does resolve problems
- Yields problems only when failed solutions are reapplied over and again
- **Second-order change**:
  - A change of a system's primary premises, rules, and patterns
  - Usually yields strikingly different or opposite interactions
  - May appear counterintuitive or paradoxical from first-order premises
  - Is the *key element* of most effective treatments
- **Vicious cycles**
  - Represent the classic description of problem patterns across most, if not all models of effective treatment
  - Involve a trigger, within a frame describing the situation, repeated failed solutions, and escalation
  - Interdicting vicious cycles is the heart of all effective treatments and is the cornerstone of I-FAST.
- **Virtuous cycles**
  - Represent positive feedback loops that move the family system away from the problem pattern and closer to the desired family goals
  - These exceptions to the problem patterns can be identified or co-created in the treatment process or can exist outside the awareness of the family and become apparent to them only through treatment.
  - Virtuous cycles can be initiated by initiating or noting some difference from the problem pattern and then building upon it with all involved.

The essence of intervention in I-FAST is the interruption of vicious cycles or identification of and amplification of exceptions to these cycles. Identifying and changing interactional patterns that support problems, two of the main components of I-FAST, are supported by the evidence-based literature and can also be considered as common factors.

LEVEL III

Practice Procedures

I-FAST assumes that all effective treatments will involve a number of key common elements:

- **Working alliance.** Explicit efforts will be made to create and maintain a *working alliance* with all involved parties and systems.
- **Vicious and virtuous cycles.** There will be an understanding of the problems and their resolutions of severely disturbed youth within the interactional context of interactional patterns that keep the problem going and creating or identifying exceptions to those patterns and building upon them.
- **Frames.** They will attend to the *culturally shaped and systemically unique frames* and ideas that influence the interactions of those systems. These *frame analyses* will be used in guiding the description of presenting problems and in framing explanations of problems and their resolution.
- **A treatment rationale.** A *therapeutic rationale* will be present to guide interveners and clients in initiating these desired changes.

- **Pattern shift.** Interventions will thus be targeted at *shifting an interactional pattern*, often involving what may be identified as second-order changes in the involved systems.
- **Multisystemic.** They will view problems as embedded in *multiple social systems* and assume that *treatment is best done by engaging those systems*.

Based on theory and evidence-based common factors, I-FAST provides meta-frames on practice techniques at different phases in the treatment process. We describe each of these phases and the practice techniques in each phase in great detail from Chapter 3 to Chapter 9. These phases and meta-frames are:

- **Engaging.** *A minimum requirement for being faithful to I-FAST is engaging and developing a collaborative relationship with at least one parent or primary caregiver.* In I-FAST the focus is on empowering the parent or primary caregiver to be the one to solve the child's presenting problem.
- **Tracking interactions.** *Whether focusing on problem patterns or exceptions, I-FAST requires obtaining an interactional understanding.* Interactions representing patterns that support the problem or those representing exceptions must be tracked and identified. To remain faithful to I-FAST, problems and their solutions must be understood in terms of the interactions of the various parties involved.
- **Goals.** *To remain faithful to I-FAST, at a minimum treatment must focus on something specific and achievable to be changed:* (1) That the parents are motivated to focus on, (2) is defined as something the parents can do something about, and (3) while the client remains in his or her natural environment.
- **Framing and rationales.** *To remain faithful to I-FAST, all frames, no matter what their therapeutic aim may be, must be accepted by the client and the family.* Frames can be borrowed from other models, but to be utilized in I-FAST the client must accept the frame.
- **Initiating change.** *To remain faithful to I-FAST*: (1) Interventions are offered only if an alliance is established with at least one parent; (2) interventions must have an obvious connection to the specific problem or goal the aligned parent has identified; and (3) the intervention requires a deviation from interactional patterns that support the problem, or an amplifying of exceptions to those patterns.
- **Building resilience and terminating.** *To remain faithful to I-FAST*: (1) Review what worked; (2) attribute the change to the clients and systems involved; (3) emphasize the strengths and resilience of all involved; (4) predict future challenges and emphasize episodes of care; and (5) link the family to resources in their natural environment.

In the following chapters we explain in more detail the key elements of I-FAST and how to successfully implement and sustain its use in agency settings.

I-FAST

INTEGRATIVE FAMILY AND SYSTEMS TREATMENT

WHAT'S IN A NAME?

There is always a risk in labeling an approach, particularly if it is intended to be a flexible and integrative point of view. The main risk is that people will eventually see the new point of view as simply another approach similar to those that it intends to integrate. This is a paradox of language and levels that is hard to escape. With this in mind, it may help to describe how this name has been chosen.

- **Integrative**
  The first term, "integrative," was chosen to represent how the point of view integrates not only several intervention protocols, but also levels of the systems involved in intervention. As explained in chapter 1, this perspective attempts to synthesize key elements of most all evidence-based approaches.
  - Integration, however, also refers to the fact that a number of different treatment rationales might be used effectively within the broad parameters of this perspective.
  - It also refers to the fact that the same principles used to address and intervene with individual and family levels of systems apply just the same to the multiple larger systems involved with these cases. This also holds true for the persons who are practitioners or interveners and for the agencies in which they work. Once more, the same concepts are used for all levels and players involved, and thus the term "integrative" takes on all of these meanings within this perspective.
- **Family and Systems**
  The terms "family" and "systems" were chosen to reflect the multilevel focus of this perspective. The term *family* needs to be defined flexibly to include all forms of caretakers who may be involved with each youth. These may be not only mothers or fathers, but also frequently grandparents, stepparents, other family members, foster parents, or other responsible caregivers in many other constellations. Similarly, the term *systems* needs to be broadly defined as all of those systems influencing each case. [One way of identifying these groups is by the term *problem-generated systems*, referring to all of those systems engaged in identifying the youth and/or family as a problem and who are engaged in trying to do something to deal with them (Anderson, Goolishian, & Winderman, 1986).]
- **Treatment**
  Finally, the term "treatment" has been chosen over the word "therapy" to open the option for multiple levels of interveners to be engaged in this practice. The term "therapy" often officially restricts the credentials of the practitioner to those who are licensed with master's degrees and above. The term "therapy"

also often carries a full range of traditional in-office procedures that also can restrict what may be effective in any multisystemic treatment approach. The intent of this perspective is to be inclusive, and consequently it explores the prospect that very effective work, especially in a home-based venue, may be done by agents without advanced degrees or licenses. Whereas experienced and licensed practitioners are often needed and effective in this work, the work itself may benefit by being opened to all levels of practitioners. Thus we chose the term "treatment" as more neutral than "therapy." We could have as easily chosen the term "consultation" (although it would not have as conveniently finished spelling the useful word "FAST" as part of the I-FAST label).

MAJOR ASSUMPTIONS OF I-FAST

The specific assumptions underlying I-FAST are an application of the theories that inform it: systems theory and social constructivism as described in Chapter 1. The assumptions that underlie I-FAST represent a special-case application to the treatment of families and children where there is risk for out-of-home placement. Specific assumptions of I-FAST include:

- **Frames are critical.** How people think about problems and what they do about them determines whether problems are resolved or develop into serious conditions that warrant clinical intervention.
- **Vicious cycles and virtuous cycles.** Problems are maintained by interactional patterns that support them, which can become increasingly rigid and redundant over time. As problems with children and adolescents develop and worsen, parents, friends, neighbors, teachers, and other community persons become involved in the patterns. Solutions represent changes or exceptions to these patterns.
- **Multiple systems.** A problem-generated system may evolve that includes all parties and systems involved in defining something happening as a problem and trying to do something about it.
- **The main task of intervention is**:
    - Interrupt, stop, or reverse the patterns of interaction that maintain problems, or
    - Identify exceptions to problem-maintaining patterns and initiate the solution-building process.
- **Alliances.** The quality of the relationship between the practitioner or case manager and the family and systems is essential to change.
- **Treatment rationale.** A treatment rationale or set of frames is provided and agreed on that explains the problem and clearly supports the goals and therapeutic tasks.
- **Collaboration.** Engagement means collaboration on problem definitions, goals, and procedures that are designed to promote change.
- **Prioritizing.** Collaboration on goals includes establishment of priorities so that it is clear what goal or goals will be pursued first.
- **Respecting client perspectives.** All goals and therapeutic procedures should fall in line with all parties' values and motives.
- **Strength and resilience.** Families are resilient and have strengths and resources that can be used in finding solutions.

- **Parental primacy.** Parents are the principal agents of change. *Engaging parents as partners in the treatment process is essential to outcome.* A major focus in this kind of work is restoration of the parent–child relationship.
- **Multisystemic.** Effective treatment requires working with the family system and other involved systems such as schools, courts, and so forth.
- **Strategic involvement.** Decisions about who should be involved are made strategically and take into account persons or agencies that have influence over the child/adolescent and his or her family.
- **Intervener support.** Effective treatment is based on recruiting, training, and retaining competent staff with expertise in intensive family treatment services.
- **Sustained supervision.** Effective treatment involves continual tracking and support of all parties' investment in the rationale, tasks, and agreed on goals of treatment.

THE I-FAST TREATMENT PROCESS

There is some risk when breaking down the treatment processes of change into discrete entities. In the real world, treatment processes can occur on multiple levels and overlap, making it difficult at times to distinguish one process from another. This can occur in treatment that is quite effective. Regardless of whatever blurring might occur, research shows that there are discrete outcomes that families achieve when treatment works. In the literature, many of these outcomes are referred to as *common factors*. Common factors include outcomes such as understanding the problem, goal consensus, and developing therapeutic procedures that make sense to the family. These outcomes, or so-called common factors, however, are not qualities that simply exist in effective treatment sessions. Each outcome or component occurs as a result of a process. This is what we call the treatment process of change.

Breaking down the treatment process of change into components can be helpful when teaching practitioners how to work effectively with the families of at-risk youth. Our view is that to facilitate change, practitioners need a map. Understanding the processes of change helps the practitioner to have confidence in the direction of treatment. There are also specific procedures associated with each change process and a skill set that practitioners need to accomplish the tasks. Figures 2-1 and 2-2 show the key processes that are used by I-FAST practitioners to trigger change. Figure 2-1 shows the six phases of the I-FAST change process. More detailed information about the different phases of I-FAST is provided in the section following this diagram.

PHASES AND PROCEDURES OF THE I-FAST PROTOCOL

The I-FAST protocol includes training in the following key phases of this integrative approach.

Engaging
In order to connect well with all clients in all systems being worked with, the practitioner should find herself:

- Collaborating well with all parties and systems
- Identifying and supporting the strengths of all parties and systems involved

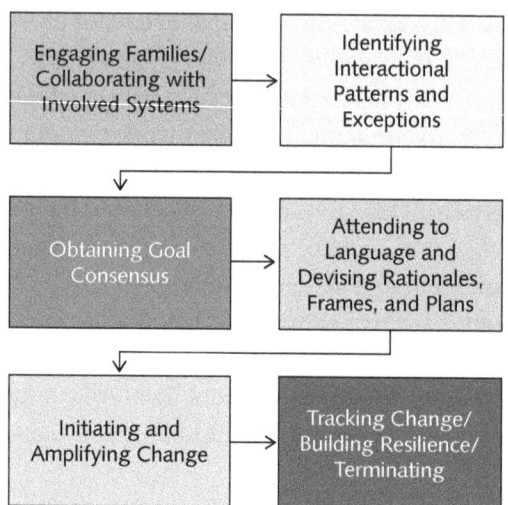

FIGURE 2-1 **offers a picture of the I-FAST Treatment Phases presented as a flow chart of the overall progression of one phase to the next.**

- Understanding and validating the perspectives and dilemmas of all parties and systems involved
- Setting clear, observable, and agreed on goals with all parties and systems involved
- Identifying and using clients' language and values, noting how they shape and drive the problem pattern and how they may help frame future interventions
- Identifying and using the major frames employed by all parties and systems, noting how they contribute to the problem and how they may be used to shift problem patterns
- Identifying, aligning with, and engaging parties who have major power and control in the problem-generated system and enlisting their efforts in redirecting the problem cycle patterns

Tracking Interactions

The I-FAST Practitioner follows the patterns of what is happening in all systems by:

- Identifying who is involved with defining the problem and trying to do something about it
- Respecting the client's definition of the problem
- Identifying a specific problem pattern
- Tracking the pattern of that problem
- Identifying the vicious cycles of the problem
- Identifying exceptions to the problem pattern and strengths of all parties
- Identifying and using all involved parties' and systems' stages of change
- The decision of whom to include in treatment is, in and of itself, an intervention and therefore is made strategically on a case-by-case basis depending on:
    - The problem being focused on

- The pattern of the problem and parties involved
- The motivation to change and position on change of the various participants involved in addressing the problem
- In I-FAST, this issue is dealt with flexibly and on a case-by-case basis depending on the goals of treatment and the pattern we are attempting to change.

Goal Development and Consensus

The I-FAST practitioner will develop a collaborative contract with all involved by:

- Setting goals that reflect the wants and needs of the family. The parents' wants and needs for the child are primary.
- Defining goals as achievable and as something the family can do something about.
- Identifying a priority focus of treatment
- Obtaining goal consensus from both family and professional

Frames, Framing, and Reframing

The I-FAST practitioner will smoothly link with all parties in all systems by paying attention to the language, values, and worldviews of all involved through:

- Skillful use of framing and reframing in all steps of I-FAST treatment:
  - Tracking and utilizing client frames to enhance engagement
  - Framing problems and goals as something families can do something about
  - Devising treatment rationales that make sense to the family
  - Offering task frames that make sense to the family
  - Framing improvement so families are given credit for change
- Determining a therapeutic rationale to explain the problem, fit with the clients, match practitioner knowledge and skills, and imply directions for treatment
- Articulating a procedure to shift the problem pattern and support strengths and exceptions to the problem pattern
- Asking questions such as:
  - What are the goals of all involved?
  - What patterns need to shift?
  - Who are the key players?
  - How shall we involve them?
  - How can we use their frames, language, and motives?
  - What will change look like as it begins?
- Identifying frames to use in delivering interventions including:
  - Client frames
  - Theoretical frames
  - Developmental frames
  - Evidence-based treatment frames
  - Other creative frames
- In summary, generating a clear rationale to explain the problem, which implies a direction toward solution, and enlisting all parties' energy in following that path

Initiating Change

While all therapeutic interaction is essentially intervention, explicitly targeting and initiating change in all systems is achieved by:

- Targeting specific aspects of the interactional *patterns* or interactional *exceptions* of families and taking into account the needs, resources, and positions that family members have on change
- Initiating interventions in collaboration with other agencies and parties that have a stake in the outcome of the case
- Once the change process has been stimulated, refocusing on amplifying and sustaining change
- Being able to affirm and validate all involved parties, and engaging their motives in the change process
- Being technically proficient in major **intervention procedures** reflecting the skill of the practitioner:
- Use of questions, frames, and tasks as intervention procedures to amplify exceptions or shift patterns
    - **Reframing.** Being able to flexibly frame, reframe, and de-frame actions, roles, or situations as needed relating to the therapeutic rationale and the language and positions of all involved
    - **Use of questions.** Being able to use questions effectively as interventions to initiate change
    - **Use of tasks.** Being able to derive and give tasks effectively as interventions to initiate change
- Being able to identify successes and changes and being able to support and generalize them within the goals and rationale of the approach being used
- Generating hope and enthusiasm in all parties

Building Resilience and Terminating

Once change has gotten under way and major goals are being achieved, then practitioners attend to relapse-prevention and building resilience in the involved systems by:

- Designing, implementing, and tracking the success of intervention directives
- Modifying interventions in response to how clients respond to the change strategy and homework
- Tracking and supporting changes as they occur and ascribing them to the efforts of the clients and involved system members
- Then, employing relapse prevention strategies such as predicting and prescribing "relapses"
- Using the "episode of care" concept in affirming success and maintaining an open invitation to clients to revisit treatment as other challenges come along

Figure 2-2 offers a flow chart of the phases and related procedures of the I-FAST intervention process. Sometimes it is helpful to see the intervention process in a graphic form to help remember the process.

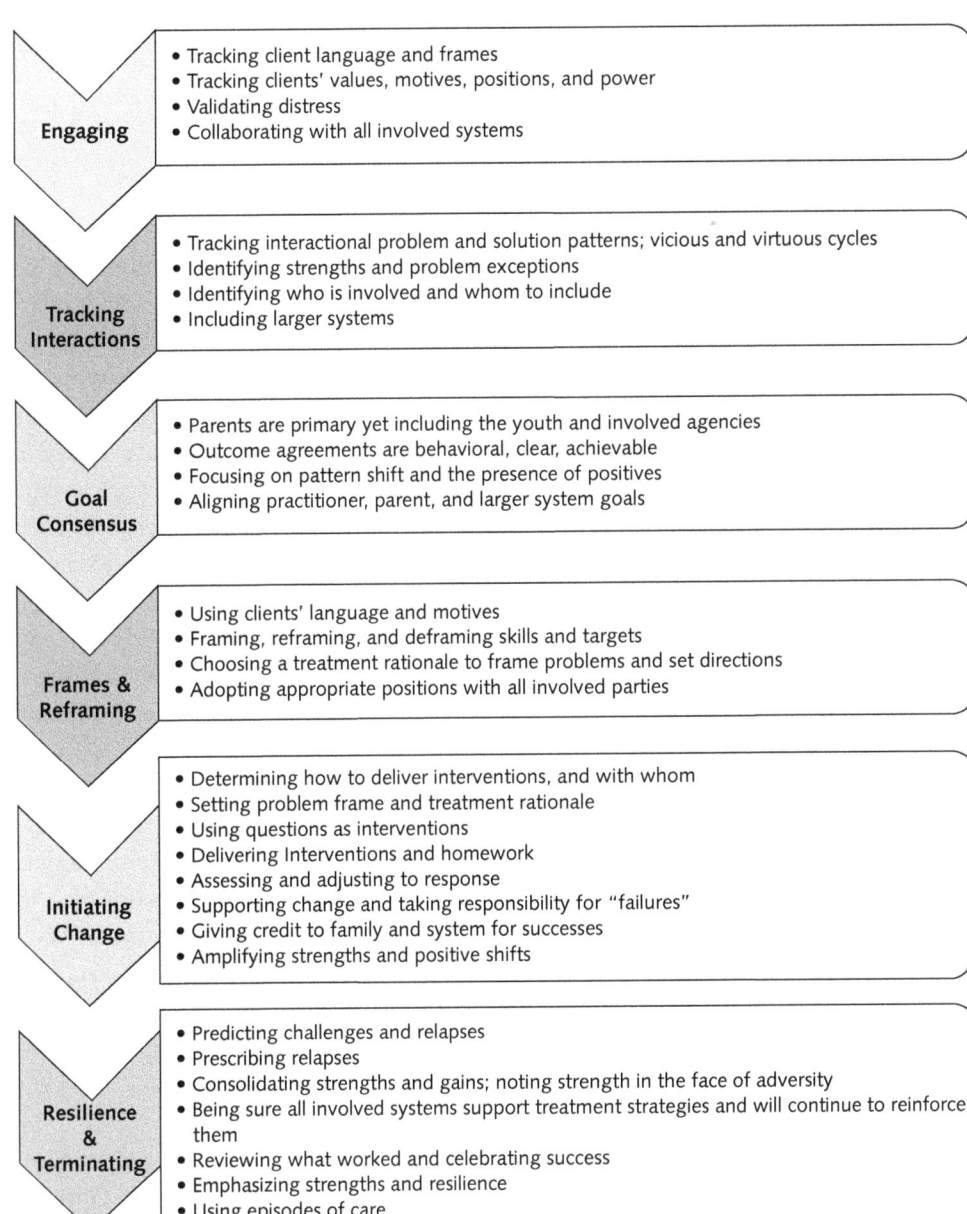

FIGURE 2-2 offers a visual flow chart linking the I-FAST phases with the main procedures in each phase to serve as memory points for the practitioner as they learn and impalement the approach.

GUIDELINES FOR THE PRACTICE OF I-FAST

I-FAST and Episodes of Care

With this said, it should be noted that we chose the term "FAST" as a representation of the structure of the perspective itself. This is a time-limited approach, usually implemented within eight- to twelve-week "episodes of care." The idea of this perspective is for it to remain focused and intensive with clear attention to resolving one major problem area. Changing a key problem area often has a positive influence on others within the system, but this is not always so. The initial successful intervention episode often opens the case to other episodes of care for other identified problems at some future time. The point of the term "FAST" is that the approach itself is to be quickly and intensely employed and as quickly brought to some form of resolution.

The Dose–Response Effect and Intensive Episodes of Brief Treatment

The acronym "FAST" used in the abbreviation I-FAST was chosen purposely. All of the current specific factor models of treatment for at-risk youth and families employ relatively rapid, intense, and time-limited intervention models. The I-FAST moderated common factors model matches this profile. A case can be made that this intensive and time-limited approach mirrors what has been found to be effective across all approaches to effective treatment. Since the publication of the seminal paper by Howard and his colleagues (Howard et al., 1986) on the dose–response effect in psychotherapy, it has become increasingly evident that therapeutic change can and does occur within the first 8 to 16 sessions, with diminishing returns after that. They found that between 10% and 18% of patients had improved before the first session of therapy, and after 2, 8, and 26 sessions of therapy, 30%, 53%, and 74% of the patients, respectively, had improved. Although there has been extensive debate and refinement of these findings (cf. Hansen et al., 2002; Howard et al., 1996; Lambert, 2007; Shapiro et al., 2003), there remains agreement on the fact that a significant amount of all therapeutic change occurs within the first 8 to 16 sessions. I-FAST practitioners initially go into the home two to three times a week for a total of up to four to six hours a week for the first four to six weeks. As families progress, sessions are spaced out through termination. This is similar to the specific factor models where, for example, multisystemic therapy practitioners go into the home two to three times a week for four to six hours throughout the duration of treatment. With multiproblem families of at-risk youth, one might argue that the standard structure of treatment emphasizing rapid and intense intervention is not only supported by the general psychotherapy literature, but may also be one of several key elements contributing to the success of all of these treatment models. Early and intense intervention is highly associated with most effective treatments.

Furthermore, the basic structure and assumptions of the I-FAST model conform to the key components of all brief therapies as identified by Budman and Gurman (1988) and by Koss and Shiang (1994). (This tends to be true as well for the implicit structure of the alternate specific models for at-risk youth and families.) These core brief therapy components include the use of a developmental life span model, rapid intervention, setting time limits available for intervention, an emphasis on working alliance, and explicit focus on presenting problems; high therapist activity level; flexibility in intervention techniques and rationales; and an explicit focus on termination and transition issues. I-FAST has been informed by both the dose–effect literature emphasizing the value of rapid and intense intervention and by the brief therapy literature that describes the range of therapy components that most highly correlates with effective episodes of care.

TREATMENT DECISIONS AND CHOICES

One major implication for practice and a way to distinguish I-FAST from numerous other manualized approaches regards key treatment choices. Most manualized approaches are very prescriptive as to what practitioners should do in treating specific families. I-FAST, however, is not prescriptive but instead is flexible in that treatment choices are decided on by the practitioner and supervisor on a case-by-case basis. For example, in most manualized models, whom the practitioner works with is dictated by the approach. The rule might be that parents may be interviewed with or without children present, but children are never interviewed individually; the model will dictate this. In I-FAST, whom to interview and whom to intervene with are choices that must be made on a case-by-case basis; this allows for flexibility and adaptability but may be more difficult to learn. The key choices to be addressed in treatment need to consider the following.

Clinical Choices in I-FAST

In I-FAST, practitioners have the flexibility and the tasks to make the following choices of how to intervene in each different case.

- Choosing the unit of analysis—determining who is involved in the interactional patterns around the defined problem and its solution attempts
- Choosing whom to work with directly
- Choosing how to define problems and choose goals
- Choosing overarching frames and therapeutic rationales that explain the problem and what to do about it
- Choosing when to focus on pattern exceptions and solutions
- Choosing frames offered to set up tasks
- Determining how to choose from a wide range of procedures available to the practitioner

IN THE MAJORITY OF APPROACHES CHOICES ARE DICTATED BY THE MANUAL

For many treatment models, the unit of analysis may be the individual client with the symptom; this would always be the case and would be dictated by the manual. For example, if a 19-year-old young woman who has been sexually abused is having nightmares and avoiding public places, her parents' knowledge and responses to her nightmares and avoidant behaviors might not be considered because the parents are not part of the unit of analysis in a particular approach.

- The manual would also dictate whom to work with and that would be the client individually.
- The problem might be defined by the diagnosis of posttraumatic stress disorder (PTSD) and that is decided on by the approach.
- The frames for offering tasks may be largely decided on. The range of tasks would be limited to what is required to remain faithful to the model.

IN I-FAST MORE CHOICES ARE AVAILABLE

The I-FAST practitioner has a wide range of choices that they can make to help to fit the intervention to the case and to their own approach to intervention.

- In the preceding example, the problem might be defined by what the client is most upset about, regardless of *Diagnostic and Statistical Manual of Mental Disorders* (*DSM*) diagnosis.

- The unit of analysis could include anyone interacting with the client regarding the problem she is upset about.
- The person(s) worked with could include a range of possibilities from the client individually, the client and her parents together, the parents without the client, with the client's boyfriend alone or with the client, and so on. The treatment possibilities are wide.
- An overarching frame or rationale would most likely be selected that fits with the client's beliefs.
- The tasks could include those that fall under the category of exposing the individual client to what she is anxious about, or they could include involving her parents and/or boyfriend in helping her.
  - For example, if she has nightmares, she could be asked to tell her parents the nightmare the morning after she has it, or she could tell them the night before so she may come to feel that she does not have to have it.
  - If she was asked to do this and she responded by indicating her parents might blame her for the abuse, a whole new very important issue would arise that would have bearing on how to define the problem.

Practitioners applying I-FAST to this type of problem have a range of choices regarding numerous therapeutic decisions that are not available to them if they are administering the typical manualized approach. I-FAST therefore has the potential to be adapted to a wider range of clients. *The issue becomes how to make the clinical choices consistent with the flexibility of I-FAST. How does one choose what unit to analyze, what group or individuals to involve in treatment, how to define the problem, and so on?*

HOW TO MAKE THERAPEUTIC CHOICES IN I-FAST

A major task in learning I-FAST involves learning how to make therapeutic choices as they arise in the I-FAST treatment process. Generally speaking, the two key variables for informing these decisions in each of the above listed areas are:

- What are the practitioner's existing skill sets in implementing treatment?
- How is the client/family responding to the practitioner statements and interventions?

UTILIZING PRACTITIONERS' EXISTING SKILL SETS

One advantage of I-FAST is that practitioners' existing beliefs and skills can be incorporated into the approach as long as those beliefs and skills fit within the larger frames that define the I-FAST treatment process. The practitioner's existing skills can be a basis for choosing what frames to offer, what family members to work with, or what types of tasks to offer.

- *When choosing whom to work with,* for example, some practitioners are very skilled at recruiting family members into treatment. Others are very skilled at working with the family members who initially seek treatment. *Either skill can be applied to I-FAST as long as the practitioner aligns with at least one parent and works within the frame of empowering the parent to solve the presenting problem of the identified child client.*

- *When giving tasks*, some practitioners are skilled at identifying exceptions and focusing on solutions; others are skilled at offering tasks that represent a change in how the parents habitually work with their child. Some family practitioners are skilled at asking families to deviate from their patterns in the session; these types of tasks are sometimes referred to as "enactments." *This way of working is consistent with I-FAST as long as the "enactments" focus on the problems the parents are defining as their major concerns.* Any of these task-giving skills can be utilized in I-FAST and can be the basis for choosing how to work with a given family.
- *In I-FAST, practitioners do not have to discard skills and beliefs they may already hold.* Practitioners just have to find ways for those skills and beliefs to fit within I-FAST's larger frames.
- *In I-FAST, treatment can be directed by the practitioner's existing skill set as long as the family is positively responding to this way of working.* If, however, the family does not respond positively to how a practitioner already works in I-FAST, practitioners must modify their approach until the family does respond positively. For example, a child's problem can be defined as neurological, with the solution requiring the child to "practice" special behaviors under a parent's guidance. This approach can fit within I-FAST as long as the parent accepts this way of defining the problem, the parent carries out the tasks that come out of working this way, and the child actually improves. If, however, the parent does not "buy" the frame, or if the parent does not carry out the adjoining tasks, or if the child does not improve by working this way, then the practitioner should construct a new approach that fits in with I-FAST's larger frame.

OBSERVING AND UTILIZING HOW CLIENTS RESPOND TO INTERVENTIONS

A meta-skill encouraged in I-FAST involves observing and utilizing how clients respond to practitioners' statements and interventions. This skill can enhance virtually every intervention and task in the I-FAST treatment process. Observing how the client is responding to practitioner interventions and how to utilize those responses is a core skill in I-FAST. Whether it is establishing rapport and empathizing, or setting goals and defining clear problems, or offering reframes, or offering tasks, all levels of intervention are greatly enhanced by the I-FAST practitioner's ability to track how the client is responding to whatever statements are offered. But I-FAST practitioner musts not merely track how clients are responding to them; they must also be able to utilize and make therapeutic use of those responses in the interest of achieving therapeutic goals.

When I-FAST practitioners are skilled at observing and utilizing how clients are responding to interventions, a three-step interactional sequence is followed:

1. The practitioner offers a statement, whether it is an empathic response, a proposed goal, a reframe, or a task.
2. The practitioner tracks how the client responds to the statement.
3. The practitioner modifies his or her statement or intervention to incorporate and utilize the client's response.

This sequence can be seen in various therapeutic techniques and in the literature associated with numerous concepts.

- In *active listening*, the practitioner is following this three-step sequence. A practitioner might offer an empathic statement, the client then corrects the practitioner, and the practitioner repeats back an empathic statement modified to fit the client's feedback.
- This three-step sequence has also been noted in relation to **reframing**. A reframe is offered, the client responds to the reframe, and the practitioner then modifies the reframe to accommodate the client's response.
- Milton Erickson, a well-respected founding father of a range of family systems and hypnotherapy approaches, followed this sequence when offering both hypnotic suggestions and therapeutic tasks. In the classic hypnotic example, Erickson suggests to the client that her arm is getting lighter. She responds by saying her arm is getting heavier. Erickson then responds by saying her arm can go on getting even heavier. Erickson is tracking and utilizing the response in the joint interest of helping the client produce trance phenomenon. In this way, Erickson and the client are in synch and working together. Erickson makes a suggestion, the client responds, and Erickson then follows her lead.
- In I-FAST, this three-step process is also followed when offering tasks.

In I-FAST, this three-step sequence can be applied to all I-FAST techniques throughout the entire I-FAST treatment process. Intensifying alliances, devising reframes, agreeing on goals, offering tasks, and tracking how clients respond to change are all enhanced by the skillful use of observing how clients are responding and then utilizing those responses. *Following this three-step sequence becomes the underlying skill that unifies the I-FAST approach.*

With I-FAST, practitioners have a range of choices with each step in the treatment process. The issue with so many choices becomes how to make them.

- In I-FAST, practitioners are free to begin a treatment by choosing from their own existing treatment repertoire, as long as those choices remain within the larger frames outlined by I-FAST.
- In addition to the skills practitioners bring into I-FAST, if the skills of observing and utilizing how clients respond to practitioners' statements and interventions are also learned, then how clients respond to whatever is being offered becomes the major force behind what reframes, strategies, and interventions are chosen in a given treatment.
- I-FAST offers a wide range of choices, and if the I-FAST practitioner is observant, how clients respond to those choices ultimately drives each I-FAST case.

It is very important to keep in mind that in I-FAST *the family's response to interventions and tasks is simply feedback to the practitioner.* If the family does not respond positively to an intervention/task their response is not seen as resistance but simply feedback to the practitioner to adjust how they are working with the family.

IMPLICATIONS FOR PRACTICE: AGENCY ADVANTAGES

Speaking practically, I-FAST has demonstrated the following advantages for agencies that are currently using the model.

Flexibility
Because the I-FAST model operates at a broader level of abstraction than treatment models designed for specific populations such as delinquent youth, it is being used with a wide range of childhood and adolescent problems. This has made it easier for agencies to respond flexibly to the needs of at-risk families and the community.

Adaptability
Though at first blush the idea of a meta-level model may sound complicated, in practice it can be taught to a wide range of professionals including indigenous helpers who may not have formal academic degrees. Because there are many ways to achieve the same end, practitioners' natural helping skills are cultivated and empowered. Good work is not defined as fidelity to a specific procedure that is enacted in a certain way. From the perspective of I-FAST, we seek adherence to a broader set of constructs. For example, there are many ways to achieve goal consensus with a family. How goal consensus is achieved is less important than the practitioner and client achieving it. In this way I-FAST consultants are accepting of a wide range of therapeutic styles.

Empowerment
With I-FAST, the consultant–agency relationship is based on agency empowerment. The overall objective of I-FAST training is to empower the agency to develop experts who can take the lead in supervising cases that involve at-risk families. It is expected that as an agency develops internal experts on the application of the I-FAST meta-principles it will need I-FAST consultants less. In this sense the overarching goal is for the agency to control its own destiny with regard to the use of outside consultants.

Sustainability
The empowerment model has implications for the relationship between I-FAST consultants and agency supervisors. It is understood that the agency is the expert on its own culture and on the culture of the community. The agency is viewed as owner of the all treatment interventions and has the right to veto any ideas offered by an I-FAST consultant. Agency supervisors are responsible for approving changes that are made to the client's treatment plan. In this sense, I-FAST consultants take on a consultative role and do not in any way alter the command and control structure of the agency.

Strengths-Based
Training takes into account the strengths that practitioners and supervisors bring to the table. It is understood that in many cases agencies already have at least some staff who are able to work within the umbrella of the meta-constructs that comprise I-FAST. As stated earlier, the fundamentals of establishing positive treatment alliances are well known. I-FAST consultation takes this into account and works on a flexible basis.

STRUCTURE AND ORGANIZATION OF THIS WORK

I-FAST is a meta-model that is flexible rather than rigid. It is adaptable to the style, strengths, skills, and needs of families and their specific problems, to practitioners and their training and personal styles, to the multiple systems involved in trying to solve the problem, and to the agency within which the work is being done. The I-FAST model gives practitioners an evidence-informed approach that is respectful to each practitioner's style and strengths. It encourages practitioners to be flexible and creative in fitting the model to clients and their problems and situations. This flexibility also presents a challenge for practitioners using the model.

Practitioners looking for the assurance and guidance of a set of invariant steps and content, skills, and format for each session and type of problem may find the I-FAST model to be frustrating. Other evidence-supported protocols do offer such detailed and structured instructions, which can be reassuring for those wanting to know exactly what to do with every case. Those practitioners wanting the assurance of a clear map of the territory and directions for what to do at each session and what skills and content to offer at particular times may become frustrated with the flexibility and choices inherent in the I-FAST model. I-FAST will not tell you exactly what procedures to do with each case and when and how to do them. Practitioners looking for such detailed and invariant directions initially may be frustrated with the I-FAST model. . . often asking, "Yes, but what exactly do I do and how do I do it?"

The model will offer a set of clear guidelines on how each practitioner can come to those detailed case conceptualizations, strategies, and therapeutic procedures *on his or her own*. Remember that I-FAST is a meta-model based on evidence-based common factors. In practice, following this meta-model will always provide the "rigor" to guide each practitioner's creativity and imagination in applying the model (Wilder & Weakland, 1982).

Rigor and Imagination

There are three implicit levels to the meta-model of I-FAST. These three levels represent the "rigor" that will allow for all practitioners to employ their own "imagination" and creativity as they approach each different and challenging case. These three levels form a hierarchy as noted in Chapter 1.

- **Level I: The Conceptual Level (Theoretical/philosophical constructs).** The top of this hierarchy represents the broadest level of ideas, premises, and assumptions on the nature of problems and their resolution. All of the choices and procedures of the I-FAST model are guided by these ideas and premises. Each of the next two levels follows from these assumptions. Therefore, the practitioner needs to have a very solid understanding and agreement with these highest level concepts. The conceptual section of each chapter discusses the chapter's topic as it relates specifically to **systems theory, social constructivism**, the use of a **strengths-based approach,** and **common factors.**
- **Level II: The Strategy Level (Evidence-based common factors).** The next step down the hierarchy represents a midrange level of structures addressing the elements of all effective treatment, how to fit the treatment to the practitioner and the client, and how to choose a therapeutic set of meta-frames and

treatment rationales to employ. These are the elements of fitting common factors to the clients and systems involved, of identifying interactional patterns and the frames and concepts that guide them, and of identifying and using the language, values, and frames that best fit with all involved, among other factors we have already noted. All of the choices at this second level will be guided by the top or **conceptual level** ideas and they will set the structure to determine the tactics, techniques, and procedures that will be used at the final **implementation level** of treatment. Once the processes of this level are completed, then the actual procedures of what will be done or implemented in treatment will follow.

- **Level III: The Implementation Level (Meta-frames for practice).** The third and lowest level of the hierarchy represents the set of procedures that will be used in each particular case. These procedures are a product of the choices made at the second or *strategy level*, and are guided by the first or *conceptual level* premises and assumptions on the nature of problems and their resolution.

    This is the level closest to the actual interaction in the treatment or intervention. These procedures, their timing and delivery, and so on are closest to what other evidence-supported models direct practitioners to do. These answer the questions of those practitioners asking "What do I do?" However, the advantage for the practitioner is that *these procedures are chosen in collaboration with the strengths and needs of the practitioner, clients, and other involved systems.* They evolve from the meta-structure of the I-FAST model used by the practitioner rather than being imposed from an external set of mandates. The rigor of the meta-model of using this three-level hierarchy of the I-FAST model supports the imagination of practitioners as they design the final strategy and implement it with each different family, with their unique problems in the unique set of systems and agencies involved.

Chapter Organization (CSI)

The I-FAST skills chapters are ordered in the manner in which we encourage I-FAST practitioners to think about their cases. We call the order **CSI: conceptualize, strategize, and implement**.

- **Conceptualizing**
    - Conceptualizing refers to the theoretical assumptions that practitioners make about what works in the treatment of at-risk youth and their families. For I-FAST, the main theories are systems theory and social constructivism. Each chapter discusses how that chapter topic relates to these two theories.
    - In the conceptualizing section of the clinical chapters of this book, the ideas and directives covered are informed by relevant research that guides effective treatment approaches. These are the common factors. Each chapter discusses common factor research related to that particular chapter.
    - This book attempts to bring the key points to the foreground for practitioners to keep implementation simple (we believe in the principle of... Keep It Simple!)

- **Strategizing**
  - As noted earlier, in I-FAST choices and decisions must be made about major aspects of treatment that are made for the practitioner in most manuals.
  - Decisions start with whom to involve in treatment and extend to decisions about how to engage various parties, what intervention approaches will be employed, how change will be measured, and so on.
  - Strategic means that the I-FAST practitioner is aware of the importance of treatment decision making and makes decisions with a treatment purpose. In the strategizing section of the treatment chapters of this workbook we identify important treatment decisions and try to provide guidelines for making such decisions.
- **Implementing**
  - The I-FAST practitioner understands that *all approaches are behavioral experiments or trial balloons*. When implementing an approach the objective is to be responsive to how well it fits with or is accepted by system members.
  - This means pursuing desired results with planned strategies that are accepted and are working while modifying strategies that are not working.
  - The I-FAST practitioner is aware that there are many approaches that may work for a given problem and so *treatment flexibility is the key*.
  - In the implementation section of this and the following treatment chapters we provide case examples that illustrate the application of conceptualizing and strategizing in I-FAST cases.
  - In all cases several alternative approaches that might work equally well for a particular family should be considered.

In Part Two, the following chapters will follow the order of the I-FAST treatment protocol.

Chapter 3: Engaging
Chapter 4: Tracking Interactions
Chapter 5: Goal Development and Consensus
Chapter 6: Frames, Framing, and Reframing
Chapter 7: Initiating Change
Chapter 8: Building Resilience and Terminating/Stepping Down
Chapter 9: Some Final Thoughts on Practice

In Part Three, the two chapters address larger issues of supervision in I-FAST (Chapter 10), and fitting I-FAST to the nature of the agency (Chapter 11).

Chapter 10: Teaching and Supervising I-FAST
Chapter 11: Fitting I-FAST and Agency Together: Creating Sustainability

Part Four includes the final chapter addressing the program of research and promising results so far on I-FAST as a unique and evolving evidence informed, flexible and effective meta-model of intervention with at-risk youth and families.

Chapter 12: Research on Integrative Family and Systems Treatment

These basic ideas are the "rigor" that will guide you as you then apply your "imagination" to designing and intervening with often highly distressed and chaotic systems and families. I-FAST is flexible in that it offers a combination of "rigor and imagination." The key to designing this book so that treatment can be flexible and adaptable for each different practitioner, in each different agency, with each different family, in each different sets of systems and communities, is to set forward a set of clear *meta-ideas* that can then be adapted to and owned by practitioners, agencies, and clients alike. Such flexibility is all based on understanding and using the above basic premises of the I-FAST approach. With this introduction and roadmap for where we are going, it is time to turn our attention to the journey of learning the I-FAST model and putting it into action.

2

I-FAST PHASES, SKILLS, AND TECHNIQUES

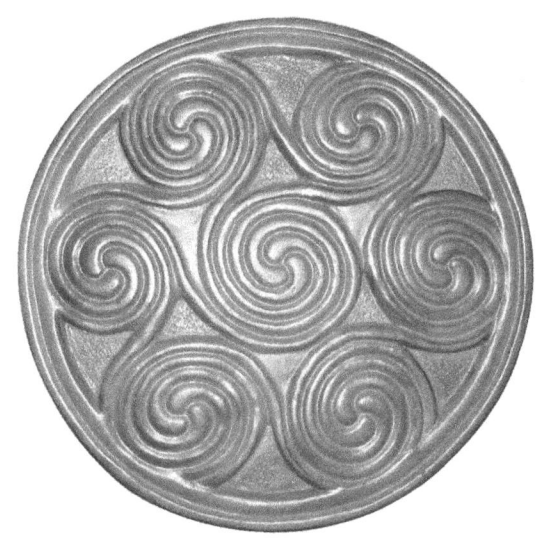

ENGAGING

3

INTRODUCTION

When I-FAST practitioners and at-risk families first meet they are strangers to one another. Often these families have had a negative experience with previous encounters with treatment providers. In their involvement with the new practitioner they now have to begin again to form a relationship with a person who is a stranger to them and to whom they are again expected to open up and reveal their emotions and shortcomings. Opening up to a stranger can be very difficult for anyone and can be considerably more so when families experience themselves as "deficient, flawed, incompetent, discouraged, and demoralized" (Greene & Lee, 2011, p. 53). At this point the challenge for practitioners is how to approach family members so they will feel comfortable and trusting enough with the practitioner to engage in and stay engaged in treatment until desired changes are successfully achieved (Friedlander, Escudero, Heatherington, & Diamond, 2011). What can the practitioner do to get the family to allow her or him into their family system in order to facilitate enough change to solve their presenting problem and achieve their desired treatment goals?

Previously, we mentioned the "therapeutic alliance" as one of the evidence-based common factors involved in successful outcomes in family treatment (Sprenkle, Davis, & Lebow, 2009). In addition to consisting of positive affective bonds, mutual agreement on goals, and mutual agreement on tasks for achieving those goals in working with families, the therapeutic alliance has also been described as involving a process of "engagement" between the practitioner and the family (Escudero, Heatherington, & Friedlander, 2010; Friedlander, Escudero, & Heatherington, 2006). When thinking about engaging families in the treatment process we are tempted to think of the noun—engagement—or a commitment made to treatment that occurs in a specific timeframe. Though this is understandable, I-FAST uses the word *engaging* because it denotes action that is ongoing throughout the process of treatment. The practitioner is continuously working on eliciting the commitment of clients to treatment throughout the process. In effect, engaging runs through each step of the I-FAST model.

TYPES OF ENGAGEMENT: INDIVIDUAL AND FAMILY

Traditionally, engagement refers to a practitioner engaging an individual client. However, in family treatment practitioners also need to be skilled at engaging the entire family (Friedlander et al., 2006); for I-FAST, the family is defined minimally as the household of the identified client. Skills for such a process may include:

- Active listening
- Empathic responding

- Tracking and utilizing client language
- Accepting and validating
- Using strengths-based language
- Adjusting to the family's response to him or her

In addition, in I-FAST practitioners need to be skilled at engaging an organization such as an entire family system and most often also engaging with individuals and groups from other organizations involved with the family and its members. Although both sets of skills are relevant, in I-FAST there is an equal emphasis and importance given to engaging an individual and engaging a family or group. Engaging an individual means simultaneously joining the group or family in which that individual belongs. On the other hand, when attempting to engage a family as a whole, key individuals must be engaged. Engaging an individual means engaging a family, and engaging a family means engaging individuals.

Also, in I-FAST we do not have a rule about whom specifically to engage in each case. In one case, we may engage a parent and a probation officer. In another case, we may engage the whole household. In another case, we may engage a parent, a grandparent, and a social worker. The decision about whom to work with is made on a case-by-case basis. Thus, when working with families of at-risk youth, engaging occurs with not only one person, such as in individual treatment, or a household, such as in some family therapies, but selectively with the at-risk youth, family members, significant others, and various community representatives.

The complexity of deciding whom to engage can offer an extraordinary challenge for I-FAST practitioners. The more parties who are involved, the more likely there will be differing and even conflicting agendas. For example, the youth may have no interest in change whereas parents, the probation officer, and others are at odds over what should be done by whom. Each party may have a different view about what is causing the problem, what should be done about it, and what will be happening when the youth is doing better. The clinical objective is to enlist the commitment of all parties, despite differing points of view. Consequently, the process of engaging requires that the I-FAST practitioner have expertise in working with families in identifying problems to be addressed, forging alliances, and collaborating on goals, while taking into account the diverse needs of all involved. There are also decisions to be made about whom to involve in treatment and whom to empower, while remaining flexible.

CONCEPTUALIZING

Systems Theory and Engaging
STRENGTHS AND A SYSTEMS VIEW OF PROBLEMS
A systems view of problems can enhance a strengths-based perspective to working with clients. A systems view emphasizes viewing identified problems within the context of current and past interactions and understood further as a result of the descriptions, roles, and traditions of the involved parties. When viewed this way, problems are seen as relative to the descriptions and interactions of all involved and less as the product of individual deficits or pathology. Change is seen as building on identified strengths of all involved, including the identified youth.

CONSTRUCTIVISM: FRAMING AND ENGAGING

Co-Constructing Frames with Clients

Both practitioners and clients come to treatment with overarching frames and beliefs about why the problems are occurring and what to do about them. How practitioners frame clients and their situations can either enhance or interfere with successfully engaging families in treatment. Although frames can be borrowed from other models, in I-FAST our preference is that an overarching frame be co-constructed with each family. Overarching frames in I-FAST are accepted or constructed on a case-by-case basis according to what the family will respond to and engage around.

How Practitioners Frame Clients and Families

To enhance engagement and treatment effectiveness practitioners should develop frames with clients in a way that shows respect and allows them to be seen in a humane light and "save face." Thinking of clients as "wanting chaos" or "living from crisis to crisis" are common examples of how practitioners come to classify their clients in ways that interfere with engagement. Clients can be seen as motivated for selfish reasons, such as getting revenge on someone, or exploiting someone, or some other unsavory motivation. Clients can be classified as "manipulative" or "rigid." Though there may be truth to these views, they are not conducive to a practitioner trying to connect with such clients. Practitioners need a positive view of their clients, true or not, that will promote the establishment of an alliance.

Sometimes diagnoses can interfere with empathy and stigmatize clients, even among professionals. A client diagnosed with "borderline personality disorder" is somehow fundamentally different from other people, for example. How does one empathize with a "borderline?" In I-FAST, practitioners are encouraged to classify and frame clients in ways that enhance respect and understanding. Examples of ways of doing this involve viewing clients and family members as:

- Being protective of one another
- Being well-intended (benevolently rather than malevolently motivated)
- Already having strengths and competencies they can use in achieving their goals and successful treatment outcome

COMMON FACTORS AND ENGAGING

Engaging and Collaborating with Parents

With I-FAST, parents are viewed as the agents of change for their child with the presenting problem. To help their child, parents are encouraged to initiate the change process. That the parents will be the ones who resolve the child's problem resulting in improvement in the child is consistent with numerous well researched approaches (Alexander & Sexton, 2002; Henggeler et al., 2002; Kazdin, 2008; Liddle, 1991; Quinn, Kuehl, Thomas, & Joanning, 1988, 1989; Stanton, 1980; Szapocznick et al., 2002).

In addition to the research, there is a clear rationale that informs the I-FAST decision to align with parents. If a child is brought in for treatment and an expert works only with the child and solves the problem, or a pill solves the problem, the parents have not been empowered as parents. Someone or something other than the parents has fixed their child for them and thus there has not been a change in the family system; this is the opposite of what is needed when parents come in feeling helpless and powerless to deal with their child. To empower the parents and render the experts unnecessary the parents must be helped to find something they themselves can do to help their child. When this is successful, the parents are empowered by whatever new approach they have discovered and thus there is a change in the family system.

Aligning with parents does not mean that the child is ignored or not seen alone; this is not a "Tough Love" approach. Research has consistently found that engaging the child or adolescent is also important to treatment success. Early in the treatment process it is usually advisable to see the child alone without the parents:

- The child's input is valued and utilized.
- During the course of treatment, the child is typically seen alone, not just to give an opportunity to speak privately but also because parents often expect their child to be seen alone.
- Because of this parental expectation, seeing the child alone then also strengthens the alliance with the parent as with the child.
- Seeing a child alone also adds weight to whatever advice is eventually given to parents about what they might do to help their child.
- Obviously, joining with and gaining the child's trust is also important.

Identifying Strengths and Engagement

Identifying and amplifying client strengths in the process of achieving goals and positive change have been increasingly emphasized in the literature (Greene & Lee, 2011). Strength has been defined as "the capacity to cope with difficulties, to maintain functioning in the face of stress, to bounce back in the face of significant trauma, to use external challenges as a stimulus for growth, and to use social supports as a source of resilience" (McQuaide & Ehrenreich, 1997, p. 203). Aspinwall and Staudinger (2002) state that strengths "primarily lie in the ability to flexibly apply as many different resources and skills as necessary to solve a problem or work toward a goal" (p. 13). Strengths-based approaches have been used successfully for a wide variety of presenting problems in a wide variety of settings such as domestic violence treatment (Lehman & Simmons, 2009), sexual offender rehabilitation (Marshall, Marshall, Serran, & O'Brien, 2011), school counseling (Galassi & Akos, 2007), mental health (Rapp & Goscha, 2011), gerontology (Fast & Chapin, 2000; Ronch & Goldfield, 2003), addictions treatment (van Wormer & Davis, 2007), grief and loss (Pomeroy & Garcia, 2008), professional and life coaching (Biswas-Diener & Dean, 2007), leadership and organizational change (Lewis, Passmore, & Cantore, 2011; Linley, Harrington, & Garcea, 2010; Rath & Conchie, 2006), and social policy development (Maton, Schellenbach, Leadbeater, & Solarz, 2004; Tice & Perkins, 2001).

An assumption of strengths-based approaches to change is that client systems already have the resources and competencies to change but they are not using them, under-using them, or forgot that they have them (Greene & Lee, 2011). Practitioners therefore should assess for and identify client strengths and work with clients to build on these strengths in the service of change. There is evidence in the literature that clients want practitioners to think positively of them (Bohart & Tallman, 2010; Gassman & Grawe, 2006; Kelly, 2000) and they have negative reactions to practitioners who make "hostile, pejorative, critical, rejecting, or blaming" comments to them (Norcross, 2010, p. 130). Practitioners emphasizing client strengths rather than deficits can help facilitate engagement and the success of their work together (Bohart & Tallman, 2010; Friedlander, Escudero, & Heatherington, 2006; Sparks & Duncan, 2010; Walsh, 2006).

> A minimum requirement for being faithful to I-FAST is engaging and developing a collaborative relationship with at least one parent or primary caregiver. In I-FAST the focus is one empowering the parent or primary caregiver to be the one to solve the child's presenting problem.

STRATEGIZING

The aforementioned points on engaging all relate to the important components of why engaging is crucial to effective treatment and some guidelines and tips on how to do engaging. This is the conceptualizing part of all treatment. It is important to know, to value, and to internalize these conceptual elements of effective intervention because they form the foundation upon which the strategies of intervening are then built. Once practitioners know how important the multiple processes of engagement are to ultimately helping clients, then they may actively move to the critical decisions of the "who," "what," "when," and "how" of the engagement process. This is the strategizing phase. When engaging families, significant others, and community members there are a series of critical decisions that the practitioner must make. These decisions center on who will be engaged in the treatment and who will be empowered as principal change agents.

Guidelines for Deciding Whom to Include in Treatment

Deciding whom to actually include in treatment is a major treatment decision and is dealt with in I-FAST on a case-by-case basis. The various family treatment models have dealt with this issue in a variety of ways ranging from including the household (Minuchin, 1974), the household plus extended family and community members (Atteneave, 1969), or one individual (Bowen, 1974). Whitaker insisted on involving whomever the family did not want to be involved (Whitaker & Napier, 1978). With child problems, some approaches emphasize bringing in the mother and problem child (Weakland, Fisch, Watzlawick, & Bodin, 1974). Other approaches emphasize including fathers (Grove & Haley, 1993; Haley, 1976).

- With I-FAST, decisions about whom to involve are made strategically on a case-by-case basis.
- Emphasis is placed on effectiveness versus a formula that prescribes a certain number or combination of persons to involve.
- The practitioner attempts to engage a constellation of participants who are most likely to keep the at-risk youth living in his or her community.
- Flexibility extends throughout the treatment process as whom to involve may change as the case unfolds.

Even with the emphasis on empowering "primary caregivers" as the principal agents of change, there are often interests in the community who play important roles in the process. For this reason empowerment is a bit more complicated than simply empowering parents. If a youth is showing improvement with following parental rules at home while behavioral difficulties at school continue then parental empowerment will not be enough. Teachers and other school personnel will also need to be able to influence the youth. Though decisions about whom to involve in treatment and whom to empower are made strategically on a case-by-case basis, there are some guidelines that the I-FAST practitioner uses to assist in the process.

Who Has What Position on Change?
Each system member's position on change will be critical to choices the practitioner will make on how to engage them. The familiar perspective of the "Stage of Change" model is often helpful and can be employed within I-FAST including the classic phases of:

- **Precontemplative.** The party or system members have not even begun to consider that there is a problem, much less something that needs to be changed.
- **Contemplative.** System members have begun to consider that maybe there is a problem to be addressed.
- **Preparation.** Systems or members have acknowledged and agreed on the issue of a problem and are deciding on exactly what to do about it and the costs and benefits of alternate options.
- **Action.** This is the phase implicitly assumed (yet by no means always present in the clients or systems involved in treatment) by many approaches to treatment. It is the point at which all involved parties have agreed on how to define the problem, what course of action to take, and are motivated and actively engaged in the change process.
- **Maintenance.** Change has taken place and attention is turned to how to build resilience, consolidate and maintain changes, and predict hurdles and prevent relapse.

Practitioners will engage very differently with clients and systems that are at each of these different stages of change to both validate their positions on change and help them move forward to the next phase. Mismatching practitioner and client or system position on their current stage of the stage of change model will likely derail the engagement process and actually risk losing the trust and collaboration of one or all involved parties. Identifying each party's or system's stage or position on change, accepting and validating it, and then helping to move those clients forward in the change process is a key element in all treatment, especially in the I-FAST approach.

Who Is Most Motivated to Make a Change?
I-FAST assessment includes determining *who is most motivated to change and enlisting them in treatment*. The aforementioned stage of change model is one way of assessing this. Some factors to consider in this process are:

- What would gain their cooperation?
- Who is the most upset about the problem and what do they want done about it?

- A mother of a problem child may be the most upset about the problem but she may want her child seen individually.
- In this approach, the child may be seen individually in order to align with the mother and eventually recruit her more direct involvement in the treatment.
- This would be important if the parent has the expectation and desire for the child to be seen alone at least some times. In this instance, not doing so would imperil the engagement of the parent.

Understand the Big Picture

Another important set of factors to look at are the elements that compose the larger context, and asking the following questions:

- Who in the family is chronically involved in the pattern that supports the problem and what do they do?
- Who in the family is chronically not involved and what do they not do? Those who are not involved represent potential resources latent within the system.
- Are there out-of-household family members who are directly involved with the child's problems?
- Are there out-of-household family members who are interacting with the care giver(s) who are directly involved with the child's problems?
- What professionals are involved and what is their impact on changing or reinforcing patterns?
- Once the big picture is understood a decision can be made on whom to work with.

Whom to Empower?

I-FAST emphasizes *empowering primary caregivers to solve the child's problem*. That could mean mother, father, stepmother, foster mother, grandmother, and so forth. In a culture where divorce is common and shared parenting has become the norm it is not clear who the primary caregiver is in some arrangements. Complex problems often involve numerous participants. When helpers with the status of "expert" interview any combination of participants in a pattern, whom helpers listen to, whom they validate, and to whom they give tasks are elevated within the group. An expert has a "laying on the hands" power, so to speak. The status of anyone who receives the helper's special attention can be elevated.

- Whom practitioners align with, therefore, is in and of itself an intervention. The issue is, who can be empowered to change a pattern, rather than reinforce one?
- One does not want to empower an out-of-control teenager whose parents are immobilized in the face of the teen's extreme behavior. Yet this is a possible consequence of seeing that teen individually week after week no matter what is being said in that office. Meeting with parents is not always a solution to this problem.
- In difficult problems a multitude of adults are often involved. Whom to empower must be chosen strategically.

Who Has Power?

Another important consideration involves figuring out who has power to exert influence. One perspective on this question is, when helping to change an organization, the rule is to go to and through power (Haley, 1996). This could be a grandmother, a noncustodial parent, or a probation officer. The power brokers on a given case need not regularly attend sessions. At a minimum, they must be in agreement with treatment goals and methods in the broadest sense. For example, everyone must agree that a child will be worked with while remaining in the home, or that the parents will be worked with and helped to develop effective ways of dealing with the child's problems.

Flexibility

Ultimately, I-FAST emphasizes flexibility regarding whom to involve directly and indirectly in treatment. Flexibility allows maximum therapeutic possibilities and therefore I-FAST can adapt to a wide range of problems, patterns, practitioners' skill levels, and settings where treatment is offered. One practitioner may be skilled at working with just a mother and a child. Another practitioner might want to work the same case by including an uninvolved father. Flexibility in I-FAST allows for either option.

A final consideration regards where treatment is being offered. It is often difficult to recruit numerous family members to the office. Working with just a mother and a child makes more sense in this setting. When going into the home, however, the whole household is often present. In this setting it makes more sense to include more participants. Again, flexibility allows for either approach. Yet, the process of joining with those parties chosen for engagement is relatively the same. One must listen, understand, validate, and learn the language, frames values and motivation of each party. Through this process, the members of the system will come to allow the intervener in and the intervener will subsequently be able to influence the process of change from within the assumptive world of those key players.

Summary

Overall, when strategizing about how to engage and stay engaged in each case, the practitioner needs to view engagement as a key element. Engagement is not only a crucial component of all subsequent change, but also is an ongoing and evolving process. Throughout each episode of engagement with all systems, from parents to child to all larger systems involved, constant attention needs to be paid to feedback. Observing how clients and families respond to practitioners' frames, questions, empathic statements, and so forth and adjusting to and utilizing these responses is a key skill for maintaining engagement. The language, motives, position on change, and frames of all parties need to be constantly attended to, valued, and utilized. Client positions on change, their view of your role as practitioner with all of your own multiply saturated roles, and their relative power and control within the system, among other things need to be continually monitored and adjusted to as they may shift and evolve. Strategizing about how to keep such multiple engagements on track is not simply a onetime task but an ongoing process and skill for effective practitioners.

IMPLEMENTING

To implement the concepts and strategies discussed earlier practitioners need to be competent in a range of skills they can draw upon as needed. In this section a number of specific skills are presented along with case material and illustrations.

Understand and Validate Perspectives and Dilemmas of Involved Parties and Systems

Core practitioner skills used in the engaging process are listening, understanding, and validating the viewpoints and struggles of everyone involved in each ease. Inevitably, the views and descriptions of problems are described very differently from the perspectives of parents or caregivers in charge versus the view of youths. Validating is a practitioner-initiated process in which the family's thoughts feelings and behaviors are accepted, and considered completely understandable, given their subjective experience of the world. The practitioner genuinely accepts the client's presentation at face value and holds the belief that the client is doing the best he or she can. In addition, the practitioner respects the family's experience of the problem by emphasizing its importance and empathically offering total justification of the family's experience.

- Often the youth identified as having problems rejects the idea that there are any problems except for the position his parents are taking and the fact that he has you and others now butting into his life.
- The youth's position needs to be understood and affirmed as compassionately as does the position of the adults in authority positions in his life.
- The same goes for the frames and struggles of all agencies and other professionals involved in each case.
- *Practitioners must see themselves as involved in the process of joining with all parties and systems engaged in defining the situation as a problem and attempting to do something about it.* This is what we have termed the "problem-generated system."
- *It is fundamental to remember that the ideas, descriptions, and viewpoints of everyone involved in the case are what channels everyone's attempted solutions and thus shapes the patterns of the problem being addressed.*

Without this, practitioners will be less able to enter into relationships with everyone, speak their language, validate their distress, gain their trust, and enlist their motives in new efforts to resolve problems. Practitioners need a clear understanding of everyone's premises, motives, language, and positions on the problem and its resolution.

- For example, if one party, such as the youth, doesn't see that there is a problem, then she may be viewed as "precontemplative" from a stage of change model.
- The task in this case is to align with her puzzle about why others are so upset and then try to determine how others are defining the problem and how their problem definition affects the youth.
- *Trying to convince someone that there is a problem when she sees none will do little more than alienate her from you as an intervener.*

One way to view effective practitioners from this perspective is to see them as *respectful cultural anthropologists* who are entering several cultures and:

- Learning the languages used
- Understanding the world views

- Identifying values and motives
- Being respectful and validating of the dilemmas encountered and the goals of all

As previously stated, collaboration with fellow professionals is also emphasized in I-FAST. Professionals, particularly those who have the power to place children out of the home, and those who have become chronically involved in a case, can unwittingly become part of the patterns supporting problems.

- In I-FAST, all professionals are treated with respect with efforts made at establishing alliances with them as well, especially if they will be requested to change how they are approaching the case.
- *Learning their frames, using their language, and identifying and aligning with their values and goals and position on change are always critical to success in these multisystem cases.*

VALIDATION AND EMPATHY

An essential practitioner skill for validating clients is empathy. For anyone who has gone through any basic training in psychotherapy, the concept of "empathy" is most often viewed as fundamental to building a therapeutic relationship and a working alliance.

- Some have simply referred to this as the process of creating a "LUV triangle," or "Listening," "Understanding," and "Validating" the positions and plight of all clients and involved others (Echterling, Presbury, & McKee, 2005). But what do we mean by *empathy*?
- The most broadly used definition of empathy is that of Carl Rogers (1980), who defined it as: ". . . the practitioner's sensitive ability and willingness to understand the client's thoughts, feelings and struggles from the client's point of view. [It is] this ability to see completely through the client's eyes, to adopt his frame of reference" (p. 85).
- As stated previously, in multisystemic treatment with distressed youth and families, this invariably involves doing this with multiple and different individuals and groups. This is no small task!

At the same time, research suggests that empathy is critical to engaging active involvement of clients in treatment and that active involvement is an important contributor to outcome.

- Bohart (2002, p. 101) cites Orlinsky, Graw, and Parks (1994), who suggest that client active involvement is the most important factor in making treatment work. They indicate that:
    - "First, empathy promotes involvement.
    - Second, empathy provides support for clients' active information-processing efforts. . .
    - Third, empathy helps the practitioner choose interventions compatible with the clients' frame of reference. . .."

We also need to be aware that this is true across approaches.

A Complication

Research on empathy indicates that there is an additional complication that I-FAST practitioners keep in mind when engaging clients in the treatment process. That is, clients probably have a different need and capacity for receiving what practitioners traditionally view as empathic communication (cf. Beutler, 1973; Beutler, Johnson, Neville, & Workman, 1972; Ham, 1987; Henry, Sprenkle, & Sheehan, 1986).

- Several sources suggest, for example, that clients who are highly sensitive, suspicious, poorly motivated, or reactive to authority tend to do worse with more empathic, involved, and accepting practitioners (Beutler, Engle, Oro-Beutler, Daldrup, & Meredith, 1986). This is often the position of youth and families involved in treatment.
- Mohr and Woodhouse (2000) found that some clients prefer business-like relationships over those judged as warm and empathic.
- These findings reinforce O'Hara's (1984) suggestion that in some cases it is most empathic for the practitioner not to express the traditional qualities of empathy!
- Clients are not only the best judge of the quality of empathy but also of the type and amount of it they desire.
- Thus empathy is really always a client-directed endeavor where *the best measure of what is empathic is the judgment of clients and others involved in any intervention.*
- *This underscores the need for I-FAST practitioners to be flexible in the way that they demonstrate empathy.*

The definition of validating and steps in the process suggests that it is directional and empathic. In other words, validating involves understanding the client's perspective in the direction of justifying his or her assumptions and corresponding actions that drive first-order change.

IDENTIFYING AND UTILIZING CLIENT LANGUAGE AND VALUES

As noted previously, it is important for practitioners to act like respectful cultural anthropologists as they enter the multiple systems involved with each case.

- Practitioners need to carefully and often literally identify the nature of the culture they are entering, the norms of the local area, and the unique ways in which each family interacts with one another.
- They need to allow the family and involved agencies to teach them their language, values, norms, and aspirations just as if the practitioners were anthropologists entering into a different culture, village, family, and the structures and groups functioning within that culture.
- *Very importantly, practitioners also need to be aware of their own language, culture, and demographic identities and biases, and become aware of how they are likely to be viewed by the involved systems as outsiders coming in.*

- Practitioners must be willing to suspend their own language and premises on the way things are in favor of learning the new language and assumptions of the family and those around them engaged with trying to help them.
- As practitioners are successful in negotiating these tasks, they will also gain access to joining into these systems, as well as gaining perspective on how the identified problems are being defined and acted on.
- Once this is achieved, then practitioners can partner with the groups and individuals to shift identified problematic patterns of solution and build on strengths and new directions to create the kind of pattern shift that will achieve everyone's goals.
- This takes skill and respect for all involved, yet once achieved, the successful process of treatment will follow more easily.

IDENTIFYING STRENGTHS AND ENGAGEMENT

The literature on working with high-risk youth and families discusses assessing for and using clients' strengths but often is lacking specifics on how to do this. Some of the specific ways to identify and amplify the strengths of at-risk youth and families used in I-FAST are the following.

Clients Identify Their Own Strengths

A first step in identifying strengths is to have clients identify their own strengths.

- I-FAST practitioners assume that clients and families already have qualities and strengths needed for successes.
- *Clients can be asked to identify their own personal qualities and strengths that led to these successes.*
- Useful questions can include: "What personal qualities and strengths have helped you to hang in there instead of giving up your children to foster care?"
- All parties can be complimented for their investment in the process of resolving the identified difficulty, framing everyone's motives positively.

Strength in the Face of Adversity and Resilience in the Face of Challenges

Undeniable strengths may be brought forward when the practitioner emphasizes how challenging the clients' lives have been.

- I-FAST practitioners assume that the family has resilience in the face of adversity.
- A useful question to ask the family that acknowledges and reinforces this could include: "How has the family been coping with dad being laid off from his job that helps you to stay together and not fall apart?"

Identifying Exceptions

Another way to redirect clients from simply dwelling upon their weakness and problems is to ask them about times the problem hasn't occurred, or has been less intense.

- I-FAST practitioners assume that there are exceptions to the habitual interactional patterns.

- Not only can the solution interactions around the identified problem be identified but also *exceptions to the problems and successes* can be noted and *clients can be asked to identify their own personal qualities and strengths that led to these successes.*
- Useful questions include: "When was last time that you thought you were going to explode and get in a fight but instead you were able to stay calm and walk away from the situation?" "How were you able to do that?"

View Family Members as "Co-Practitioners"

In a strengths-based approach, family members are viewed not as part of the problem but as part of the solution. When recruiting family members, practitioners should approach them as helpers, or co-practitioners, regardless of whatever problems they themselves may have, or how they may be described by others. In a strengths-based perspective, no matter what, or how severe the personal problems of family members may be, it is assumed that if family members can become organized around solving specific problems latent resources within the family can be mobilized.

A CASE EXAMPLE

A 27-year-old mother had a serious and chronic drug addiction. Her two children were removed from her care and placed in foster care. Her parents, who lived separately, had serious problems. Her father was a chronic alcoholic and had been violent toward her mother. In addition, there was serious and ongoing conflict in her parents' home involving her and her siblings. She described one occasion when visiting her parents during which she and her brother had conflict and the brother chased her off the property with a loaded gun aimed at her. Despite these serious problems, her parents were recruited into treatment to help her end her drug use. The parents were able to put their chronic difficulties aside and work together. They successfully helped their daughter get off of drugs, reorganize her life, and eventually be reunited with her children.

In this strengths-based approach the woman's family was viewed as a potential resource, despite their serious and chronic problems, and how negatively they were described.

FRAMING AND POSITIVE REFRAMING

Initially practitioners usually have their own frames based on their training and life and professional experiences. At some point the practitioner may offer a frame to the family to see if it resonates with them. In I-FAST, if the family does not accept ("buy") the frame the practitioner must adjust and find a frame that the family will accept. This flexibility allows for engagement with a wider range of families than is allowed by approaches locked into their own idiosyncratic overarching frame.

Case Examples

In both of these cases, engagement in treatment was dependent on the practitioner accepting the overarching frame of the client. Both clients believed strongly in their frames and would not have engaged if the practitioner had not respected and worked with their frames.

> **CASE 1**
>
> A woman experienced bizarre sensations in various parts of her body. She felt as if her uterus was floating around inside of her. She believed her pelvic bone was collapsing and that her spine was protruding up the back of her head, pushing her brain forward. She had been to several prestigious clinics and several specialists but they found no medical problem. She was then sent to a psychologist. The psychologist worked with her trying to help her realize that she was having psychosomatic delusions. The psychologist was working outside the client's frame. As a result, the client fired the psychologist. A second practitioner accepted the client's frame that perhaps there was an undiagnosed medical problem. The problem, the second practitioner pointed out, was the client's life was falling apart and she would have to find a way to improve even in the absence of a clear medical diagnosis. She agreed with this and engaged in treatment focusing on improving her functioning. A way to work within her frame was found and she engaged in treatment.
>
> **CASE 2**
>
> A woman came to treatment after her drug addicted husband detoxified and went into Narcotics Anonymous (NA) for treatment. He was gone five nights a week, dutifully following traditional substance abuse treatment. The problem from the wife's point of view was that he had withdrawn completely from her and the family. The man accompanied her for her second appointment and stated that he had been a serious prescription drug addict. NA had saved his life. He was totally sold on the disease model of substance abuse. The practitioner pointed out that at his stage of recovery, he had achieved abstinence but now had to reintegrate back into his family. He agreed but was unwilling to give up any NA meetings. The practitioner suggested he and his wife find NA meetings that include both addicts and their spouses, and for them to attend together. Both husband and wife liked this idea. Again, the husband's frame was accepted and a treatment approach that was in alignment with his thinking was constructed.

Positive Reframing

Positive reframing is one technique I-FAST practitioners can employ to frame clients in a positive light, which can intensify family engagement.

- Positive reframing involves the practitioner taking the "facts" of the presenting situation the client and/or significant others have defined negatively and providing a positive meaning to them; this usually involves moving some

behavior or personal attribute from a problem/deficit frame to a strength/resource frame.
- Positive reframing is one intervention that focuses on changing the client's narrow world view by redefining the client's reality to include more alternatives, to perceive their concerns as being resources rather than deficits.
- Reframing enlarges the client's frame, or widens the perspective, around the facts.
- Positive reframing requires mentally shifting a "problematic" behavior, feeling, or thought into a different frame (category) that is meaningful and acceptable to the client.
- The positive reframing process involves offering a client a plausible, alternative positive frame (category) for something the client has defined as negative and thus undesirable.
- Once clients accept the plausibility of the new and more positive "reality" represented by the new frame, they cannot go back to using only their former, more narrow "world view" that contributed to the problem maintaining vicious cycle of first-order change.
- For positive reframing to be successful, the practitioner must offer a new frame that is compatible with the client's way of thinking and categorizing reality.
- In positive reframing, it is important for the practitioner to offer the plausible, alternative meaning in a tentative manner with a questioning tone of voice.
- Presenting a positive reframe in this manner allows the client to either agree with the practitioner and accept the reframe or to correct the practitioner and then accept it or take it in a mull it over; this also avoids an unnecessary power struggle with the client over its rightness or wrongness.
- The suggested positive reframe may introduce enough novelty to the client's assumptive world that it will start to put a small "chink" in the client's habitual problem maintaining patterns resulting in second-order change.
- When offered effectively, positive reframing can also serve to help clients and parents save face, further intensifying engagement. One objective is to frame what could be viewed as negative or hostile statements or behaviors by parents as benevolently motivated.

SOME EXAMPLES OF POSITIVE REFRAMING

- Mothers whose children are in foster care and who are not visiting or completing their case plans can be framed as making the ultimate sacrifice for their children. Typically, children and professionals frame the mother's withdrawal as abandonment. These mothers are often described as caring more about their boyfriend or taking drugs than their children. It is possible, and possibly closer to the truth, to frame their withdrawal more positively. They may be viewed as sacrificing their own relationship with their child so their child can be in a better place.
- Often these mothers actually feel they do not have anything to offer their child and that their child is better off without them. Despite their own

(continued)

> love and desire to be with their child, from the mother's point of view it would be better for the child to be with another family. The child and perhaps other family members and professionals, however, can misinterpret this as abandonment.
> - When attempting to engage such a mother in treatment, which practitioner would the mother more likely connect with, the one who frames her as caring more about her drug habit than her child, or the one who frames her as making a sacrifice for her child?
> - The motives of parents who want their children placed in foster care can also be framed positively. If a child's behavior has been out of control and the parents have failed to help their child, often the parents want the child placed in a setting where they (the parents) think there are professionals who will know how to help their child. The parents feel helpless and want what they think is best for their child. When framed this way, the parents will often agree that is their intention, and will also agree that ultimately their goal is to be reunited with their child.
> - Parents with overly restrictive rules can be framed as protective.
> - Parents who become angry can be framed as caring intensely.
> - Parents who are uninvolved can be framed as not wanting to interfere.
> - Noncustodial fathers who have withdrawn from visits can be framed as loving their children too much. It is too painful for them to be reduced to a part-time parent so they have withdrawn.
> - A six-year-old child's acting out may be a result of caring for and protecting a depressed parent. When the child acts out the parent gets angry at him or her, and thus the child's misbehavior mobilizes the parent out of his or her depression. The parent being angry is also reassuring to the child because usually children would rather have their parents angry at them than to see their parents as being depressed.

Parents, and most frequently mothers, are often blamed for the problems their children are exhibiting due to perceived neglect, or other poor parenting practices. Interveners are invariably drawn to frustration with parents as clients, blaming them and often alienating them from therapeutic influence in the process. Aligning with parents and finding positives in them is crucial to forming the type of positive working alliances that are crucial to success in treatment.

Framing motives positively can serve to reduce hostility between family members and offer face saving to the parents. Parents are viewed as caring, wanting what is best for their child, and as loving. Parents are more likely to engage in treatment when their motives are framed in a more positive light and children are less hurt by defining their parents as trying to engage in something positive. To the extent that this view can be extended to the perspectives of others involved with the case such as child protective workers, probation officers, teachers, and others, the positive outcome of the cases are enhanced even more. Similarly, the perspectives, motives, and struggles of all involved systems such as schools, courts, child protective services, and so forth also need to be understood, validated, and their strengths built upon in the process of joining with them to create jointly desired goals.

TRACKING POWER

A family member with power is defined as being the one who:

- Determines what actually happens in the family
- Has power to get the family to treatment
- Has power to make or break the treatment
- Is able to influence the group and get something accomplished

The possibility that treatment will succeed can be greatly enhanced when a practitioner understands who in the family has influence and that family member is either engaged directly in treatment, or at a minimum, their blessings of treatment goals and methods are obtained. Ignoring or missing such a powerful family member can result in that member sabotaging treatment, or at worst, firing the practitioner altogether. Assessing who has such influence is often difficult to do by asking directly. Who the family states has influence may not be who actually has it. The most reliable way of assessing who has power and influence is to track family interactions. To do so, practitioners must put their social stereotypes aside and observe who in the family does or says what and how other family members actually respond.

Tracking and respecting who in the family has power and influence can be an important tool within I-FAST to promote engagement into treatment. Tracking and engaging powerful family members has been an important task in both traditional family treatment models (Haley, 1987, 1996; Minuchin, 1974) and home-based treatment models (Kinney, Booth, & Booth, 1991; Lindbald-Goldberg, Dore, & Stern, 1998; Szapocznik et al., 2002). Both Haley and Minuchin stressed conducting what they called a "hierarchical interview" in which the family power structure was observed, respected, and engaged (Haley, 1987; Minuchin, 1974). Szapocznik places such emphasis on engaging powerful family members that within this model, treatment is not thought to have even begun until those powerful family members have been identified and are engaged directly in treatment. Perhaps Haley describes the idea most succinctly by stating to engage a family "one must go to and through power" (Haley, 1996).

For the purposes of I-FAST, tracking and engaging powerful family members, like tracking language, is an option for enhancing engagement, not a requirement. In I-FAST, this does not necessarily mean powerful family members must come to treatment. An understanding who has influence, what their positions are about the problem brought to treatment, and what to do about it must be acquired, along with their approval of both treatment goals and of treatment methods. By methods, we mean methods in a broad sense, such as parents will be helped to resolve the child's problems, placement will be avoided, and so forth. These understandings and agreements can be obtained either directly by engaging powerful family members in sessions or indirectly by interviewing those who do come to treatment and coaching those individuals on how they interact with powerful family members.

Tracking Power by Observing How Decisions Are Made and How Conflict Is Resolved

Often the question of who has power in a family can be observed in direct interaction in session. The following are some of the ways this may be done.

- Often, who has power can be determined by tracking how important decisions are made or by how conflict is resolved.
- At the end of a session, who decides when to come next?
- Whose schedule must be adjusted and who accommodates whom?
- If parents have to decide how to respond to a serious infraction by their child, how is this decision made?
- If parents disagree with how to deal with a problem their child is presenting, how is the disagreement resolved?
- Does one parent dominate the discussion and impose his or her view, or do the parents each present an idea and reach compromises?
- If a child is guilty of an infraction do the parents follow through on agreed responses, or does one parent side with the child, resulting in agreements not being upheld?

Observing these interactions directly or getting a detailed description of the discussion can often reveal who has power.

A CASE EXAMPLE

A man requested treatment for himself individually. The man lived with his second wife, had two sons, ages 19 and 12, from his first marriage, and a 15-year-old stepdaughter. He explained that his 19-year-old son no longer lived with him because one year earlier it had been discovered that the son had been molesting the man's stepdaughter. When this discovery was made, his wife banned the son from the house and forbade the man from ever seeing him again. The son was sent to live with his paternal grandmother. The courts became involved and ordered the son into treatment, which he had now successfully completed. The man then wanted his son to be able to become part of the family again, preferably by moving back home. His wife was adamantly opposed to any family involvement with the son. The man disclosed that to avoid problems with his wife, he was secretly seeing his son on a regular basis. He wanted his relationship with his son to be in the open and preferably at home. This man's wife had much power. She had the power to ban the man's son from the home and to forbid him from seeing his son. The man had to conduct a secret relationship with his own son. More importantly, the man's goal for treatment could obviously not be accomplished without a minimum engagement from his wife. She had to become involved either directly in treatment or indirectly by coaching the man on how to negotiate with her on this issue.

In this case, with the man's permission, the wife was invited to treatment. A negotiated agreement was reached between the parents. The wife stated that if the son was truly repentant and sorrowful over what he had done, she could agree to the boy visiting the house under adult supervision, and to the husband seeing the son as much as they both wished. The boy was remorseful and since he was now 19 and wanted to have his own place, the father agreed that the proposed compromise was fair.

RECRUITING FAMILY MEMBERS TO TREATMENT

A major skill emphasized among approaches that engage whole families is that of recruiting family members into treatment who do not initially attend. This skill can be useful in many I-FAST cases. To recruit additional family members into treatment, those who do attend must first be persuaded of the need to involve additional family members. The emphasis should be placed on the help additional family members can provide at resolving the problems the family is seeking help on. Additional family members are defined as additional helpers. Their views about the problem can be of benefit as well as their efforts to solve the problem. In some cases it may be obvious and must be emphasized that the additional family being recruited can play a vital role in helping to solve the problem.

When family resist the idea of recruiting additional members into treatment it is often useful to assume they are being protective of those family members. They are uncertain and may not trust how the practitioner will treat them. They may fear the practitioner will blame them. When operating from the assumption that family members are protective, practitioners will be more likely to frame other family members with respect and emphasize the sincere need for their help.

COLLABORATING WITH ALL PARTIES (SYSTEMS COLLABORATION)

I-FAST assumes that the effectiveness of any intervention is wholly dependent on the quality of the therapeutic relationship. For treatment to be successful the practitioner must demonstrate caring for the client, and in return the client must care about what the practitioner thinks. At its most abstract level, engaging consists of a two-step process that involves *first establishing a bond* and *then requesting change* (Fraser & Solovey, 2007).

- Generally, to establish a therapeutic bond, practitioners must demonstrate genuine interest in the client, engender hope, and win faith and trust that they can indeed help. The I-FAST practitioner must also demonstrate that clients are understood and validate their dilemmas and beliefs about the problems.
- When dealing with multiple participants of a pattern, the rule is for practitioners to engage all participants using this two-step process.
- This includes parents; at-risk youths; significant others; and community representatives such as children's service workers, probation officers, teachers, and so on.

THE ESSENTIAL BEGINNING ELEMENTS OF ENGAGING

In summary, the essential elements of engaging may be condensed as follows.

- The practitioner initially accepts and maintains the family's way of interacting.
- The practitioner uses the family's language (e.g., figures of speech, metaphors, theory of problem formation and change, frames of reference, beliefs).

(continued)

- The practitioner adapts to the family's or individual's style of nonverbal behaviors.
- The practitioner uses strengths-based language that implies positive intentions.
- There is an easy flow of communication between the clients and practitioner back and forth.
- Communication demonstrates a process in which the practitioner listens to clients and clients listen to the practitioner.
- The practitioner adjusts responses consistent with the way that family members experience empathy, noting the presence of validating client distress, empathic postures, language and voice tone, and so forth.
- The practitioner aligns with parents or caregivers who are the primary agents of change.
- The practitioner joins with involved individuals who have different perspectives (positions) on the presenting situation.

TRACKING INTERACTIONS 4

INTRODUCTION TO TRACKING INTERACTIONS: TYPES OF INTERACTIONS

Interactions can be habitual and promote stability or exceptional, or outside the pattern of habitual interactions, and promote transition. During the life cycle of any family periods of both stability and transition occur and therefore neither type of interaction is inherently positive or negative. At times when problems cannot be resolved, interactional patterns can maintain them. Also, at times when developmental processes demand transitions, interactional patterns can interfere with those transitions and serious problems can then develop. It is during these times that families need to move away from habitual interactional patterns and find or emphasize new exceptions to those interactions.

Traditionally, family treatment approaches that track and focus on interactions tend to fall into two categories: those that track and identify interactional patterns and those that track and identify interactional exceptions. Approaches that focus on identifying patterns track and identify sequences of interactions that are habitual and support the problem. Numerous traditional family treatment approaches have focused on interactional patterns (Bowen, 1978; Haley, 1997; Minuchin & Fishman, 1981; Weakland, 1981). Terms such as family structure (Minuchin & Fishman, 1981), sequence of interaction (Haley, 1987), problem maintaining behavior (Weakland, Fisch, Watzlawick, & Bodin, 1974), and triangulation (Bowen, 1978) all refer to what we call interactional patterns.

Approaches that focus on exceptions track and identify sequences of interactions representing how participants interact when the problem does not occur. Identifying exceptions (Berg & Kelly, 2000; De Jong & Berg, 2008; de Shazer, 1985) and identifying new stories (counter-stories; White & Epston, 1990) are two examples of working this way.

In either way of working, sequences of interactions are the focus. An interactional understanding of either what keeps the problem going or what solves the problem is the goal. It has been noted that problems and solutions are "two sides of the same systemic coin" (Fraser, 1995b). For every interactional pattern there is an exception to that interaction.

Although I-FAST practitioners are free to work either way, we strongly support and teach the use of both. Learning both skills allows for numerous ways of combining the two. At a minimum, I-FAST practitioners who are skilled at tracking exceptions are encouraged to also develop the skill at identifying interactional patterns. The skill of identifying exceptions is strongly enhanced when the pattern the exception relates to is understood. By identifying the habitual interactions, the practitioner focused on exceptions has a better grasp of the context in which the exceptions are occurring. I-FAST practitioners who are skilled at tracking patterns must also attend to changes that may occur at any point in the I-FAST treatment process. They must also follow up on how families respond to intervention procedures. When doing either, exceptions must be tracked. Skillful use of exception questions must be utilized at these points in the treatment process to identify changes that have occurred.

CONCEPTUALIZING

Systems Theory and Tracking Interactions

Systems theory provides the concepts for understanding how problems are maintained and how change occurs. To maintain itself or change, a system fluctuates between stability and change through feedback. Feedback involves part of a system's output being reintroduced from its environment back into the system as information about the output (Keeney, 1983; Watzlawick, Beavin, & Jackson, 1967, p. 31). Feedback can be positive or negative. In *positive feedback* one event (A) produces a change in another event (B) in the same direction, that is, an *increase* in A produces and *increase* in B (Capra, 1996). Positive feedback is involved in "the commonly known runaway effects, or vicious cycles, in which the initial effect continues to be amplified as it travels repeatedly around the loop" (Capra, 1996, p. 59) (see Figure 4-1). In negative feedback an increase in A produces a *decrease* in B. In human systems feedback involves verbal and nonverbal communication. According to Watzlawick et al. (1967), a single unit of communication is a *message* and an *interaction* is the exchange of a series of messages between two people. Over time, communicational feedback processes become redundant and patterned and these *patterns of interactions* become the *rules* (frames or assumptions) of the system. In using a systems framework with families we are not looking for causes of a system's current level of functioning but only at how it is currently functioning.

An additional aspect of systems theory that informs intervention in I-FAST is that all systems interactions are interconnected. Because all elements in a system are interconnected, a change in one part of the system can cause the entire system, in

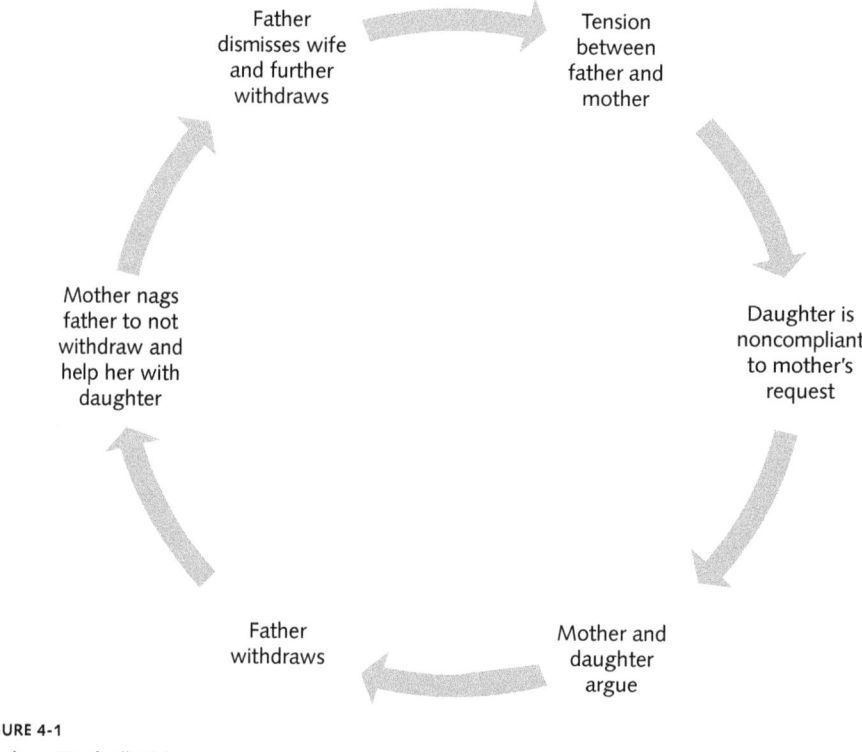

FIGURE 4-1
Simple positive feedback loop.

this case a family, to change. Change one interaction and the entire cycle can change. In the preceding example, if the mother and the daughter fight less, the father may not withdraw and conflict between mother and father may diminish. Likewise, if the father supported the mother, the mother and daughter may stop fighting. Changing one set of interactions can change all sets of interactions in the cycle.

Finally, one basic assumption of a systems perspective is that change is constant. Though there are some repeated sequences in all systems (especially those caught in escalating vicious cycles) there are always points when there are different interactions or exceptions to the rule of those escalating and repeating cycle patterns. As such, every problem pattern includes some sort of exception to the rule (de Shazer, 1985). Such a view underlies our beliefs in the strengths and potentials of families (Berg & De Jong, 1996). Despite the multi-deficiencies and/or problems families may perceive they have, there are always times when they handle their life situations in a more satisfying way or in a different manner (Lee, Sebold & Uken, 2003). These exceptions can often provide the clues for solutions (de Shazer, 1985) and represent the family's "unnoticed" strengths and resources.

CONSTRUCTIVISM AND TRACKING INTERACTIONS

The Role of Language

The role of language in sustaining or creating reality reinforces the importance of helping the family to identify exceptions and solutions. Social constructivism suggests that language serves as the medium through which personal meaning and understanding are expressed and socially constructed (Gergen, 2009). Further, the meaning of things is always contingent on the contexts and the language within which it is described, categorized, and constructed by families (Gergen, 2009; Wittgenstein, 1958). Because the limits of reality that can be known and experienced by an individual are framed by the language available to him or her to describe it, and these meanings are inherently unstable and shifting, a major question for the practitioner to consider is how to use language in treatment to assist the family in describing and constructing a "beneficial" reality. Because language is inherently powerful in creating and sustaining realities, it is beneficial to utilize treatment conversation to help construct meanings and solutions by describing goals, observable behaviors, and progressive lives in new, more beneficial ways (de Shazer, 1994; Miller, 1997). Language requires that when labeling a pattern of behavior as problematic that exceptions to the rule are omitted. The child who usually throws tantrums when asked to do something he finds is unpleasant may readily comply at other times.

Thus, a counterpart to tracking and identifying interactional patterns that support problems is the tracking and identification of interactions that resolve problems, that is, exceptions. The use of pre-suppositional language in questions can focus family attention on exceptions.

Questions such as "What are you doing when the problem is not occurring?" assumes there are times when the problem is not occurring:

- The task for the practitioner is to assist families in noticing, amplifying, sustaining, and reinforcing these exceptions regardless of how small and/or infrequent they may be (Berg & Kelly, 2000).

- Often, families focus so much on their problems that they "miss" noticing or not recognizing the times when they are doing better. "What we notice becomes reality and what is not noticed does not exist" (Lee, Sebold & Uken, 2003, p. 31).

Strengths and Identifying Interactions

It is tempting to become blaming when identifying interactional patterns. Parents who habitually engage in hostile exchanges with teens can be blamed by practitioners who identify those interactions. Many beginning family practitioners respond this way when identifying interactional patterns. Blaming, however, is not consistent with I-FAST. A strengths-based way of viewing habitual interactions is that they are empowering. Defining problems interactionally defines them as changeable. Participants can change how they habitually respond. When family members are empowered to think and behave outside the box, they are empowered to solve problems. I-FAST practitioners are encouraged to understand the empowering aspect of identifying habitual interactions and to assume that families are capable of producing interactions that are outside of the box of their habitual responses.

Regarding exceptions, clients and families can make rapid and beneficial changes if the focus is on what they can do and what strengths they have if they decide to do so (Berg & Dolan, 2001; Greene & Lee, 2011). The focus on strengths to achieve change is also supported by a systems perspective (Bateson, 1979) and the role of language in creating reality (de Shazer, 1994). Within I-FAST, we are offering multiple methods of utilizing client strengths. One method is to put a major emphasis on identifying exceptions to when the problem occurs and amplifying these exceptions.

- Once families are helped in noticing their strengths and resources and the times when they are engaged in non-problem behavior, they are on the way to a solution-building process (Berg & De Jong, 1996).

> Whether focusing on patterns or exceptions, I-FAST requires obtaining an *interactional understanding*. Interactions representing patterns that support the problem or interactions that represent exceptions must be tracked and identified. To remain faithful to I-FAST problems and their solutions must be understood in terms of the interactions of the various participants in response to those problems.

STRATEGIZING

Problem Defined

The first step to identifying interactional patterns or interactional exceptions is to define a specific problem. To track interactions there must be a specific problem to associate them with. Although it might seem elementary, it is important that we define what we mean by a problem as a first step in discussing how we engage families in discussions around problem identification.

Notice that there are two criteria for a problem to be a problem. The first is the behavior itself and the second is persistence in spite of change efforts. The idea of persistence is critical for two reasons.

- I-FAST practitioners are strengths-based and so presume that families solve many problems on their own. The objective of treatment is not to uncover and

change every strange, unusual, or inappropriate behavior that goes on in a family. Instead, the objective is to give credit where credit is due and work on behaviors that the family and/or engaged other systems are struggling with.
- Persistence despite efforts to change provides insight into patterns that support and maintain problems. As was mentioned earlier, efforts to bring about change or failed solutions comprise the stuck cycles (positive feedback loops of vicious cycles) that perpetuate a problem. In pattern assessment we are concerned with who is or is not involved in solving the problem, and what is being done or not done to bring about change.

Multiple Problems

Families with at-risk youth usually have many problems in multiple domains. The objective of the I-FAST practitioners is to work within the multiple domains identifying key stake holders and their views on what problems need to be addressed. I-FAST practitioners are aware of complexities involved in the change process and are aware that problems are reciprocally linked. This means that change in one problem can have either a positive or a negative influence on another. Because problems are linked, the I-FAST practitioner works with stakeholders to prioritize problems while advocating small steps.

VIEWING AND DOING

The nature of the problem and supporting patterns is that they occur on two levels:

- *Viewing* has to do with the concepts or frames that stakeholders use to describe the problem and how it has come about. Parents, teachers, probation officers, and so on may view the youth as being bad or as mentally ill. There may be confusion such that the youth is seen as both:
  - If the youth is viewed as mentally ill, solutions may be seen as falling in the domain of psychiatric medications.
  - If the youth is viewed as bad, then the family may push for placement in the court system.
  - If there is confusion, the family may be stuck and go back and forth on what to do about their child.
  - A key task for practitioners is to modify the views of family members and child helping professionals so that problems can be addressed in treatment.
- *Doing* is the behavior that is labeled as problematic and answers the question:
  - "What is the youth doing to whom that is considered to be a problem"? When describing what behaviors are problematic many families and child helping professionals will mix theories of causation with the problem.
  - For example, when talking about a youth who is skipping school, there may be discussion about his low self-esteem. Self-esteem is not a behavior. It is a theory of causation about behavior.
  - I-FAST practitioners endeavor to assist family members and child helping professionals describe problems in behavioral terms. This assists with the later processes of establishing goals and therapeutic tasks.

- In I-FAST we are not focused on labels such as low self-esteem, mentally ill, or various diagnostic labels such as conduct disorder, oppositional defiant disorder, bipolar disorder, and so forth but rather we want to know what behaviors does the youth engage in that indicate to observers the assigned label(s). *In I-FAST we find it is easier to change what a person does rather than who he is.*

UNIT OF ANALYSIS

Understanding interactions suggests identifying them among groups. Consequently, practitioners need to decide how many individuals are to be included in the group being observed. Habitual or exceptional interactions can include one, two, three, or more individuals. Interactional patterns or interactional exceptions can be observed in any of these units. Unit of analysis has a major influence on how cases are conceptualized. Deciding whom to include in one's tracking and analysis of interactions is a major treatment decision that will have substantial impact on the practitioner's understanding of patterns and exceptions and on what to do about those patterns or how to amplify those exceptions.

I-FAST practitioners should attend to two types of interactions: Interactions between various adults and the problem child and interactions between various adults *about* the problem child. How a parent or other adult interacts with the child about the problem should be tracked and noted. The adult may habitually get drawn into a hostile argument, or habitually lecture or plead, or stand their ground only to cave in after determined resistance from the problem child. The focus of interactional assessment and intervention can be on changing adult–child interactions. Exceptions to these interactions can also be tracked and amplified.

A second type of interaction that can be part of a larger problem can involve how adults interact with each other about the child. A father may withdraw from habitual fighting between the mother and the problem child. The mother may habitually nag the father to become more involved and the father can respond to the mother by habitually criticizing her. These adult-to-adult interactions about the child can be part of the interaction cycle that includes how the mother and problem child interact. Another common example can include a professional and a parent. The professional may habitually blame or criticize the parent and the parent then is more determined to continue his or her habitual interaction with the child. Again, the adult-to-adult interaction is part of the cycle that includes the adult in problem child interaction.

In I-FAST, tracking both types of interactions is encouraged. Intervening in one or both types can change the entire cycle. A father who withdraws when the mother and daughter fight may not continue to withdraw if the mother and daughter stop fighting. On the other hand, the mother and daughter may stop fighting if father is more supportive of mother.

Guidelines for Deciding Unit of Analysis

How to decide what unit to focus on can be aided by the following considerations:

- **Utilize what the practitioner is already skilled in doing.** The practitioner may already be skilled in thinking either in dyads or triads or larger groups. It is totally permissible in I-FAST to begin conceptualizing a given case in either unit. As stated, neither unit is considered better or worse. In I-FAST it is assumed both ways of conceptualizing interactions have equal potential to help resolve the problem. If conceptualizing in either unit helps resolve the case that is fine. If, however, the case cannot be resolved by conceptualizing either in dyads or triads, for example, the supervisor may consider changing the unit of analysis as a way of resolving a therapeutic impasse.

- **Understand the big picture**. Before offering interventions, it is often wise for practitioners to understand the big picture when deciding who should be involved in treatment. Serious child problems typically involve multiple adults in the family, as well as multiple professionals. Despite this, an initial session may be attended by only a mother and the problem child. In this situation, the views of other adults in the family and of key professionals such as case workers, probation officers, and others must be ascertained. Failure to do so can result in mobilizing resistance from key persons not included in the practitioner's observational field, or on focusing on goals that do not make sense given the larger picture. At a minimum their contribution to the pattern must be understood and incorporated into the practitioner's thinking about the case and into the interventions offered.
    - Family members outside of the client's household can be actively or passively involved in patterns that keep the problem going. It is often helpful to understand these contributions at the outset of a case, before deciding whom to work with directly. In addition, family members not actively participating in interactional patterns that directly support the problem can represent latent family resources that could be called on to help solve the problems. Further, extended family such as grandparents and sometimes others may have views, beliefs, and thoughts about how to solve the problem that allow openings for how to make progress that immediate family members may not be offering. Taking a wide lens and understanding this larger family picture can often inform choices of an I-FAST practitioner that more efficiently and effectively resolve the problems.
    - The danger in selecting a wider lens is the I-FAST practitioner can become overloaded with information. Attempting to understand patterns with large numbers of participants can sometimes confuse and immobilize a practitioner. He or she can become paralyzed and confused about where to start, or be run around in circles bouncing back and forth between multiple problems and their patterns without obtaining change in any of them. The result can be a treatment without a focus.
- **Keep it simple and focus on something specific.** Though it is important to understand who all the key participants are on a case and to understand their respective views of the problem, ultimately it is important to select a unit of analysis that makes the problem both comprehensible and generates ideas for how to solve it. A balance must be struck between understanding the larger picture of a particular case and focusing on something specific. Selecting smaller units allows for the treatment to be more focused and increases the chances that something will actually get done.

- **Pros and cons of small units.** Though the pros of selecting small units allows for cases to be more easily comprehended and thus are more focused, the cons of selecting smaller units can be that change in a smaller unit may not result in sufficient pattern shift to bring about meaningful change. Focusing on too small a unit can sometimes result in first-order changes only. Another con regarding smaller units is that the practitioner can end up focusing on problems that do not make sense to focus on given the larger picture. A family may be referred due to one of the children not going to school. The practitioner can engage the family in trying to get the child to school while being oblivious to the fact that the mother has serious health problems and the child is staying home to help her with her infant who the mother is unable to care for. Smaller units can result in important patterns and family problems being off the practitioner's radar.
  - One can overthink a problem or one can oversimplify a problem. One way to avoid either pitfall is to understand the wider picture first and then focus in on a smaller unit and specific problem. The decision regarding what smaller unit to focus on is informed by an understanding of the larger picture.
- **Changing unit of analysis in response to how a case is unfolding.** Whatever unit of analysis a practitioner starts with in conceptualizing the case, inevitably, in some cases, the practitioner will be faced with a decision about whether or not to change their unit of analysis. When this occurs, the unit of analysis can either be enlarged or narrowed. The question is when to do which. If a practitioner is confused and unfocused, as noted this may be due to information overload. Their unit may be too broad. In this instance, it may be helpful to focus on a smaller unit. Doing so may help the practitioner set a direction and focus to the treatment where before they were confused and disorganized.
  - On the other hand, when an alliance is struck with a caregiver, goals are agreed on and tasks are given and carried out, but change is either not occurring or is not being acknowledged. This can be due to important participants and patterns being outside of the practitioner's observational field. The practitioner may be unaware of important individuals involved in the interactional pattern that supports the problem. These individuals do not necessarily need to be worked with directly, but at a minimum their contribution to the pattern must be understood and incorporated into the practitioner's thinking about the case and into the interventions offered. In this instance, enlarging the unit can make the case understandable and lead to a focus on something that the family will more likely consider meaningful change.

In all cases the goal will be to determine how the involved parties are describing the problem, how they are viewing the problem or whether or not they feel there is a problem, what their position is on the need to change things, and what they are and are not doing about the situation. In all cases, the target in this phase is to identify patterns of interactions around the problem as defined. Where are the potential vicious cycles, exceptions to that cycle, and potential strengths and solution patterns?

SAFETY AND INTERACTIONS

Intensive in-home treatment is by design focused on cases when there is a high risk of a child being removed from the family and placed out of the home. Often, the authorities will require a safety plan. Any safety plan is more likely to succeed if it is based on an *interactional* understanding of the unsafe behavior. I-FAST practitioners understand the specific unsafe behaviors within their interactional context. A number of key points in these cases include the following:

- Inevitably the safety of the child is in question and that is why the child is at risk to be placed.
- Strong safety measures are often imposed by the courts or children's services to allow the family to remain together while the home-based worker presumably is working with the family to resolve the issues producing an unsafe situation.
- Those safety measures can include placing an ankle bracelet on an out-of-control teenager, putting a teen on a 24/7 line of sight supervision plan, or court ordering no contact between family members.
- Executing these procedures often can guarantee safety. The problem is they can also simultaneously interfere with change.
- When safety is a serious issue, the problem is how to devise a safety intervention that simultaneously promotes change, rather than interfering with it. To achieve this, the specific interactions associated with the unsafe behavior must be discovered. Knowing these interactions allows for designing a safety intervention that both provides safety and changes the pattern.
- Not knowing these interactions raises the possibility that the safety intervention will reinforce the very patterns that are producing unsafe behavior.
    - For example, a teenage boy who has sexually offended a younger neighbor boy is placed on 24/7 line of sight supervision to ensure the safety of children in his community while he receives treatment. It is learned that he is uninvolved with peers his own age and interacts exclusively with much younger children.
    - However, he is interested in girls his own age, but has no clue how to interact with them and so avoids them. As he improves and becomes more interested in same-age peers, he wants to ask a girl to the upcoming homecoming dance at his school.
    - The safety plan, however, requires that he be accompanied by an adult who will guarantee he will not be out of line-of-sight supervision.
    - If part of the problem for this boy was his inability to appropriately interact with girls his age, the safety plan is now interfering with him, changing that aspect of the problem. Having an adult never allow him out of his or her sight can seriously interfere with natural peer interactions with other teens, particularly girls.
    - The 24/7 line-of-sight supervision promotes safety but interferes with change.
- As with all other reasonable goals of a family and the systems related to each case, solutions may become, escalate, or exacerbate the problem they are designed to resolve.

- Identifying these problem-supporting interactions around ensuring safety and reframing issues of safety to allow for more positive interactional shifts is often one of the critical skills of effective intervention.

IMPLEMENTING: SKILLS FOR TRACKING INTERACTIONS

Tracking Interactional Patterns

Part of clients' stories are the ways they and/or other people have tried to solve the presenting problem but thus far have not been successful in their efforts. Identifying interactional patterns indicates how the client and/or significant others are caught up in a problem-maintaining cycle. Working this way, the practitioner wants to know what the client and significant others have been doing in attempting to solve the presenting problem and reach the desired goal. By identifying what the family has habitually tried, the practitioner learns what types of interventions to avoid using; Fisch, Weakland, and Segal (1982) refer to this as the "mine field" (p. 114). According to Fisch et al. (1982), the habitual interactions that support the problem may have nothing to do with what got the entire process going in the first place. Therefore, it is not necessary to investigate a client's intrapsychic world or past history in searching for the cause of the problem initially but instead focus on what is probably maintaining it and preventing clients from achieving their goals (Nardone & Watzlawick, 1993, p. 52).

Obtaining information about unsuccessful attempts to solve the presenting problem and attempts thought about but not tried is helpful in a multiple ways. First, it provides more information about the client's existing mental models and frames. In addition, when clients become aware that their existing frames are not working and their current situation is not where they want to be they will experience some discomfort (Fairhurst & Saar, 1996). This awareness and discomfort will then tend to loosen up and make more permeable their existing frames and they will then be more open to novelty, expanding their frames, and thus second-order change (Fairhurst & Saar, 1996). This process is referred to as *deframing*, which O'Hanlon (1984) defines as "abolishing or casting doubt on current frames or meanings" (p. 1), which is another way of describing the effects of the process of deconstruction.

All approaches that seek to identify interactional patterns associated with the problems presented for treatment can be integrated into I-FAST. Examination of the various approaches concerned with interactional patterns yields three basic methods for their identification. Before engaging with families the I-FAST practitioner makes a strategic decision as to which method will be used. The choice made is based on the practitioner's knowledge and skills. Because each method is effective, I-FAST practitioners are encouraged to bring previously learned skills to the table. Regardless of the method chosen, the I-FAST practitioner is intensely curious and observant about the details of who does exactly what when the problem occurs, and/or when it does not occur. It is understood that the ultimate objective is to identify chains of interaction that begin when the problem is exhibited and end when the problem ceases.

Assessing Interactional Patterns by Interview

The first method of assessing patterns involves obtaining a behavioral description by interviewing one or more of the participants in the pattern (Watzlawick, Weakland, & Fisch, 1974). Obtaining a description of the problem and what everyone does as if it were on film (de Shazer, 1985), circular questioning (Selvini-Palazzoli,

Boscolo, Cecchin, & Prata, 1978), a Dialectical Behavior Therapy "chain analysis" (Linehan, 1993), or Bowen "process questions" in which an individual is encouraged to describe his or her own part of the pattern are examples of this method. Specific interviewing skills are required to obtain such a description.

- Typically when asked to describe what happens, clients do not describe what actually happens, but will tell their theory about why they think what is happening is happening.
- Practitioners must be aware when this occurs and patiently and steadfastly inquire into what actually happens. Practitioners must also be aware when only a partial description is being offered and be willing to doggedly pursue the details until a full description is obtained.

The following list of interviewing questions for tracking habitual interactions and exceptions may help to make initial interviewing to track problems simpler. These questions include the following:

- What is the problem as you see it?
- Do others see this problem differently? If so, who and how do they see it differently?
- How or in what ways is this a problem and for whom?
- What effect does the problem have on you? On your relationships with each other?
- What have you done about this?
- What do you usually do about things like this? Have you done that?
- What have others told you about this and have they suggested things to do?
- If you have done some of these things, how have they worked?
- Can you give me a recent example of what you have done when this problem has occurred? (Ask for several more similar examples.)
- Who is present when the problem happens and what are they doing and saying?
- When the problem occurs, what does each person involved do?
- If I were a "fly on the wall" what would I see as this goes on?
- If I were doing a documentary and following you all around making a video of this all taking place, what would I see?
- So... what happens... then what... then what?
- What advice have you received for how to handle the problem and who have you gotten advice from?
- Do you agree with the advice?
- If you do not agree with what others have suggested, has that caused difficulties between you and them?
- What concerns you most about the problem?
- When does the problem occur... where does it occur... how often... how long does it last?
- What happens that stops it?

Assessing Interactional Patterns by Direct Observation

A second method of assessing patterns is by directly observing them when they spontaneously occur. The concepts of "tracking" and "accommodating" exemplify this (Minuchin & Fishman, 1981). Using this method is a possibility with in-home sessions in which all of the participants of the interactional pattern are present and the problem occurs during the interview. When this occurs, the family will often spontaneously go through their habitual interactions.

Special skills are required to employ this method. The practitioner must be able to simultaneously conduct an interview while staying alert to observe what is happening. The pattern can occur in seconds and involve several participants. An alert practitioner must be able to observe the entire chain of events and not intervene and interrupt the process. Practitioners must be open to the possibility that what actually happens may not fit with what clients may have reported in previous interviews.

A CASE EXAMPLE

An in-home practitioner was interviewing a mother who was accused of medical neglect. Her 12-year-old son went to school with a serious and untreated cut on his leg. The school reported the family to the authorities. The boy lived with his mother, father, infant sister, and 9-year-old brother. While the practitioner was interviewing the mother in the living room, the infant, who was lying near the mother, soiled her diaper. The mother went on talking as if nothing had happened. With no words spoken, the 12-year-old went over to the infant and changed the diaper. The mother went on talking with the practitioner as if nothing had happened.

Next, the 9-year-old brother came home, went back into his room, and began making loud noises. Again with no words spoken, the 12-year-old went back into the brother's room and a large thump was heard followed by the ceasing of any noises coming from that room. Again the mother just continued talking with the practitioner as if nothing had occurred. By simply observing and not interrupting, the practitioner learned that the 12-year-old boy was parentified and in charge of himself. He went to school with an untreated wound because he himself did not think it needed attention. It is doubtful the mother would have revealed this in an interview.

When a practitioner observes such interactions in the engagement stage, no requests for change should be offered. Changes are not asked for during engagement. Nor is it advisable to comment on these observations. Practitioners should just take note of their observations for use in latter stages of I-FAST treatment.

Assessing Interactional Patterns by Observing Responses to Tasks

A third method for tracking habitual interactions is to track responses to tasks given either in the session or between sessions. Tracking interactional responses to in-session tasks has been the major method of assessment for structural and strategic family practitioners (Haley, 1985; Minuchin, 1974; Minuchin & Fishman, 1981). An in-session task like this is referred to as an *enactment* (Minuchin & Fishman, 1981).

When using this method, I-FAST practitioners must focus the in-session tasks on the problem on which the parents are requesting help. In the engagement stage of treatment, I-FAST practitioners should observe and note privately how the family responds but not comment or ask the family to deviate from their habitual interactions, even if those interactions do not follow the requested in-session task. Requests to change interactions come later. During the engagement stage, interactions are simply noted by the practitioner. In general, there are no requests for change until an alliance with a parent is clearly obtained and goals have been agreed on.

> **A CASE EXAMPLE**
>
> A teenage boy was brought to treatment for defiance. The boy's mother and father were asked to talk to each other in the session regarding what they will do that evening if the boy becomes defiant. This in-session task can be given in the presence of all three family members. How they respond will often reveal their habitual interactions. The father may look at the mother and suggest the boy receive some punishment. The boy then interrupts, saying something provocative, and the mother and son then engage in an intense, hostile exchange while the father sits by and says nothing. The parents were asked to talk to each other, but instead the boy and mother quickly became intensively involved with each other while the father was disengaged. How the family responded to this task revealed their habitual interactions around the boy and his problem. Note that the requested task focused on the presenting problem of the boy's defiance.

Tracking Interactional Exceptions as a Focused Skill

The skilled I-FAST practitioner is preferably adept at focusing on both habitual interactions associated with the problem and interactional exceptions. When skilled at both, interviews can switch from conversation focusing on tracking interactional patterns that maintained the problems and interactional exceptions that signify times when the family is doing something different and helpful. When practitioners do engage with the client in dialogues around the presenting problem, it is part of listening to their story, which contains the problem, and allows validation of their distress in the process of co-constructing a collaborative relationship with them. Allowing clients to vent about their problems and validating their difficulties sometimes helps them to be more receptive to identifying exceptions that may already be occurring. A useful question to follow up with is:

- "What have you thought about trying in attempting to solve the problem but have not tried so far?"

Sometimes the successful solution to the presenting problem is the very thing they have thought about trying but have not yet done so. People are much more likely to do something they have thought of on their own but have not yet tried than doing something very different and new offered by someone else.

Time spent on treatment dialogues on strengths and interactional exceptions to the problem is also done to de-construct their problem and problem-saturated story.

This can destabilize their experience of reality as unchangeable and not containing options to one that has possibilities (strengths, resources, competencies) and is changeable. This helps to increase the client's sense of hope. Treatment dialogues focusing on strengths and interactional exceptions, in which the problem is externalized and de-constructed, opens up space in the therapeutic conversation for possibilities, strengths, and exceptions to the problem to emerge, is validating to clients, and helps co-construct a collaborative relationship.

- I-FAST practitioners can interview for exceptions by seeking to learn about what happens when the problem sometimes does not occur
- I-FAST practitioners can pursue this line of questioning and empower families to focus on exceptions as successes when this method builds rapport
- I-FAST practitioners can drop this line of questioning when there is resistance

The skillful tracking of interactional exceptions can be employed in multiple ways and at multiple points in the I-FAST treatment process. Tracking exceptions can be employed:

- In the traditional solution-focused manner as a major tool in identifying and amplifying pattern shifts that may be already occurring
- Throughout treatment to check what changes, if any have begun as a result of any contact between I-FAST practitioner and family
- To follow up on interventions intended to promote pattern shifts such as reframes or tasks offered

Regardless of when tracking exceptions is employed, the I-FAST practitioner seeks to obtain a behavioral description of what each participant is doing differently when the problem is not occurring. A core set of questions are utilized regardless of what point in the treatment process tracking exceptions is employed:

- What did you do differently?
- How did you do that?
- How did you decide to do that?

In keeping with the assumption of a systems perspective that there are fluctuations in how families experience the problem, the practitioner asks questions of families to learn when the problem does not exist or is at least less frequent or intense (De Jong & Berg, 2008; de Shazer, 1985). In regard to this Kral and Kowalski (1989) state that the practitioner's job "is not to initiate change, but to punctuate the differences between the complaint pattern and the pattern of the exceptions (change) thereby making explicit the 'naturally' occurring variations which are in the direction of the desired solution" (p. 105). From an I-FAST perspective, this amounts to tracking interactions that constitute exceptions to the patterns that support the problem and are in the direction of desired change.

Though assessing for exceptions to the problem pattern as well as strengths and resources of the families should be an integral part of treatment, there are times when focusing on exceptions alone can constitute the primary intervention to help the family resolve their problems. The guideline is: if a family can successfully resolve presenting problems by the practitioner helping them to notice, expand, and amplify times when they are able to better handle the problem then go with that focus because this is the least intrusive intervention and it utilizes what the family can do well. Some useful guidelines are:

- Family members are able to identify exceptions and the practitioner is able to help family members in developing useful treatment directions and goals based on this line of therapeutic dialogue.
- The practitioner observes that family members are energized by these questioning sequences and become more hopeful and engaged in treatment.
- A process of change is triggered by this line of change dialogues, as evident by positive, specific, and behavioral changes in the problem pattern.
- If intended as a primary intervention, interviewing for exceptions should be dropped if clients resist the idea that change is already occurring.

Exception questions inquire about times when the problem is either absent, less intense, or dealt with in a manner that is acceptable to the family (de Shazer, 1985). This type of question is called an *exception question* because it asks the family to look for an exception to the problem (de Shazer, 1985).

- This type of question is often a "when" question: "When was the last time you and your son felt things were going well?"
- Assuming that during these times the family is usually doing something to make things better, the practitioner then follows up by asking families questions to identify the specific strengths, resources, and competencies they use to make these *exceptions to the problem* occur.
- The practitioner can then use additional follow up questions to further facilitate amplifying and reinforcing the families' use of these strengths, resources, and competencies in order to make these exceptions times occur more frequent and to become more the rule.
- Therefore, instead of asking families "When do you have the problem and what are you doing then?" the practitioner can use such questions as the following:
  - "When are there times that you are feeling just a little less depressed than usual?"
  - "When are there times the two of you do get along?"
  - After families identify exception times the practitioner should then use follow-up questions such as the following to discover specifics about those times in order to amplify the family's strengths and expand the solution picture:
    - "What's different at those times?"
    - "What are you doing differently at those times"
    - "How were you able to get that to happen?"

There are other questioning sequences that can be helpful to access times when the family is more successful in addressing the problem situations.

IDENTIFYING PAST SUCCESSES (EXCEPTIONS)
Sometimes families initially have difficulty identifying exceptions to their presenting problem in their current lives. When this situation occurs the practitioner can ask

the family about times in the past when they successfully handled the same or similar kinds of situations and how she or he was able to do so (Berg & Gallagher, 1991). Identifying past successes is essentially identifying past exceptions. In regard to the presenting problem the practitioner can even ask the family about exceptions that occurred years earlier. If the family cannot come up with any exceptions ever occurring in the presenting problem, the practitioner can ask the family about an exception to similar problems in the past. The idea is to find out what solutions have worked in the past and to apply them to the current situation if at all possible.

IDENTIFYING CURRENT SUCCESSES

Sometimes the family's presenting problem will involve some issues of a child's impulsive, compulsive, and/or other behaviors that may seem completely out of their control. We assume that there have been times when the family has been successful in exercising some self-control. The task here is to focus on control, not on the lack of it. This task implies that the family will overcome the urge by doing rather than passively waiting for things to happen. When he or she overcomes again implies that it is only a matter of time until the family will overcome again in the future. The question no longer is built around if she or he will overcome but rather *when*. For example:

- For a family that has problems with anger: "When have there been times that you felt like going off on each other but you were able to stop yourself?"
- For a family presenting an adolescent with an eating disorder: "When are there times when you are able to ignore or resist the temptation to binge?"

After the family identifies the current successes times then the worker can follow up with questions to identify how they were able to control themselves successfully at those times, such as:

- "How are you able to do that?"
- "How are you able to get yourself to do that at those times?"

COPING QUESTIONS

Often families in crisis will state that nothing is going right, can find nothing positive in their lives, and are unable to identify any exceptions—present or past. Families such as this can feel very hopeless about themselves and their future and there may be legitimate reasons for feeling this way (Berg & Miller, 1992). The worker needs to recognize the negativity in the family as a sign of great desperation and a signal for empathetic help. In such a situation, the family could perceive the practitioner's focus on the positive as being artificial and imposing.

- *Coping questions* ask families to talk about how they manage to cope with and endure their problems, especially when the family is not able to identify exception times and/or when their life circumstances are overwhelming.
- Coping questions help families to notice times when they are coping with their problems and what it is they are doing at those times they are successfully coping. The coping question can be quite effective with families who see little possibility for positive changes (Berg & Miller, 1992).

- Coping questions can be an impetus for families feeling a sense of empowerment and hope because they start to become aware of resources they did not know they had or had forgotten (Berg, 1994). When a family reports that nothing is going right or positive and persists in this view the practitioner can accept the family's negative appraisal by asking variations on the coping questions, which families should experience as further validation.

The following examples are designed to point out to family members that they have the resources and strengths to manage and improve their situation. For example:

- "Your situation seems to be really very overwhelming. How do you cope with it? How are you able to keep yourself going and your family together?"
- "It sounds like the problem is very serious. How come things are not worse?"
- "What are you (or your family) doing to keep things from getting worse?"
- "How has that been helpful? Would your parent (or adolescent) agree?"
- "What are you doing to keep going when things are so bad?"
- "What would tell you that things are getting a little better?"
- "What would it take to make that happen?"
- "What do you imagine yourself doing then?"
- "How have you been able to keep going despite all the discrimination you've encountered?"

THE ESSENTIAL ELEMENTS OF TRACKING INTERACTIONS

The practitioner obtains an understanding of the interactions among family members of how they have tried to cope with the problem as they see it, either by conducting a well-organized interview or by observing interaction patterns directly.

Interactional Assessment
The following list is a summary of the basic skills for tracking interactions:

- The interactional patterns that are maintaining the problem are specifically and behaviorally described and identified.
- The practitioner asks the family to explicitly articulate the sequence of what goes on between them as they engage to deal with the problem.
- The practitioner asks detailed interaction questions around what happens:
    - "If I had a video of what went on, what world I see?"
    - "If I were a fly on the wall, what would I see?"
    - "He said, she said . . . etc."
    - Recognize "no action" as an attempt to solve the problem.
- The practitioner tracks the interactional pattern in terms of who, when, where, what, and how.
- The problem is understood as part of the context of family patterns.
- The practitioner identifies whom to include in treatment that will create change in family interactional patterns.
- The practitioner requests family members to interact with each other about the problem and observes and notes how those interactions maintain the problem.

Problem Definition

The following is a summary of the basic skills of problem identification:

- The major frames that shape the problem pattern and/or the exceptions to the problem are identified.
- A problem that can lead to change is defined as the presence of a positive and not simply the absence of a negative.
- The problem is specifically and behaviorally defined.
- The list of identified problems is clearly prioritized.
- The practitioner and the family/child mutually agree on the defined problems.
- The problems fit within an agreed on set of frames and/or within an agreed on therapeutic rationale.

Identifying Exceptions

The following is a list of the basic skills for identifying exceptions:

- The practitioner helps the family identify and amplify their strengths, competencies, and resources, for example,
    - What is going right?
    - What is different about those times when things were better?
    - How does the family cope with the stresses in their lives?
    - What were some past or current successes?
    - What are the things that the family is proud of?

- The practitioner helps the family notice exceptions to the problem, for example,
    - When was the last time that the problem was not happening?
    - When was the last time that the problem happened but was less severe?
    - When was the last time the problem happened and the family handled the problem more satisfactorily?

GOAL DEVELOPMENT AND CONSENSUS

5

INTRODUCTION TO GOALS AND GOAL SETTING

In working with at-risk families it is not enough to just identify and define the primary presenting problem and track interactions around the problem. For progress and change to occur everyone involved needs to have a clear idea as to what they are progressing and changing toward; that is, what is the family's goal in treatment. Mutual agreement on goals (goal consensus) is another key ingredient in developing and maintaining positive treatment alliances with families. In addition to providing direction for the work together, collaborative goal setting also enhances the family's motivation (Michalak & Holtforth, 2006; Ryan & Deci, 2008; Tryon & Winograd, 2011) and sense of hope, helps in monitoring progress, and is an intervention itself.

Goal setting invites the family members to begin envisioning what a desirable future will look like for them in which the problem is no longer present or at least with acceptable improvement in the problem behaviors of the identified client and functioning of the family. Goal setting increases the family's awareness of options and choices and actively engages them in the treatment process (Elliot & Church, 2002; Lee, Sebold, & Uken, 2003). Well-formed goals provide clear indicators of what change will look like, the progress the family is making, and how they will know when it is time to terminate treatment. Without clearly defined goals treatment can get off track and/or progress can easily go unnoticed or minimized by the client, his or her significant others, or practitioners (Berg & Kelly, 2000).

A *goal* is the object or aim of an action (Locke & Latham, 1990, 2002; Ryan, 1970). A person or family having goals:

- Directs attention and effort toward goal-relevant activities and away from goal-irrelevant activities (Locke & Bryan, 1969)
- Serves an energizing function
- Affects persistence
- Affects action indirectly by leading to the discovery and use of task-relevant knowledge and strategies (Wood & Locke, 1990)

Goal commitment, self-efficacy, feedback, and task complexity affect goal setting and performance (Locke & Latham, 2002).

- High *commitment* is achieved when individuals are convinced that the goal is important and attainable. People defining and setting goals for themselves have been found to be effective in gaining goal commitment (Latham, Winters, & Locke, 1994).
- It is important for people to have a sense of *self-efficacy* in that they believe the goal is within their capacity (Bandura, 1986).

- People also need ongoing *feedback* on their progress toward the goal (Locke, 1996).
- The *complexity of the task* also affects goal achievement. People are not as effective in goal achievement if they have no prior experience or training on the task, there is high pressure to perform well, and there is high time pressure to perform well immediately.

CONCEPTUALIZING

Framing and Goal Setting

EPISODES VERSUS ILLNESSES

The way we frame the presenting problem has important implications for goal setting and treatment. As was briefly mentioned previously, in I-FAST we frame the family's presenting situation as an episode of care rather than an illness and a problem rather than a diagnosis. Specifically, framing the family's presenting situation as an episode versus illness as well as a specific problem versus a diagnosis significantly influences how the practitioner and the family set the goals for treatment. Serious problems can be defined as ongoing illnesses requiring continuous care once they are diagnosed. Or, problems can be defined as episodes that may or may not repeat, requiring intervention when they do occur and not requiring intervention when they subside. Within the field of mental health, especially considering cross-cultural methods of treatment, both of these approaches are represented.

EPISODES VERSUS DIAGNOSIS

An interesting study that unwittingly offered some comparison data of the relative effectiveness of these two broad approaches was conducted by the World Health Organization (WHO) in the mid-1970s and then repeated again by WHO in the mid-1990s. Treatment of serious mental health problems was studied in 12 different countries, 6 in the developed world including the United States and 6 in the Third World. WHO was attempting to compare the overall quality of life of clients diagnosed with a serious mental health condition in each set of countries. Surprisingly, contrary to expectations, in both studies it was found that clients diagnosed with serious mental health conditions had a higher quality of life in the Third World countries than in any of the developed countries including the United States. Both studies were definitive, yet differences between the two groups of countries have not been thoroughly studied.

One ethnographic study conducted in Zanzibar, Africa attempted to uncover the differences between the two sets of countries (McGruder, 1999). To summarize McGruder's findings, it was discovered that in areas uninfluenced or little influenced by Western medicine, what the West would refer to as mental illness was treated as an episode to be gotten through followed with a return to the previous level of functioning. The client's family and community were organized around this principle. McGruder's study suggests that treating serious mental problems as episodes offers the potential for greater quality of life, so much so that the effects of serious poverty are outweighed by the benefits of approaching the problem this way.

Although the use of episode of care models is in the minority in the West, Mosher reports over one dozen "alternative" approaches to severely mentally disturbed clients in the United States (Mosher, 1999). Warner offers a review of outcomes of "alternative" care programs (Warner, 1995). One such program is the Soteria project first developed in San Francisco, California and later replicated in Bern, Switzerland (Mosher, 1999). Both programs treated psychotic youth and young adults. In both programs the client and family were not organized around the idea that the client had an incurable lifelong illness, but instead defined the problem as an episode that may or may not return and set the goal as total return to previous level of functioning with no medication. Outcome studies reported results superior to those of traditional approaches that define the problem as an illness.

The best known recent program is the Open Dialogue Treatment of Dr. Jaakko Seikkula in Finland (Seikkula, 2006). This treatment also defines the problem as an episode and sets the goal for total return to previous functioning with no medications. Ongoing outcome studies show 80% treated return to work or school and 75% show no psychotic symptoms. Although all these programs employ different treatment models, what they have in common is that the problem is treated as an episode that can be fully recovered from and may not reoccur. In most of these programs, medications were either not used at all or only temporarily used and withdrawn before the end of treatment.

One project in which the treatment model can fit into I-FAST was conducted by Haley (1980). This project was one of the pioneer projects to employ a *parent empowerment model*. A total of 42 clients, all age 16 to 25, were treated after an initial hospitalization. Of the 42 clients, 30 had been diagnosed as psychotic or schizophrenic, 5 were severely suicidal, 4 were drug or alcohol addicted, and 3 had anorexia. Regardless of diagnosis, the problem was defined as an episode and the goal was set as returning the client to his or her previous level of functioning. The medical personnel on the program supported this frame. A parent empowerment model was employed in which the parents were powerfully joined and helped to help their youth regain his or her prior functioning. Interactional family patterns that contributed to the problem were identified and changed. All treatment was outpatient. The average number of sessions was 11. All 42 clients were taken totally off medications. All were followed for an average of two years after termination. As with Seikkula's Open Dialogue Treatment, 80% of the clients in Haley's project regained their previous level of functioning with no medications and no additional hospitalizations.

I-FAST IS AN EPISODE OF CARE MODEL

If at all possible, serious problems are treated as episodes. An emphasis is placed on avoiding defining problems as chronic conditions requiring continuous care and a marginalization of the client into long-term institutions that define them as incurable and or abnormal. This presents a special challenge when the larger mental health treatment community is operating primarily from the illness perspective. Nonetheless, as a parent empowerment model, defining serious problems as episodes allows the difficulty to be defined as something parents can do something about, a primary prerequisite for I-FAST.

SPECIFIC PROBLEMS VERSUS DIAGNOSES

A second variable regarding how problems are defined that has major implications for directing treatment is whether or not the problem is defined as a diagnosis or something specific. A diagnosis could be thought of as a group of specific symptoms that occur together. Parents are now becoming aware of mental health diagnoses through various avenues of U.S. culture and in many instances are seeking treatment already having self-diagnosed their child. From the point of view of parent empowerment, this presents a problem. Only professionals can do something about diagnoses. Defining the problem this way puts it outside the domain of parents to do something about.

Interestingly, many of the evidence-based specific factor manuals focus on specific problems not diagnoses. Although many manualized treatments advertise themselves as addressing diagnoses, they actually focus on specific symptoms. Exposure therapy for posttraumatic stress disorder (PTSD) is one example. Although the treatment is for the diagnoses of PTSD, treatment actually focuses on specific PTSD symptoms, such as the most upsetting nightmare, or the most frequently avoided location. The data accumulating regarding outcomes of these treatments are supportive of the effectiveness of treating specific problems versus treating diagnoses.

From the I-FAST perspective, focusing on something specific is empowering. It defines the problem as something the client, or in the case of I-FAST, parents can do something about. A parent can do something about a child who has a nightmare, or cannot get out of bed, or who throws a serious fit. But professionals must do something about a traumatized child or a depressed child or a bipolar child. As with the episode versus illness issue, the problem becomes how to shift families and fellow professionals into the category of solving specific problems when the larger culture is operating from the diagnosis model.

Common Factors Research and Goal Setting

SET CLEAR TREATMENT DIRECTIONS

Establishing and maintaining a focus throughout treatment has been found to be essential to successful outcomes especially with multiproblem clients. Goal setting establishes a clear direction for the larger treatment process. Once goals are clearly framed, families may jump out in front of the treatment process and begin making positive changes on their own. Because I-FAST is rooted in empowerment, practitioners are prepared to put aside their own agenda and support desired change whenever it begins to occur.

INTRINSIC MOTIVATION AND SELF-DETERMINATION

In working with clients, practitioners are concerned with the clients' level of motivation. An accumulation of research has found that goal setting is a critical factor in client motivation. Research has found that people are much more motivated to work on and more likely to be successful in achieving goals that they have defined for themselves rather than those defined for them by others (Brown & Ryan, 2004; Deci & Ryan, 2002; Ryan & Deci, 2000a, 2000b, 2008; Zuroff et al., 2007). Goal setting in this way helps people develop a sense of mastery and competence that humans are naturally inclined to seek (Deci & Ryan, 2002; Ryan & Deci, 2000a, 2000b).

- To develop mastery and competence a person needs to have appropriate challenges and positive feedback about his or her performance, and not receive demeaning feedback (Ryan & Deci, 2000a, 2000b).

- To develop a sense of competence a person needs to also experience a sense of autonomy and self-determination, referred to as *intrinsic motivation* (Ryan & Deci, 2000a, p. 70).
- In addition, intrinsic motivation is greater when the context provides a sense of security and relatedness (Ryan & Deci, 2000a, 2000b).
- Intrinsic motivation is diminished by negative evaluations (feedback), the use of rewards, and use of a controlling approach (threats, deadlines, directives, competition, and imposed goals) (Ryan & Deci, 2000a, p. 70). Such approaches are perceived as not being supportive of autonomy but rather as external sources of causality and control (Ryan & Deci, 2000a, 2000b).
- On the other hand, "recognizing others' unique perspectives, acknowledging their feelings, refraining from pressuring them, providing as much choice as possible within the context, and providing meaningful rationales when choice is not possible" are ways of enhancing autonomous motivation (Zuroff et al., 2007, p. 138).
- When trying to motivate someone to engage in an activity (perform a behavior) it is helpful to provide the person a *rationale for the activity* (behavior) and *support their autonomy* within a *positive relationship* in which the person experiences a sense of relatedness (the person feels respected, listened to, cared for) (Brown & Ryan, 2004).

DEVELOP A COMMON SENSE OF PURPOSE

In the beginning of treatment, with most families there is finger pointing and blaming others for the problems in the family. Different family members often have different ideas as to who and what is the problem and who and what needs to change. For example, parents frequently focus on the adolescent as the person needing to change because of his or her acting out and noncompliant behaviors while the adolescent focuses on the parents as needing to get off his or her back with their rules and consequences.

- This being the case, it is very important for the practitioner "to frame the treatment in a way that validates these disparate perspectives" (Friedlander, Escudero, & Heatherington, 2006, p. 125).
- The practitioner may start initially with defining problems and goals regarding the adolescent's behaviors.
- As soon as possible the definitions of the problem and goals need to be broadened to include all the family members as having common goals and their seeing the importance of working together to achieve these goals and to experience overall benefit as a family (Friedlander et al., 2006; Friedlander, Escudero, Heatherington, & Diamond, 2011).

PROMOTING HOPE

As mentioned previously, when beginning treatment, families usually feel hopeless and demoralized. They have tried everything they know, often numerous times, to solve their problem(s) but nothing has worked. Many families may have gotten to the point where they have stopped trying, perhaps thinking something like "what's the use of trying anyway?" and have given up hope of things changing for the better. It has been established that hope is important to both clients and practitioners in treatment outcome

(Coppock, Owen, Zagarskas, & Schmidt, 2010; Larsen & Stege, 2010a, 2010b; Reiter, 2010; Ward & Wampler, 2010). Goal setting plays an important role in people having a sense of hope. Hope has been operationalized as having three interrelated components:

1. Establishing goals
2. The extent to which people believe they have the "ability to produce one or more workable routes to their goals" (Snyder, Michael, & Cheavens, 1999, p. 180)
3. The extent to which people believe they have the "ability to begin and continue movement on selected pathways toward those goals" (Snyder, Michael, & Cheavens, 1999, p. 180)

The first aspect of hope is referred to as "agency thinking" and the second as "pathways thinking" (Irving et al., 2004; Rand & Cheavens, 2009; Snyder, Ilardi, Michael, & Cheavens, 2000; Snyder & Taylor, 2000; Valle, Huebner, & Suldo, 2006).

In many situations, clients know that things are not the way they want them to be in life, but at the same time they are not sure as to what it is they really want. In "hope treatment" Snyder et al. (1999) state that often the task begins with careful "detective work" with the client to figure out what it is she or he really wants.

- Often people forget the skills and success they already have that they can use in resolving their presenting problem and accomplishing their desired goals, and one way of intervening is to ask clients questions whereby they are able to remember and identify these skills and successes (Snyder et al., 1999).
- In practice, one way to activate and slowly build a sense of hope is to focus on client strengths and small successes (Cheavens, Feldman, Gum, Michael, & Snyder, 2006; Snyder, Feldman, Taylor, Schroeder, & Adams, 2000).

To remain faithful to I-FAST at a minimum treatment must focus on something specific and achievable:

- That the parents are motivated to focus on
- Is defined as something the parents can do something about
- While the client remains in his or her natural environment

STRATEGIZING

Goal Consensus

Although the content (the definition) of a goal is important, the process of goal setting is equally important. After engaging parents, and identifying interactions that maintain the problem or identifying interactions that are exceptions, mutually defining goals and obtaining goal consensus is crucial and can point treatment in a direction that will allow for second-order shifts from these patterns. An essential and effective element of the relationship is *goal consensus* and *collaboration*; as previously noted, this element is also an explicit part of Horvath and Bedi's (2002) definition of the working alliance. *Goal consensus* is defined as client–practitioner agreement on the goals and expectations of treatment (Orlinsky, Grawe, & Parks, 1994). As noted earlier, goal consensus understandably correlates well with outcome. This concept also correlates with empathy because clients regard collaboration on goals and tasks as a sign of empathic understanding (Horvath & Greenberg, 1986). Research shows further that responding to clients' goals, intentions, and values is equally as important to empathy as it is for the practitioner to resonate with their feelings. In other words, an important aspect of empathy is goal consensus and collaboration with the client (Watson, 2002).

Engagement, goal consensus, and collaborative involvement are pan-theoretical concepts applying to all types of treatment and contexts (Tryon & Winograd, 2002).

- *Engagement* is defined as the degree of involvement of the practitioner and client in the therapeutic process, often measured by clients returning to practitioners after initial and successive sessions. They also cite research that suggests that client engagement in the first session is critical to their continuing treatment.
- *Collaborative involvement* refers to the degree of mutual engagement of the practitioner and client in treatment, usually measured by completing between-session tasks, measures of cooperation and resistance, and involvement in the client role.

Such an understanding and agreement about the goals and conditions for treatment and the ways clients and practitioners mutually engage in it is called a *therapeutic contract* (Orlinsky et al., 1994). It intuitively makes sense that such mutual collaborative involvement in the tasks of treatment should be well related to positive outcome. Not surprisingly, the more that clients and practitioners agree on goals, actively engage in treatment, and are collaboratively involved in the process of treatment, the greater client satisfaction and the more positive outcomes are to be found (Tryon & Winograd, 2002). Client–practitioner goal content agreement is important for the client success in treatment (Busseri & Tyler, 2004; Long, 2001). Negative treatment outcomes in terms of decreased client's satisfaction, treatment noncompliance, and premature termination were associated with incongruity of goal content between client and practitioner (Goin, Yamamoto, & Silverman, 1965), or client's request is ignored or overruled (Lazare, Eisenthal, & Wasserman, 1975).

In their most recent update of their meta-analyses of studies on goal consensus and collaboration, Tryon and Winograd (2011) conclude: "The results of the primary meta-analyses indicate strong links between client-practitioner goal consensus and positive treatment outcomes, as well as between patient-practitioner collaboration and positive treatment outcomes" (p. 55). Just as problems need to be defined interactionally, as previously discussed, goals should also be defined in interactional terms (Walter & Peller, 1982).

Guidelines for Setting Goals
GOALS ARE CHOSEN THAT THE PARENTS ARE MOTIVATED
TO ACCOMPLISH
Client motivation is always an issue in any type of treatment. The following guidelines can enhance the motivation for treatment with at-risk families:

- I-FAST focuses on changing what families want changed.
- Goals are useful and make sense to the family.

- Family and client are self-motivated and committed to goals that are personally meaningful and make sense for them.
- Choosing goals that reflect what the families want serves to strengthen therapeutic alliances. To these ends, I-FAST encourages practitioners to use the family's language when describing the problems and their beliefs about why the problems are occurring.
- Challenges can arise when some family members want one thing and others want something else. The task becomes finding a frame that enlists everyone's cooperation when goals of various parties conflict. When parents bring in their defiant teen for help and the teen just wants the parents off his or her back a deal can be struck. The parents can first be helped to gain their teen's cooperation and then the teen can be helped to get the parents off his or her back.
- When setting goals, include both parents if possible.
- This same pattern can be followed when families are referred by protective services or the court system owing to serious safety concerns. For example, if there has been violence the family can be asked what *they* want help on. Whatever they identify, a deal can be struck that the family will receive help on those problems, but first there can be no violence.

GOALS SHOULD BE WITHIN THE CLIENT'S CONTROL
- The action should be able to be started and/or maintained by the family members. Clients often want someone else or some other situation to change that they have no control over (They want their child to change, their partner to comply, or the teachers to change).
- The key question here includes the term "YOU." So, for example, you will say, "What will YOU be doing when that happens?"
- People have more control over what they do and can change themselves, but not others.

GOALS SHOULD BE INTERPERSONAL IN NATURE
- Because the problem is interactional in nature, the goal should be such that when the family or a person is working on the goal, another person will be able to notice the changes and potentially be affected by the change.

THE GOAL SHOULD BE A BEHAVIOR THAT CAN BE PRACTICED ON A REGULAR BASIS
- Clients can practice their goal behaviors and efforts on a regular basis so that constant feedback can be provided. Feedback helps clients develop clear ideas as to whether or not they are moving in the right direction. If progress is not being made then the strategies for achieving the goal or the goal itself made need to be changed based on feedback.

ALIGN THE GOALS WITH STAGES OF CHANGE
- A crucial factor in goal identification and engagement regards aligning with the "stage of change" positions of all parties involved with the identified problem. These stages were outlined in the engagement chapter.
- Each system member's position on change will be critical to choices the practitioner will make on how to engage them and how to identify clear and agreed on goals.

- Practitioners will engage and interact differently with clients and systems that are at different stages of change. Specific goals may differ depending on where each system member is in relation to his or her stage of change.
- Mismatching practitioner and client or system position on their current stage of change may interfere with or even derail engagement and goal attainment by losing the trust and collaboration of one or all involved parties.
- Identifying each party's or system's stage or position on change, accepting and validating it, and then helping to move those clients forward in the change process by identifying their related goals is a key element in all treatment and especially in the I-FAST approach.
- It must be remembered that clients in early phases of engagement will most likely have the overriding goals of getting you and all involved others out of their life. This is a perfectly acceptable goal, and one that may be built upon in finding out what others need to see from the family or youth before they are willing to leave them alone.
- In some cases, early stages of change are likely also to call for the practitioner to take the position of "devil's advocate" in noting the challenges, sacrifices, and potential down sides of changing. This is often experienced by clients as validating and affirming. The goals that emerge from this kind of discussion are likely to have strong client buy-in, and help them to move to other successive steps in the change process.

Agreeing on a Priority Goal

As mentioned previously, many if not most of the families we work with have multiple problems and it is important for the family to prioritize the problems for the focus of treatment. Just as problems need to be prioritized then so do goals. Prioritizing problems and goals usually involves asking the family which one they want to focus on first. One simple way of viewing this is the goal should represent what the changes will look like once the problem is solved.

A common situation involves a parent who is over-intervening locked in a struggle with a defiant youth. The parent who is over-intervening is typically trying too hard to obtain compliance from the child. There is a loss of perspective as parents attempt to coerce compliance *on a wide range of issues* that range from trivial to major. Because the parent is essentially attempting to bend the will of the child, all issues may be treated with the same amount of intensity. For example, the same level of importance may be assigned to picking up toys as to playing with knives. In other situations priorities may be hierarchical but highly faulty in terms of their relative importance. Here more attention may be paid to picking up toys than playing to with knives.

- Effective parent–child treatments counter these problems through the process of goal setting. In I-FAST we want to place parents in charge of developing a plan that establishes specific parenting priorities while ignoring issues that are of lesser importance. Here we see two subtle second-order changes: Prioritizing goals can be done verbally or in writing.
- What is important is that it is clear what problem and thus the corresponding goal is the family's priority and that that problem/goal is worked on first.
- This is especially important with multiproblem families that are typically referred for in-home treatment. With these families, not having a priority

problem to focus on usually means treatment goes around in circles from week to week. On the other hand, it is a major intervention in and of itself if one specific problem and corresponding goal can be identified that a chaotic family will get organized to solve.

Systems Collaboration: Aligning Client, Family, and Larger System Goals

One challenge that often accompanies working with families with children at high risk involves reaching agreements on treatment goals with various important parties on the case. Often, aligning goals involves a focus on safety issues usually being pushed by agencies such as children's services and juvenile court. This becomes a challenge when the family themselves are not concerned about those safety issues, or have other concerns altogether. On a typical case, a Children's Services case worker may have one goal, the parents of the child may have another goal, and the child herself may have yet another goal. Aligning all of these goals and reaching agreements from all parties on goals that everyone is motivated and willing to pursue becomes a major objective.

A CASE EXAMPLE

A family may be referred to in-home treatment by children's services after it was discovered that the father has physically abused his teenage daughter. When meeting with the family it is discovered that there is serious conflict between father and daughter over how late she stays out at night and whom she associates with. The conflict has escalated to seriously hostile verbal battles between father and daughter and recently to the father becoming violent. In this case, Children's Services goal is for the violence to stop. The father's goal may be for the daughter to be more compliant and the daughter's goal may be to have more freedoms. The problem becomes, how can all of these goals be aligned? The most common scenario involves both family problems and safety issues. There are both problems the family wants help with and problems that pose serious safety risks.

In I-FAST, parents are primary; therefore the father's goals must be respected and worked with. Children's Services, however, has the power to remove the girl if the father does not bring his temper under control. On a case like this, safety must also become a primary goal whether that goal is shared by the father or not. Finally, although in I-FAST the adults ultimately decide goals, it is often preferred and advantageous to include and incorporate an adolescent's goals to enlist both hers and her mother's cooperation in the treatment. The problem becomes, how can all of these goals be aligned?

Three Methods for Obtaining Goal Alignment Among Different Parties

Obtaining goals with multiple parties can be challenging. The following guidelines can be helpful in goal setting when multiple parties are involved:

- **Choose a goal that simultaneously addresses all parties' concerns.**
  Sometimes it is possible to choose a goal that simultaneously addresses

multiple issues. First, the practitioner must inquire into what the parents want help with regardless of safety issues. The family then may voluntarily ask for help on a problem that is or can be connected the safety concerns. The treatment can then focus on parental goals while simultaneously dealing with safety issues.

In the preceding case, for example, the practitioner can agree with the father that the daughter's behavior is a serious problem and must change. He may also agree that his method of dealing with his daughter's problem behavior is not working and that he needs a new approach. He can then be coached in using nonviolent ways of addressing his daughter's behavior. In this strategy, the goals of both the father and those of Children's Services are simultaneously addressed. The treatment is focused on what the father wants, but with safety issues also dealt with.

- **Make deals.** In some cases it is not possible to select a goal that simultaneously addresses family and safety issues. What the family wants help on may not provide avenues for simultaneously addressing safety issues. In these cases, it is sometimes possible to make deals. A deal can be struck with a parent that his or her concerns will be addressed if safety issues are dealt with first.

A CASE EXAMPLE

A couple brought their 10-year-old daughter for treatment due to serious behavioral problems she was having at school. It was obvious in the first session that the father was very fond of the girl and very concerned about her behavior. During this first interview, the mother asked to speak to the practitioner privately. She then disclosed that her husband had a serious drinking problem and when he was intoxicated he became violent and had hit her (the mother) on numerous occasions. With the mother's permission, the father was brought back into the interview room and a deal was offered. The practitioner agreed to help the parents with their daughter's school behavioral problems, but only if the father agreed to not become violent with his wife. The father was very concerned about his daughter and so he agreed to the deal. The parents were offered help at getting their daughter's behavior under control, and the father kept his agreement and did not hit his wife.

The method of striking deals to address concerns of multiple parties who have conflicting goals can be applied to a variety of therapeutic circumstances. A teen who wants more freedom can be offered help at negotiating with his or her parents after the parents' concerns are addressed first.

- **Help get the authorities off the families' backs.** In both of the above methods, in addition to safety issues, the families themselves wanted help on something and what they wanted help on was utilized in an approach that also addressed safety issues. A difficult situation arises when authorities who have power to remove children have serious safety concerns but the families are not concerned with safety and also do not want help on other family problems. In this situation, the practitioner can offer to help the family get the authorities out of their lives. The practitioner can offer to advocate for the family in exchange for the family addressing safety issues.

IMPLEMENTING

Characteristics of Useful Goals

DEFINE GOALS CONCRETELY, SPECIFICALLY, AND *BEHAVIORALLY*

Clients do not typically come to treatment with clear goals in mind or wanting to focus on specific problems. Typical adult complaints are that the child does not show "respect" or has poor self-esteem. Starting with a global nonspecific complaint and ending with a specific problem and goal requires skill. The client must agree that the specific goal or problem selected actually reflects what he or she came in upset about. Key questions can be asked to tease out something specific from something global (Walter & Peller, 1982).

- The more specific the description of the goal the more compelling it is for the clients to be motivated to work toward achieving (O'Hearn & Gatz, 2002; Weissberg, Barton, & Shriver, 1997).
- Emphasize concrete behavior that describes what the client will be doing and thinking; this may take some coaching. Clients often have been so focused on the problem that they have rarely given thought to what they *do want* for their family and what they *will be doing when* they are doing what they want. The best way to get this is to *be direct*.
- To obtain a sufficient level of specificity the practitioner needs to ask family members open-ended questions such as: Who? What? When? Where? How? How often? What will that look like? The most useful goals have as many behavioral indicators as possible of the desired changes.
- In asking such questions it is often useful to include the term "specifically." So, for example, you may ask:
  - "How *specifically* will you know your child is being respectful to you?"
  - "*Specifically*, what will your child be doing differently once she is being respectful to you?"
  - "*Specifically*, what will be the first small change in your child's behavior that will be sign indicating to you that he is being respectful to you?"
- Concrete and behaviorally specific goals are required to evaluate the effectiveness of treatment.
- Keep asking family members, especially parents, follow-up questions to get as many behavioral indicators from them as possible of the desired change; that is, from their perspective what will their future behavior look like once the problem is solved.
- Clear, specific goals usually are more likely to be attainable.
- Having clear goals can help to empower the parents. Problems must be defined as not only solvable, but also as ones that parents can do something about. Identifying clear and specific goals can serve this purpose. Parents cannot do anything about depression. Experts must deal with that problem. But, parents can do something about a child who will not get out of bed or take a shower.

- Ask the client to give a specific example of an incident. "What is a specific example of an instance where your son did not show respect?" The parent may then produce an example of a hostile argument with the son during which the son escalated and used more and more bad language and became more and more insulting. The parent describes a "fit" and that becomes the problem. Interactions related to the "fit" can then be tracked. One goal of treatment becomes helping the child not have a fit.
- Ask how the problem interferes with the client's life. "How does low self-esteem interfere with your child's life? What can the child not do because of low self-esteem?" In response to this question, the parent may list several specific activities such as going to a school dance, accepting an overnight visit of a friend, asking questions in class, and so on. Helping the child accomplish these activities becomes the treatment goal.
- For example, a mother described her 15-year-old son as depressed. When asked how his depression interfered with his life and what he could not do because of depression, the mother said he did not get out of bed in the morning and go to school on a depressed day, and he did not take showers on depressed days. A doctor and medication are required for depression, but a mother can do something about a son who does not get out of bed, go to school, or take showers.

STATE GOALS POSITIVELY (APPROACH RATHER THAN AVOIDANCE GOALS)

After families have defined the primary presenting problem practitioners ask them what has to change in order for them to feel that they no longer need to continue in treatment. The family's initial response to this question usually is stated in terms of what they do not want to see happening anymore. It is often helpful to define what *will* the client be doing or thinking rather than what they *will not* be doing or thinking. This is the presence of a positive, rather than the absence of a negative. Stating goals positively is another way of saying that it is better to set *approach* goals rather than *avoidance* goals. Numerous studies have found that knowing what one wants is more effective than knowing what one does not want or wants to get rid of. Thus, goals stated in a positive form will allow the family and client to have a clear idea about what they will be doing versus what they won't be doing (Elliot & Church, 2002; Elliot & Harackiewicz, 1996; O'Hearn & Gatz, 2002; Rooney, Higgins, & Shah, 1995; Weissberg, Barton, & Shriver, 1997; Wollburg & Braukhaus, 2010).

When the family initially defines the desired goal in such a negative way, that is, "I want my child to stop throwing temper tantrums," or "He will stop being so disrespectful," or "She will stop running away and skipping school all the time" then it is important to follow up with questions to get them to define their desired goal in terms of what will be present rather than absent once the change occurs. Some follow-up questions practitioners can ask are:

- "What will be the first thing you will notice that will show your son is respecting you?"
- "So when your daughter is no longer running away or skipping school, what will she be doing instead?"

USE THE FAMILY'S LANGUAGE IN DESCRIBING AND DEFINING GOALS

Goals should be stated in the client's language. The I-FAST practitioner wants to be working toward *what the family wants*, not what he or she wants or thinks the clients should want. To ensure this, it is often helpful to track and use the clients' own words in describing the problem or goal.

- A related benefit is that using the clients' language will help us to operate within the clients' *frame or world view*.
- When you or a colleague becomes stuck in working with a case or in constructing or achieving an attainable goal, ask, "Is that what the client says that she wants?" of or "What is the client a customer for?"
- The final form of what the clients say they want may be quite different from what they initially say. The final form that you and the client agree on should be something specific and attainable. However, make sure that the final form is put clearly in the clients' own words and is in line with their values and world view.

STATE GOALS IN A PROCESS OR ACTIVE FORM

Given that *it is easier for people to change what they do rather than who they are,* define goals in process or action form. That is, aim to state goals as verbs and rather than nouns. The following guidelines can be helpful in defining such goals with clients:

- Aim for a description as if the family were in a movie, not a still picture.
- A key indicator is when clients are using verbs ending with "-ing." For example, *"I will be listening to my child"* (future); or *"I would be setting limits and staying consistent with my partner"* (conditional); or *"I will be paying attention and complimenting my daughter as she does her work"* (current).
- The key word to evoke this process description is HOW. The clients are more likely to give "-ing" descriptions, or a sequence of actions in response to "how" questions than if you use "what" questions, which tend to produce nouns.
- Aim to state goals in the present. The implication is that the clients can start the solution immediately, or continue with solutions that are already working now.
- Use pre-suppositional language when asking questions in the goal setting and talking about the future. Pre-suppositional language presupposes that the change has already occurred or will occur. Thus, for example, use "when" instead of "if" (see the question below).
- The goal should be stated in a process way, as something they can be on track with immediately. So, you might ask, *"So, when you are ON TRACK with changing the rules in the house, what will you be doing or doing differently?"*
- Goals need to be moved from the remote future, where they are less in the client's control, and put instead into the now, where they may be done or perhaps are already happening.

- Goals stated in the present allows the family to begin doing something NOW.
- A goal stated in a process form is indicative of specific steps and tasks that will provide feedback to the change process.

Negotiating Impasses Between Professionals

When impasses occur in cases between professionals, there is a common interactional pattern between professionals that can block the resolution of the impasse. Often disagreements are over each professional's theory about why the problems are occurring, or disagreements over respective treatment philosophies. The discussions end up being about respective theories, not about the facts of what is actually occurring. Professionals will typically dig in their heels and be unwilling to collaborate

> **A CASE EXAMPLE**
>
> A teenage boy was placed in residential treatment after, among other things, running away from home repeatedly. The boy lived with his father, stepmother, and two younger siblings. While placed, it was discovered that the father had used physical discipline with him on numerous occasions. During the placement, the residential staff had minimal interaction with the family and worked predominantly with the boy. They were aware of the father's discipline methods and were against the boy being released to the parents. When his release from residential placement was imminent, a home-based worker was assigned to begin family sessions. The home-based worker met with the family as a group and did not interview the boy individually. The home-based worker and residential practitioner ended up in serious conflict over whether the boy should be returned to his parents. Both worked for the same agency, but they each recommended diametrically opposed plans to children's services.
>
> During staffing on the family, the two workers would argue about their treatment philosophies and their theories about the family. The residential worker's position was that it was unsafe for the boy to visit his home overnight. The home-based worker's position was that the family was cooperating with him in treatment and therefore it was safe. Neither inquired or volunteered any facts about the case that supported his position. When asked about any specific incidents that caused him concern about the boy's safety on visits, the residential worker described an incident he observed directly. He observed the father and son arguing in the parking lot and the father grabbing the boy's shirt and shoving him up against a tree. When the home-based worker was asked why he described the family as cooperative, he explained that they had openly discussed the father's discipline methods and the father had agreed to not get physical with the son. Both workers had facts supporting their positions but neither had shared these facts with each other. They just argued with each other about their theories. When they did share the facts with each other, both gained a new respect for why they each had their positions as well as some new ideas for how they each needed to intervene. Sharing the facts broke their impasse and allowed them to collaborate.

if it means giving up a cherished theory. On the other hand, if the facts of who is doing or saying what can be focused on, compromise and collaboration can more easily occur. *Struggles between professionals can often be resolved when the focus of dialogue between them is on the details and facts of the case as opposed to theories about the case.* Focusing on facts and details is a skill that can be employed to resolve the impasse.

ESSENTIAL COMPONENTS OF GOAL SETTING AND GOAL CONSENSUS

The practitioner and the family/child mutually agree to the described goals. The following guidelines are helpful in developing such consensus:

- Goals are connected to a therapeutic rationale that is accepted by the client and the practitioner.
- The goals match with client values, motivations, and frames of reference.
- The goals are defined in specific, observable, and behavioral terms.
- Goals are defined as outcome-oriented.
- Goals are defined in the positive (the presence of the desired outcome) rather than in the negative (the absence of the problem).
- Goals are agreed on that satisfy different constituencies including collaborating professionals.

FRAMES, FRAMING, AND REFRAMING

INTRODUCTION TO FRAMING AND REFRAMING

As mentioned previously, the families we work with are stuck in patterns in which their attempts to solve the presenting problem are maintaining that problem. Usually, these patterns involve the family members repeatedly interacting about the problem in the same ways without success in solving the problem. Of course, we are focused on intervening with the family in a way whereby they change their patterns of interaction around a problem. Usually, a necessary step in pattern change is talking differently with the family about the problem and their unsuccessful attempts to solve it. In previous chapters (1, 3, 4 & 5), there is some discussion of the importance of language in the social construction of reality, framing, and reframing. In this chapter, we elaborate on these topics and further discuss using them in working with families to bring about second-order change.

In Chapter 5, we discussed the importance of framing and reframing in engaging families in the treatment process. Framing and reframing are also involved in facilitating pattern change in families. Concepts similar to and often used interchangeably with *frame* are assumption, premise, schema, and mental model. A common use of the word "frame" is found when we say to someone "My frame of reference for this is _____" or when we ask someone for their "frame of reference" for a decision they made or an action they took. Framing is what we do when we classify and categorize our experiences as we go about everyday living (Bateson, 1955; Goffman, 1974). Frames help us make sense of the world and make it as predictable as possible (Borah, 2011, p. 248).

CONCEPTUALIZING

Constructivism and Frames

Frames are socially influenced and co-created. In everyday life we tend to pay attention primarily to those experiences that are consistent with our frames and ignore those that are not. However, that does not mean that once we create our frames they never change. For example, through our social interactions with others, we continue to influence one another. In fact, people often change their behaviors and beliefs to conform to the expectations of others:

> In social interaction, people often use their preconceived beliefs and expectations about others to guide their behaviors. Their behavior, in turn, may influence their interaction partners to act in ways that confirm the initial beliefs. This phenomenon, in which belief creates reality, is known by several names—the self-fulfilling prophecy, expectancy confirmation, and behavioral confirmation. (Snyder & Stukas, 2000, p. 216)

Behavioral confirmation is "a process in which one individual's preconceived *beliefs* and prior *expectations* about another person channel their interactions in such ways that these initial beliefs (even when they are based on erroneous stereotypes or hypotheses of dubious validity) come to be *confirmed* by the other person's *behavior*" (Snyder & Thomsen, 1988, p. 127). When we meet someone for the first time we tend to quickly form an opinion about him and then proceed to interact with and treat him as if that first impression were true.

Common Factors and Reframing

MASTER FRAMES: TREATMENT RATIONALES

Treatment rationales are larger frames that guide the direction of treatment. Fairhurst refers to these types of frames as master frames (Fairhurst, 2011). Master frames provide any kind of an organizing vision, philosophy, or ideology (Fairhurst, 2011, pp. 99–100). Treatment rationales are master frames that organize treatment and set treatment directions.

- In family treatment, treatment rationales are found in the various established theoretical approaches. These various approaches provide treatment frames (rationales) that set treatment processes and directions.
- Specific treatment frames are not provided by I-FAST but must be decided upon on a case-by-case basis. In this regard I-FAST is influenced by the work of Jerome Frank and his contextual model to treatment that describes a two-step process that is crucial to intervening (Frank & Frank, 1991):
    1. The practitioner first provides an explanation or rationale for the client's symptoms (a myth).
    2. Then the practitioner offers a procedure that is designed to change the way that the client is trying to solve the problem (rituals).
- Evidence supports this two-step process as having healing potential whether or not the client carries out the treatment procedures and tasks.
- The client's hope in getting better is elevated when the client believes that the procedure will work. This then feeds back to the relationship and increases the practitioner's credibility in a virtuous cycle.

In addition I-FAST is influenced by research (Wampold, 2001, 2010a, 2010b) that shows that what is most important in effective treatment are the following:

- Practitioners need to use a coherent approach to treatment.
- Practitioners need to have competence in using their preferred coherent approach.
- Practitioners need to believe and have confidence in the effectiveness of their preferred coherent approach (practitioner allegiance).
- Practitioners need to regularly monitor how clients are responding to their preferred coherent approach.
- If clients are not responding positively to the practitioner's preferred coherent approach the practitioner needs to make a change in the approach he or she is using with the client.

STRENGTHS AND FRAMING

Each person is born with varying levels of physical, emotional, and intellectual strengths; abilities; and possibilities unique to him or her. People with high levels of strengths have good coping abilities, positive self-esteem, a sense of self-efficacy, empowerment, resilience, and so forth. All people have strengths.

- One core concept of I-FAST is that effective intervention will always be based on assuming that all involved parties within all involved systems have strengths to be discovered, elaborated, and engaged in resolution.
- To do so, practitioners need first to attend to their own assumptions about strengths and then translate those assumptions into language, priming, and framing with clients.
- Given that families usually are feeling demoralized, disempowered, and deficient when they first begin treatment, asking them questions whereby they identify and amplify their strengths (competencies, resources, assets, successes) can cultivate and create a new frame in which view themselves in a more positive and empowered way.
- Identifying their strengths can help families rediscover and increase their awareness of what specific actions they took in the distant or more recent past to successfully address any problems they may have had.
- In this process the families can realize and become motivated to do more of what has worked before but they are no longer doing.
- Decreasing their sense of demoralization and becoming more empowered can result in their increasing their sense of hope and goal achievement.

> To remain faithful to I-FAST, all frames, no matter what their treatment aim may be, must be accepted by the client and the family. Frames can be borrowed from other models, but to be utilized in I-FAST the client must accept the frame.

STRATEGIZING

Flexibility in Approach/Frame/Rationale

As mentioned previously, I-FAST is a meta-model based on evidence-based common factors. However, the common factors can be operationalized by using any one of the established coherent approaches to family treatment (Wampold, 2010a, 2010b).

- I-FAST practitioners are welcome to familiarize themselves with a wide variety of treatment frames to maximize their flexibility in applying these frames to various cases as they fit best.
- In addition, I-FAST practitioners should be aware of their own treatment frames and are free to use them in cases where they fit with the family.
- However, I-FAST practitioners must be ready to adopt another better fitting treatment frame when families do not appear to be responding positively to their preferred treatment frame.
- Ultimately, I-FAST practitioners will be best served by developing the skill of devising frames to fit each unique case.

- Whether an I-FAST practitioner borrows a treatment frame from another model or devises one for a particular case the client must accept the frame, and the frame must ultimately be useful for interventions aiming at changing habitual interactions among those involved in each case.

Types and Purposes of Frames

TREATMENT FRAMES AND RATIONALES

In I-FAST, classification in general is conceptualized not only as a cognitive function but also as a social organizing principle within and between groups. Classification constructs social realities and organizes social behavior.

- Working with and changing how clients understand their world is a common technique across therapies.
- Terms used by some of the established approaches to family treatment for doing this are *reframing* (Haley, 1976; Minuchin & Fishman, 1981; Weakland, Fisch, Watzlawick, & Bodin,1974) *changing perception* (Ellis, 1962), *changing cognitive distortions* (Beck, 1976), *positive connotations* (Selvini Palazzoli, Boscolo, Cecchin, & Prata, 1978), *noble ascriptions* (Stanton, Todd, and Associates, 1982), and *changing narratives* (White & Epston, 1990).
- To be effective all treatment frames should be constructed within how clients understand or frame things and how those frames may be changed.
- Treatment rationales perform the organizing and classifying function to help all involved with each case understand the problems, the roles of all involved, and the reasons for their actions in the service of resolving the identified problems.
- The idea that many treatment rationales can potentially be equally useful should not be taken in any way as discounting established treatment change frameworks.
- The aim is for the I-FAST practitioner to have a method that is developed specifically for the client's problem, and that the practitioner conveys confidence in using the framework despite difficulties that may arise in the treatment process and links hope with clients' expectations that they will improve.
- From the perspective of I-FAST, treatment frames do not have to be scientifically true to be effective.
- Treatment frames must provide an explanation of the client's symptoms in ways that make sense to all involved. In other words, the explanation must be plausible to the participants in treatment and therefore believable.
- Because the practitioner must be congruent and sincere as part of the relationship building process, the explanation or rationale for symptoms must also be plausible and believable to the practitioner.
- Procedures that are designed to change the client's problem-solving approach must be linked to the explanation of symptoms in a way that likewise makes sense to the client and the practitioner. In other words, the logical connection between the frame and the procedure must create a belief in the client that the procedure will be effective.
- Research shows that practitioners must also believe in the efficacy of psychological procedures if they are to be effective. In fact, Wampold's

meta-analysis shows that it is more important for the practitioner to believe in her procedure than to perform it in a way that is in perfect conformance with a manual (Wampold, 2001).

- The practitioner and client being actively engaged in a coherent and organized approach to treatment alone has been suggested in more recent literature to be potentially one of the most potent elements in the effectiveness of most current evidence-based approaches to at risk youth and families (Sprenkle, Davis, & Lebow, 2009).
- For frames, conceptual schemes, and procedures to be effective they must be aligned with the belief system, values, and culture of the client as well as make enough sense to the practitioner that he or she will deliver that treatment both genuinely and skillfully.
- The frame must define a process that allows for the parents to be primary change agents of their child's problematic behavior.
- The frame must define the problem as something parents or client can do something about.

Treatment Rationales and Strategies

Ultimately, treatment rationales should provide frames for strategizing about how best to work with the family. A strategy is defined here as the collection of several treatment decisions regarding a given case. Those decisions include what goal to pursue, what unit of analysis to use to conceptualize the case, whom to include in the treatment, and what frames and interventions to offer. A treatment rationale should lead to all of these decisions in a way that those decisions make sense to and are agreeable to the family. In I-FAST the skillful use of framing and reframing is utilized throughout each stage of treatment. In the intervention stages, framing is used to provide rationales for various interventions and tasks or to suggest action indirectly by the skillful use of questioning.

How Practitioners Use Framing with Clients

How practitioners frame clients and the resulting impact on engagement has already been discussed in Chapter 5. As noted, framing clients in ways that promotes empathy and an ability to view clients humanely is required in I-FAST. In addition, how we frame problems can significantly influence how we frame the family and thus how we intervene with them.

FRAMING GOALS

Faming goals was discussed in Chapter 5. To review, in I-FAST, goals must represent what the family is motivated to focus on and must be achievable. In I-FAST, goals, like problems, must be defined as something specific that the family can do something about while the client remains in their natural environment. Also, overall, defining goals in the positive (approach/gain frame) is more effective than defining them in the negative (avoidance/loss frame).

POSITIVE REFRAMING

Positive reframing was discussed in some detail in Chapter 3 on engaging, as were the processes in framing and reframing. In addition to helping to engage the family successfully, reframing is an intervention itself in that it can introduce novelty and second-order change to them. Reframing can result in second-order change because it deals with how families construct their reality and thus it operates at the level of meta-reality.

- One reason families can get stuck in habitual interactional patterns is they have a limited number of frames for categorizing and making sense of reality.
- Often families have only two frames for making sense of their child with the problem such as good vs. bad, mad vs. bad, desirable vs. undesirable, defiant vs. compliant, oppositional vs. compliant, and so on. Having only two categories lends itself to families getting stuck in "either–or" habitual interactional patterns. Positive reframing can offer families a third plausible frame for their child and his or her behavior that broadens their reality and options.
- As mentioned previously, for the reframe to be effective it has to be plausible and acceptable to the family.
    - One way to increase its plausibility and acceptability is to utilize the family's language, values, and beliefs in constructing and delivering the frame (Jones, 1986).
    - Sometimes a practitioner may not be sure of the family's language, values, and beliefs but may think of a frame that could be useful if they accept its plausibility. When this is the case the practitioner can still propose the reframe as a "trial balloon" to see how they react. If they accept it then the practitioner can continue further using the frame with the family. However, if the family does not seem to accept the frame then the practitioner should drop it and move on to something else.
    - Once the family accepts the plausibility of the positive reframe they can no longer view the child with the problem the same way, which can then set the stage for them to change how they interact and intervene with the child.
- In family treatment a potent reframe is to connect the problem of the identified child to others in the family. Connecting the problem this way reframes the problem as not being just that of the individual child but now involving the family system (see the section on Implementing).

Framing Tasks (The Task Frame)

In I-FAST, between-session and sometimes in-session tasks are used to change the habitual interactional patterns or increase exception interactions to solve the presenting problem and achieve the mutually defined goal.

- These tasks usually ask the parents to deviate from their habitual ways of attempting to solve the problem.
- Because we are asking them to do something different it is important for them to be motivated to do the task.
- Engaging families and developing a therapeutic alliance with them helps increase the likelihood that they will do the task.
- For people to be willing to engage in a task it is important to frame it in a way that fits with the values and beliefs of people (Gore & Cross, 2011). Thus, families also need to make sense of the therapeutic tasks for them to be willing to perform the tasks and/or continue in treatment.

- The practitioner therefore needs to provide the family a plausible rationale for the task that makes sense to the client.
- Task frames (rationales) are constructed using the client's values, beliefs, and language (metaphors and figures of speech).
- A practitioner may "cultivate" a frame throughout the session for use in providing an acceptable rationale to the family for doing the task (Jones, 1986).

The task frame is usually used at the end of a session when coming up with between-session task with the family. The task is usually part of an end-of-session message that begins first with complimenting the family for their strengths (competencies, skills, assets, successes), then comes the task frame, and finally the task. The task frame links the initial compliments to the concluding suggestions or tasks by providing a rationale to the family for the task. The task frame should flow naturally from the compliments and will provide a bridge from where they are currently to where they want to be as indicated in their goal. As with compliments, any tasks the practitioner might suggest to clients must make sense to them in order for them to carry out the task partly or completely.

- Whenever possible it is also a good idea to incorporate and use the client's own words and phrases.
- The task frame provides the *rationale* for the task. The content of the task frame is usually drawn from client goals, exceptions, strengths, or perceptions.
- Commonly, the practitioner will begin the task frame statement by saying something like:

    - "I agree with you that . . . . . ."
    - "Since you want to. . . "
    - "Because you think that. . . "

Framing Improvement

Framing improvement will be discussed in detail in Chapter 10. The main point here is that improvement is framed in a way that gives credit to the client and family. Improvement must be viewed as something the family, especially the parents, were directly involved in bringing about.

IMPLEMENTING

Guidelines for Developing Frames and Reframes

CONSTRUCTING FRAMES AND REFRAMES

Constructing effective frames and reframes involves skill. There is an art and science to framing and reframing (Fairhurst, 2011). For frames to be effective they have to connect with other people. However, there is not a precise fail-safe formula for how to come up with effective frames and reframes. People who are effective in framing and reframing are strategic communicators in that they "have a heightened sensitivity to language" and are precise in using it. . . they "nearly always see alternative possibilities for 'the situation here and now'" and feel "confident in pursuing them" (Fairhurst, 2011, p. 19).

- Effective framers and reframers are very familiar with culture and different systems of thought (discourses) and use them as resources (Fairhurst, 2011).

- People who are effective in framing and reframing seem to come up with them almost effortlessly.
- Fairhurst states that people can become more effective in framing and reframing by "priming for spontaneity" (p. 63).
  - According to Fairhurst, "*priming* involves activating something in our short- or long-term memory, which then triggers an in-kind response in either what we say or what we do" (p. 64).

FRAMES ARE CO-CREATED

The creation of frames in treatment can be thought of broadly as a three-step process:

1. The practitioner offers a frame or reframe.
2. The client or family responds to the frame.
3. The practitioner adjusts the frame to the family's response.

The practitioner provides a frame. Perhaps the key and primary skill required to construct frames is listening. The practitioner must first immerse herself in the client's thinking. The practitioner must gain a deep appreciation for what the client wants, the language he uses and what his core values are. When a practitioner is truly listening, and is immersed in the client's thinking, often frames will come spontaneously. This is perhaps the best way to construct frames. Become engrossed in the client's story, his struggles, and what he wants from treatment, and then have faith that frames will come. If the practitioner is interested in key aspects of the client and what he wants, the practitioner will think of frames. In the end, listening and trusting one's judgment on what frame the client might like may be the most reliable method of constructing frames.

The client responds. Once a frame is offered, the client can respond in one of three ways:

- He can accept the frame as offered.
- He can accept it with his own modifications.
- can reject it.

THE PRACTITIONER ADJUSTS TO CLIENT RESPONSES

It is essential for family members to accept (buy into) the frame the practitioner identifies or suggests. If the family does not accept the frame or only part of it, then the practitioner needs to adjust accordingly:

- If the client and family accept the frame then it can be used.
- If the family partially accepts the frame a give-and-take dialogue should ensue between the family and the practitioner until a frame is mutually accepted.
- If the family rejects the frame a discussion should occur that promotes a deeper understanding of the family by the practitioner. After this a frame can again be offered.

FLEXIBLE FRAMING

Although it is permitted and encouraged to employ frames used in other approaches, and experienced practitioners often bring frames to treatment that they have successfully employed in other situations with other clients, I-FAST does not offer set frames to be used in case after case. As with several other I-FAST concepts and treatment procedures, the choice of frames to offer is decided on on a case-by-case basis. How to decide what frames to offer largely depends on understanding the client's beliefs, language, and motives regarding the problem or problems as well as what overarching frames and rationales the practitioner may be familiar with that appear to fit the problem and systems involved.

TRACKING AND UTILIZING CLIENT LANGUAGE AND FRAMES

Client frames (as well as our own) are created within language-based social interaction and importantly shape and guide our subsequent interactions:

- Our frames define and channel how we view and interpret events and others in interaction.
- They both focus and limit our interpretations and actions, particularly as we encounter problems.
- Our language and frames not only will determine whether we decide something is a problem but also will define what we should appropriately do to solve the problem as defined.
- Once stuck within a particular frame for an intractable problem, the logic and structure of the frame itself will reinforce habitual interactions focused on repeated and escalating efforts to try more of the same solutions.
- Thus frames and their accompanying language are directly related to the process of first-order change and sustaining problems with habitual interactions that represent the same method of attempting to solve the problem.
- Resolving problems is thus closely reliant on building a relationship and dialogue within the language and frames of all involved parties and through that alliance developing meaningful goals and related tasks that will change habitual interactions.
- Framing, reframing, and deframing become important therapeutic tasks for the practitioner.
- Attending to the kind of language being used by clients and others involved parties and adapting our interaction to use that language becomes important.
- First this helps building strong relationships where involved parties feel understood.
- Just as important is that it offers valuable insight into how that language and its related frames are guiding interaction with the habitual interactions of the identified problem.

According to the discrepancy model (Claiborn & Dowd, 1985), plausibility and believability directly apply to the use of these skills. In other words, effective frames, reframes and deframes must match the client's view of reality closely while offering a slightly different twist on the situation. At the same time, frames, reframes and deframes must be plausible and believable to both the practitioner and the client to be effective and ethical.

TRACKING HOW CLIENTS FRAME PROBLEMS

Part of clients' stories are the ways they and/or other people have tried to solve the presenting problem but thus far have not been successful in their efforts.

- *Identifying attempted solutions* indicates how the client and/or significant others are caught up in a vicious cycle of *first-order change*.
- Asking the family members how they think the problem developed and how it is the problem is continuing to happen is a very important question aimed at understanding how family members view the problem. That is, finding out from the family member their theory about the development and maintenance of the presenting problem? Tracking and utilizing how they respond to this question can be very useful in constructing frames that will make sense to the family.
- At this point the practitioner wants to know what the client and significant others have been doing in attempting to solve the presenting problem and reach the desired goal.
- After asking clients questions about what they have done to try to solve the problem it is useful to then ask them, if the client has not already mentioned this, to what extent any of them have worked. Most likely they will indicate that none of them are now working.
- By identifying the attempted solutions of first-order change the practitioner initially learns what types of interventions to avoid using because they are already a part of the habitual interactional pattern around the problem.
- Another useful question to follow up with is to ask them the following question: "What have you thought about trying in attempting to solve the problem but have not tried so far?"
  - Frequently, the successful solution to the presenting problem is the very thing they have thought about trying but have not yet done so. People are much more likely to do something they have thought of on their own but have not yet tried than doing something very different and new which is the idea of someone else.

Obtaining this information about unsuccessful attempts to solve the presenting problem and attempts thought about but not tried is helpful for several reasons:

- For one it provides us more information about the client's existing mental models and frames.
- In addition, when clients become aware that their existing frames are not working and their current situation is not where they want to be they will experience some discomfort.
- This awareness and discomfort will then tend to loosen up and make more permeable their existing frames and they will then be more open to novelty, expanding their frames, and thus second-order change.
- This process is referred to as *deframing* which involves abolishing or casting doubt on current frames or meanings and is another way of describing the effects of the process of deconstructing the problem pattern as it is currently being defined and acted upon by all involved.
- As all involved are heard describing the problem as they see it, the I-FAST practitioner gains in effect a window on the frames and assumptions and the associated language being used by all parties. This language and set of

frames can then be used to both understand what is channeling everyone's interactions, allow the practitioner to "speak the language" of all involved, and begin the process of framing, deframing, and reframing central to the I-FAST approach.

When devising and offering reframes, the primary skill involves observing and utilizing how clients respond to what is offered. A frame is offered. The client responds with an affirmation, or an affirmation with some twist of his or her own, or a rejection. A back and forth process can ensue in which the practitioner is tracking and utilizing what is offered until an unqualified affirmation is received.

LANGUAGE AND FRAMING

The language of the practitioner is critical to helping initiate and sustain change. The following points are useful for practitioners when they attend to the language they use with clients and involved others as they interaction with them in interventions:

- Do use language that implies the family wants to change.
- Do use language that implies that the family is capable of change.
- Do use language that implies change has occurred or is occurring.
- Do use language that implies the changes are meaningful.
- Do use language that encourages the family to explore possibilities for change.
- Do use language that suggests that the family can be creative and playful about life.
- Do use language that conveys recognition of the family's evolution of their personal story.
- Do limit energy expended in unproductive areas such as negative, blaming, or self-defeating descriptions.

TRACKING AND UTILIZING CLIENT AND FAMILY FRAMES (POSITIONS)

Tracking and utilizing client and family frames (positions) can enhance the construction of frames that will make sense to the family. For example, the parents of an acting-out teenage son may unintentionally be engaged in a pattern of over-functioning for the teenager with the rationale that they must do for their son because he is so incompetent. They further describe themselves as being devoted to their son and self-sacrificing for his benefit. Thus, they are involved in a repetitive pattern of first-order change in that the more they over-function for him to try to make him more competent the more incompetent he perceives himself and the more he continues to under-function. Facilitating second-order change can be done by doing the opposite of the problem maintaining interactions then one way for them to make a pattern shift resulting in second-order change is for them to start behaving incompetently relative to their son. One way to frame the rationale for this task is for the practitioner to emphasize how much of a "sacrifice" this will require them to make.

> **A CASE EXAMPLE**
>
> A young man complained to Milton Erickson (the well-known hypnotherapist) that his life was a waste and he felt suicidal. The young man was an illiterate, school dropout, homeless migrant worker. He had very low self-esteem and viewed himself as incapable of succeeding in school or work. He described himself as worthless and stupid. Erickson convinced him to go back to school by asking the man how badly he thought he would fail his classes if he did enroll again. The man said he would fail miserably. Erickson said to really find out he would have to go back to school and try his hardest. If he failed but did not try his hardest it would not prove he was a stupid worthless man. Erickson suggested a task of taking night classes. It was framed utilizing the man's position that he was stupid. Framing the task as an experiment to prove how stupid the man was made sense to the man. He did go back to school and tried his hardest. He received a B– in his first class and was confused. Erickson suggested the instructor may have been fooled by the man and that he should take two more classes the next term, which he did, passing them both, and received his high school diploma.

UTILIZE THE FAMILY'S BELIEFS AND THEORIES ABOUT THE PROBLEM

The rational for tasks given to clients must be framed in a way that makes sense to the client. One way to accomplish this is to link the changes requested to the clients' beliefs about the problem.

> **A CASE EXAMPLE**
>
> A 15-year-old girl became violent with her mother, threatened suicide on multiple occasions, did not go to school. All she did was see her boyfriend. The parents were immobilized by her violent and suicidal behavior. They were afraid to set limits on her fearing a violent reaction. The father responded to the problems by withdrawing. The mother responded by getting in intense and hostile verbal fights with the girl in which the mother threatened to institutionalize or hospitalize the girl if she did not behave. On numerous occasions when the girl erupted the parents called the police and had her taken to a hospital, or attempted to have her placed out of the home. The parents felt helpless and the girl felt rejected. Both reactions intensified the terrible fighting between mother and girl. When asked why they believed the girl was acting this way the parents explained that she just wanted to get her way. She was stubborn and if she wanted to see her boyfriend they better give in or "all hell was coming." *They believed the girl was stubborn* but were attempting to help her stubbornness by having her hospitalized. The practitioner agreed with the assessment that the girl was stubborn and just wanted her way. He pointed out that a positive aspect of being stubborn was having determination. If she could get over her problems, that could serve her well. The problem was she was actually having her way with them. The tail was wagging the dog. The problem was framed as a power struggle. For the girl to change the parents would have to demonstrate to her that they, not a hospital staff member, could deal with her. The parents agreed and were receptive to any suggestions the practitioner had at how to get the girl to cooperate with them.

> **A CASE EXAMPLE**
>
> The following example illustrates several uses of frames and reframing mentioned in the preceding text, including utilizing the client's way of framing the problem, setting up a treatment rationale for this specific case, and framing the tasks offered. A mother kept her seven-year-old son home from school believing him to be afflicted with anxiety. The school felt the boy was manipulating his mother and filed truancy on him. The mother was convinced her son was really sick and that the school misunderstood him. The mother's belief that the boy really did have school phobia and that he needed to be treated as sick rather than bad were affirmed. The question was: How does one help a school phobic boy over his phobia? The rationale was offered that a method for overcoming anxiety was to be repeatedly exposed to the anxiety-producing stimuli until the boy was no longer bothered by those stimuli. This is a major frame offered in exposure, which was adapted to fit I-FAST. The rationale would be used to put the mother in the key position of helping the boy, and to set up the tasks that would be given to her. After his mother agreed to the larger treatment rationale that repeated exposure to the anxiety-producing stimuli offers a way to help the son, reversing her attempts to protect him from stress makes sense. In this case it was decided that he would have to be exposed to school a little bit at a time until he could go a full day without anxiety. This procedure made sense to the mother. It also represented a second-order shift from how she was dealing with the problem. Reframing was used to approve of her intentions and beliefs, and link them to a request for her to change her past pattern of keeping her son home. This also set up the procedure in which the mother would be the person to expose him to school a little bit at a time. She was put in the key position to help him over his anxiety.

Once problems have been defined as solvable, goals have been agreed on, treatment rationales have been accepted by the family that places the parents in a key position to help their child, and reframes setting up tasks have been accepted, the treatment process can proceed to the assignment of tasks.

THE ESSENTIAL ELEMENTS OF FRAMING AND REFRAMING

- The practitioner identifies premises, beliefs, and classifications that drive the problem-maintaining patterns.
- The practitioner identifies frames and rationales that fit with the clients and their language, values, frame of reference, and world views.
- The practitioner develops a frame for that problem that'll allow a pattern shift.
- The practitioner introduces a new perspective that helps families to see things from a new perspective that is built upon the earlier work in the session.
- The practitioner tracks how well initial statements of frames and rationales are received by all family members.

- The practitioner adjusts his or her behavior and frames in response to the client so that client rejection of a frame or idea is absorbed and redirected to a new action or frame, and client acceptance of a frame or action is reinforced and continued.
- The practitioner ultimately comes to an agreement with the clients on:
  - A frame or rationale that fits with everyone's understandings
  - Offers a reasonable and relatively positive description of the nature of the problem
  - Implies a direction to go to resolve the problem
  - Enlists clients' motivations to go that way to resolve the difficulty

INITIATING CHANGE 7

INTRODUCTION TO INITIATING CHANGE

All human interaction has interpersonal influence. The logic-based axioms on therapeutic communication make the relationship between communication, behavior, and influence very clear (Watzlawick, Beavan, & Jackson, 1967). Communication theorists interested in systems of human interaction put forward the following premises about human communication:

- What we say or do not say to ourselves and in interaction with others shape what we attend to and how we come to understand ourselves and others.
- Behavior has no opposite. There is no such thing as non-behavior; a person cannot *not* behave.
- If it is accepted that all behavior in an interactional situation is communication, it follows that one cannot *not* communicate.
- Activity or inactivity, words, or silence all send a message: they influence others. These others, in turn, cannot *not* respond to messages sent and are thus communicating in response to the first person's words or silence.
- All behavior, all communication has interpersonal influence; therefore one cannot *not* influence other people (Watzlawick et al., 1967, pp. 48–49).
- In the therapeutic interchange, all actions of the practitioner and client or clients have influence.
- What interveners choose to inquire about shapes the kind of information they receive from their clients. Whether they choose to confront or teach or simply remain silent all have profound influence on the moment-by-moment course of treatment, as do the way clients choose to respond or not.
- Change can be initiated at any point in treatment after the first contact between practitioner and client. Developing rapport can set a change process in motion, whether the practitioner is thinking this way or not. I-FAST practitioners would be wise to be alert for and inquire about any changes from the outset of treatment.
- The key treatment implication for I-FAST is that problem interactions and related assumptions or frames are interrelated; change either one and the other can change as well. When this is successful, the perceived problem will *shift or be resolved.*

CONCEPTUALIZING

Systems Theory and Initiating Change
All parties involved on a case form an interdependent and interacting system. It is impossible to change one individual in a system without the entire system changing. This provides I-FAST practitioners with options regarding whom to work with and

what problem to focus on. The preferred treatment approach is to construct a strategy that follows a path of least resistance.

- Change one person by changing another. Changing one member of a system can result in changing the entire system. If one person changes and can be held to that change, the rest of the group must adjust and thus also change.
- A system can be changed either by introducing a small change and amplifying it, or even by producing a crisis in the system resulting in a reorganization of the system (Haley, 1963). For I-FAST practitioners, this means that helping a family overcome one problem can produce a *domino effect* and result in multiple changes.
- Provide treatment in stages. Introducing a change and amplifying it, or producing a major change that puts the system in crisis implies a treatment that will progress in two stages. The first stage requires getting a change going. The second stage requires amplifying changes or helping the system adjust to a major change.
- The family members most upset about the problem, and therefore those most motivated to change can be engaged in treatment. If those who can be engaged in treatment can make changes, the rest of the group may also change in response. Also, the problems the client most wants help on can generally be the focus. Stakeholders may have other concerns, but by focusing on producing a change in the areas the client wants help on, a domino effect can be initiated and the stakeholder goals may ultimately end up being addressed indirectly.
- Change can be occurring constantly and all interaction has influence; change can occur at any point in the treatment process in response to any interaction including those intended to establish alliances and identify goals.
- Change may begin with a shift in the relationship of the practitioner with the client(s) involved. This shift may itself represent a second-order change for the clients, or it may be a precursor for it to follow.
- I-FAST practitioners may facilitate changes in client assumptions, frames, or premises.
- I-FAST practitioners may choose from a multitude of intervention techniques from numerous treatment approaches to change interactional patterns or amplify interactional exceptions that support the presenting problems.
- Finally, I-FAST practitioners can look for and support new frames and successful solution patterns and reinforce and amplify them as they are found or initiated, or help families adjust to major changes treatment may help produce.

Constructivism and Initiating Change

Practitioner frames affect what we look for in working with families and thus how we intervene with them. As mentioned in Chapter 1, I-FAST is based on the master frames of social constructivism, systems theory, the strengths perspective, and the process of change model as well as research evidence supporting the common factors. These master frames are points of view that influence how we work with families. All interaction and intervention by a practitioner is *based on a point of view* on the nature of human kind, the nature of change, and thus the nature of problems and their resolution. Thus as practitioners of family treatment, we cannot *not have a point of view, values, assumptions, or premises about problems and change.*

- This can bring up a sort of "chicken or the egg" question of which comes first, the assumptions or point of view or the actions and interactions that both flow from those assumptions but also that shape those assumptions.
- We view these processes as reciprocal or circular. Both influence and shape each other.
- This is the essence of the *constructivist* assumptions accepted in I-FAST. Our world views are co-created by our interactions.
- I-FAST *expands the constructivist context* to include the influence of social, language, and cultural context in the interaction formula.
- Our frames, language, values, assumptions, and related interactions cannot *not* be influenced, embedded within, and shaped by our sociocultural contexts (as those contests are also a product of our historical and collective interactions over time).
- All of the preceding points apply to our clients and the systems involved with them *as well as to us as practitioners*. Our frames and interactions as interveners with youth, families, and systems are influenced by our own language, values, motives, and assumptions.

Frames on the Nature of Change and Focus of Intervention

The following are a set of general assumptions of the approach:

- We assume that change is inevitable and constant. The question is whether the change that is occurring is reinforcing the problems brought to treatment, or resolving them, or going unnoticed.
- Families are not static with inertia or innate resistance to change, but instead are always evolving and changing their interactions, whether noticed or not.
- Problems are viewed as resulting from repeated failed attempts to change a perceived difficulty.
- Those attempts are shaped by (and in turn shape) our frames about our roles, the nature of positive behavior, our motives, our values, our frames on the best paths to resolution, and so on.
- Perceived difficulties or differences are often resolved through what might best be described as a process of either *assimilating* the difficulty into our current systems of interaction or *accommodating* or adjusting those interaction patterns to the perceived difficulty.
- Lack of resolution is characterized by habitual interactional patterns (HIPs) (vicious cycles) that represent repeated failed resolution attempts by all involved only further exacerbate or escalate the very problem they are attempting to solve. (We have called this *first-order change*.)
- [Note that the phrase "*all involved parties*" is being used here to refer to all of those involved with defining the situation as a problem and who are engaged in doing something about it. This thus often includes the youth, family members, schools, courts, social agencies, helpful others, and so forth, as well as us as practitioners being called in to do something to help resolve the perceived problems. This is a multisystemic view.]

- This view of problems as habitual interactional patterns (vicious cycles) of often well-meaning solution attempts by all involved parties is at the heart of the I-FAST approach to problems and their resolution.
- It follows that the essence of intervention or initiating desired change within the I-FAST approach is the interruption or redirection of these interactional patterns as they occur within the multiple systems that are inevitably involved with at-risk youth and families (initiating *second-order change*).
- The focus of change in the I-FAST approach is to change or redirect the way all parties involved with a given case are trying to change or resolve the problem as perceived and described from their own points of view. Their solutions have become the problem and those interactional patterns are the target of change.
- The goal is to introduce a difference that will make a difference in the identified interactional patterns.
- This process involves identifying all involved parties' language, motives, values, and frames and noting how they influence the interactional patterns that perpetuate the problems.
- This process also is predicated on assuming that all involved are simply doing their best to try and do the right or best thing from their own perspective. It does not assume malevolent or pathological motives and avoids assigning blame to any involved party. In this respect, among others, I-FAST is a strengths-based perspective.

Strengths and Initiating Change

A first step in facilitating change is often embedded in the strengths-based assumptions of the I-FAST approach. Historically, most approaches to psychotherapy in general have been based on a deficit-based approach to seeing clients and their problems as examples of pathology or deficits in skills, emotional bonding, and so on needing to be corrected. Interestingly, this same negative lens on problems is often one shared by both client families and the agencies with whom they are involved.

- Often an ongoing intervention facilitating a second-order change itself is the point at which the I-FAST practitioner adopts a strengths-based position.
- Here the practitioner assumes good intensions are shared by all, validates the distress and pain shared by everyone, assumes that everyone has the ability and will to change things, asks what is going right, and identifies when things are working.
- This position is the basis of those questions that not only identify the problem patterns but also note *exceptions* to that pattern when things are going well.
- When engaged with intense, painful, frightening, or frustrating problems with at-risk youth, all participants can be seen as involved with what might be described as a "problem-saturated story" of their situation with plenty of negative labels to go around.
  - Parents will often view their child as sick or just bad or defiant.
  - Involved youth usually see their parents as simply jerks or not understanding them or as power hungry disciplinarians to be resisted, and so on.

- Agencies and practitioners often end up faulting the mothers or both parents for the youth's problems or end up labeling the youth with some diagnostic label such as the greatly overused attention-deficit/hyperactivity disorder, oppositional defiant disorder, or bipolar disorder.
- The validating, normalizing, and collaborative strengths-based position of I-FAST puts the dilemma in context and directs clients and involved others in new directions.
- Rather than seemingly "fighting their way into the paper bag" of their problem, clients must redirect their attention and the direction of their conversation toward strengths and exceptions when they are asked: "So, what is happening when this problem isn't going on. . . what do you notice when things are going well?" or "What do you do to get that to happen?" or "How are you able to make that happen?"
- This seemingly small shift in direction and tone of the relationship often has a watershed effect on all involved.
- I-FAST is grounded in acknowledging, honoring, and respecting the multiplicity of often very useful and yet different ways that individuals, families, practitioners, and agencies have come to organize themselves and function. I-FAST applies the same premises to respecting the strengths, values, world views, and goals of the practitioners and agencies employing the I-FAST perspective as it does to the youth, families and involved agencies of each case. Flexibility is at the core of I-FAST and yet to be genuinely flexible practitioners need to be aware of their own views and biases and be willing to move outside of them to match those of the individuals and systems with whom they are engaged.

TO REMAIN FAITHFUL TO I-FAST:

- Interventions are offered only if an alliance is established with at least one parent.
- Interventions must have an obvious connection to the specific problem or goal the aligned parent has identified.
- The intervention requires a deviation from interactional patterns that support the problem, or amplify exceptions to those patterns.

STRATEGIZING

As we noted earlier, all effective treatments begin with establishing a relationship and working alliance with all involved parties and systems, collaborating on agreed on goals of all parties, and setting a rationale for treatment that makes sense to all parties. How the I-FAST practitioner achieves each of these steps involves strategy in itself. In sum, though the therapeutic relationship is at times powerful enough to facilitate change on its own in many cases, particularly with at-risk youth, specific intervention approaches are necessary. Developing interventions emerges from relationship building. It should be remembered that:

- Intervention techniques are an outgrowth of the therapeutic relationship and are effective only when the practitioner has proven herself to be worthy of the clients' trust.

- Within the context of the relationship, the practitioner must convey understandings of the clients and their problem that are close enough to the clients' world view, so as not to appear threatening, but different enough to give the client hope that change will occur.
- Relationship building elements are client determined and must be maintained throughout the treatment process. All effective practitioners maintain the relationship by adjusting their approach to fit the client's understanding of how a practitioner should be. However, there are additional strategies and interventions that can be employed in I-FAST that are commonly associated with engagement yet can also enhance targeted interventions in later stages of treatment.

Initiating versus Joining Change

Often change does not have to be initiated because it is already occurring. When this is the case then the practitioner can simply join with it:

- The I-FAST approach assumes change is a continuous process. In the case of identified problems of at-risk youth and families, that process is part of interactional patterns that escalate or reinforce the problem or change.
- Unsuccessful attempted solutions to problems are perpetuating unwanted change.
- The process of joining with the multiple parties and systems already engaged with desired change can further influence those interactional patterns toward desired change and problem resolution.
- This involves accepting, respecting, and utilizing the language, motives, frames, and related solution attempts of all involved and matching them with who we are and how we can adapt to their frames in the process of helping them shift toward resolutions.
- The therapeutic techniques presented in this chapter have been borrowed from a multitude of family treatment and behavioral approaches. They can all be employed in I-FAST as interventions aimed at resolving problems by promoting deviations from the interactional patterns that support them.

Facilitating Change

Given that our frames help to shape our actions as they do with our clients and the agencies involved with them, we need always to check and recheck our frames before and at many points during each case. Before formally offering interventions, all previous I-FAST steps must be complete. Those steps are:

- All parties involved in the treatment are respected and accepted.
- An alliance is established with at least one caregiver.
- A decision is made regarding whom to work directly with.
- Major frames, values, and motives of everyone involved are identified, along with how these influence their approach to addressing the problem.
- Specific problems and the potential interactional patterns that support them or exceptions to those interactions are identified.
- Clear frames and rationales to explain the problem and imply a direction for resolution have been agreed on.
- When offered, interventions align with the goals of key parties.

- Key parties are engaged with procedures that will reframe their problem or interactions, and/or redirect their interactions, or identify and enlarge interactional exceptions.
- Once new directions begin, they need to be noted, reinforced, and success attributed to the involved parties.
- As success and new patterns are achieved, they need to be celebrated, solidified, and reinforced against potential future challenges or perceived "relapse."

Guidelines for Choosing How to Intervene

I-FAST allows the integration of a vast array of intervention approaches as long as they are offered within the larger I-FAST frames. The focus should be on the problem the parents want help on and promote deviations from interactional patterns or amplifications of interactional exceptions. What follows are some of the major possibilities. With so many options available, the question becomes how to decide which option to pick. By offering a wide range of choices regarding types of interventions, I-FAST allows for any given problem to be worked with in a variety of ways. We do not generally assume that one type of intervention is more effective than another. With so many choices, how does a practitioner decide? We offer the following considerations for making this decision.

READINESS TO CHANGE: WHAT IS THE FAMILY A CUSTOMER FOR?

Previously we discussed the importance of assessing the family's readiness to change, also referred to as *stage of change*: pre-contemplation, contemplation, preparation, action, maintenance, and relapse. Knowing the family's readiness to change can guide us to choosing interventions and tasks that will be the best fit for the family at a particular time in the treatment. Another simple framework is assessing for whether the family are customers, complainants, or visitors.

When families are *customers* they are able to define goals jointly with the practitioner and each other they see that they will have to do something different if a solution is to emerge. As *complainants*, families are able to jointly identify a problem or concern do not yet see any steps they might take toward a solving it. Families are considered to be *visitors* when they do not identify a problem or concern and thus are unwilling to make any changes. It is not helpful to think of families who are visitors or complainants as resistant. Rather, when this is the case it is more helpful to acknowledge that you and they still have work to do in identifying what the family is a customer for.

Families that are visitors often have been mandated into treatment and thus their participation in treatment is involuntary. What they are usually a customer for is something like "getting the courts off my back" or "getting my kids back." When this is the case we need to accept their definition of the problem and follow up with asking something like "What do you have to do to get the court off your back?" or "What do you have to do to get your kids back?" and then work with the family from that as a starting point.

WHAT IS THE PRACTITIONER'S SKILL SET AND KNOWLEDGE?

With a few exceptions, the main consideration for deciding what type of interventions to offer is the practitioner's skill level and familiarity of the various types of interventions. I-FAST aims to empower both families and practitioners. Practitioners often bring their own skill set into I-FAST that includes knowledge of the effective use of one or more of the types of interventions. The flexibility of I-FAST allows for practitioner to utilize their own skill set, or learn new ones while remaining faithful to the I-FAST model.

HOW ARE THE CLIENTS RESPONDING TO INTERVENTIONS?

Whatever approach to intervention an I-FAST practitioner begins a case with, the crucial issue is how the family and client are responding to the approach. Does it make sense to them? Do they actually try something new in response to what is offered? If they do try something new, is it helping?

Employing the skill of observing how the family is responding to interventions and adjusting to those responses, the I-FAST practitioner should maintain or change his or her approach in accordance with how the family is responding. For example, an I-FAST practitioner may be skilled at using a solution-focused approach. This approach can easily fit within I-FAST. If the approach is offered and the family responds positively, that is fine. If not, I-FAST offers a range of alternatives. In I-FAST, alternative approaches are offered until one is found that the family responds to.

IN-HOME VERSUS IN-OFFICE APPROACHES

It can sometimes be advantageous when working with families in the home to offer in-session interventions. When working in the home, it is common for most of the household to be present for the session. When this happens, often the client will enact his or her symptom and the family their interactional responses spontaneously during the session. If this occurs, the practitioner has the opportunity to help the family change how they are dealing with the problem right then and there. The family can then be given suggestions that require them to deviate from their patterns during the session. This should be done only if a proper alliance already exists. If not, practitioners are wise to simply observe how the family deals with the problem.

IMPLEMENTING

Given that all interaction has influence then all treatment procedures have the potential to produce change. Procedures therefore are a part of each I-FAST stage, including joining and forming alliances. Procedures include empathizing, validating, aligning with parents, normalizing and acceptance, setting goals, asking questions, and offering tasks. Although we are presenting I-FAST as a set of procedures each intended to fit with a treatment that progresses in steps, the reality is there is no boundary between treatment steps and procedures aimed at specific ends. Steps can be blurred and unfold in unique ways in each case. For example, techniques designed to promote engagement can actually result in change. Each treatment procedure therefore can simultaneously serve multiple purposes. This applies to offering interventions as well. In addition to promoting deviations from patterns, interventions can end up intensifying engagement or deepening the practitioner's understanding of interactional processes and client frames. There is no boundary between processes.

Intervene in the Least Restrictive Way

I-FAST emphasizes intervening in the least restrictive and intrusive way. We therefore offer intervention strategies listed in order of least to most intrusive, starting with simply validating and ending with offering tasks that require change. Although we list these interventions in this way to illustrate our emphasis on intervening in the least intrusive way possible, the list is not meant to be a series of steps to be completed on each case in the order offered here. I-FAST practitioners must match interventions they offer to the circumstances and family receptiveness on each case. In cases in which the family is in crisis and presenting with serious safety issues, for example, the practitioner may have to begin treatment with offering tasks to promote safety and stabilize a crisis. In this instance, although beginning with offering tasks, keeping the family together and preventing a placement is least restrictive. In other cases, where there are not immediate safety concerns and the family is less receptive to intervention, validating or some other less intrusive intervention can be offered first.

Validation Revisited

Validation may be understood as a crossover intervention that lies at the intersection of relationship building and intervention. (It is a crossover because validation simultaneously builds the relationship and intervenes.) It is related to the concept of consensual validation and is one of the threads that connect the therapeutic relationship and interventions, making one common pathway.

In some cases validation is an intervention that produces second-order change by itself. It is not unusual for problems to develop in a manner that the client is not validated by people in his support system. Simply hearing the practitioner demonstrate how the clients' actions reflect inner wisdom can become an effective intervention in itself. Parents who have been blamed by family, friends, and helping professionals for the behavior problems of their child may make a significant shift in their parenting approach when validated by their I-FAST practitioner.

Some practitioners are troubled by the idea that the validation process involves justification of what they view as "incorrect premises." They claim that such justification is insincere or manipulative, if the practitioner truly believes that the client is operating from incorrect premises from the practitioner's view.

- We argue that validation of "incorrect" premises is genuine, by definition, when the practitioner is mindful of the context; that is, when the practitioner is aware that incorrect premises are an artifact of the client's world view.
- When understood this way it is clear that the client is literally doing as well as possible under the circumstances. There is no insincerity or manipulation here.

Validation is also relevant to the idea of offering a selected rationale for the problem. We argue that clients have a need not only to understand the nature of their problem but also to feel that they are justified for having the problem in the first place. Therefore, from the perspective of second-order change, effective rationales not only explain the client's dilemma but also *validate* the client for having the dilemma, by justifying it.

Finally, validation of all involved parties' assumptions and distress serves to establish the key elements of encouraging all involved to experience being listened to and understood. Such compassion sometimes facilitates desired change in itself, yet always at least sets the foundation for further facilitation of change through other treatment positions and interventions.

Empowering Parents

When a professional aligns with a parent, this alliance alone can empower the parent and result in a pattern shift within the family. For example, a parent who is habitually tentative and unassertive may become certain and assertive when validated and in alliance with a practitioner. The parent is able to intervene differently with his or her child when in league with a practitioner. Direct or indirect suggestions to change something need not be offered. By affiliating and aligning with a professional, the parent now has a "teammate," an ally. They are now two, not one. The rest of the family may then reorganize around this.

Normalizing and Acceptance

Normalizing is a way to place clients at ease by conceptualizing their difficulties as normal reactions, given the constraints of their situations. Normalizing is very closely related to validation. It is different in that the implication is that no special actions are needed to make a change. If the client lets go of a problem it will resolve itself.

- Normalizing is likely to be helpful when clients are unsure if they have a problem and are seeking reassurance. This is another variant of a position of *acceptance*.
- Normalizing can also be helpful when families or family members are experiencing stress or symptoms while the family is going through a major life transition such as divorce, remarriage, or the death of a loved one, or have just experienced serious traumatic events. In such instances, it may be premature to define symptoms as problems. As the family navigates the transition, the stress and symptoms may abate.
- The position that divorce is a transition, not pathology, illustrates this idea (Minuchin, 1984). Both adults and children can exhibit serious symptoms such as anxiety, depression, behavioral problems, and/or problems at school or work during and immediately after divorce. When this occurs any or all can be diagnosed or labeled. Minuchin is suggesting that normalizing is the proper response. Everyone, including professionals, must consider that the symptoms are a response to a large transition in life and not a fixed pathology.
- Allowing clients to relax their self-pressured efforts to solve a perceived difficulty, normalizing helps them depathologize themselves and whatever they are struggling with. They don't need to close a perpetual "generation gap" between themselves and their child, for example. Or, it may be a relief to learn that what parents were concerned about is a normal element of adolescent transitions in their culture.
- With normalization the practitioner does not deny that the client is feeling or acting badly. Instead the client is told that acting or feeling badly is expected under the circumstances.
- To emphasize this point the practitioner might indicate that it is surprising that the client isn't functioning even worse given the set of circumstances that she is facing.
- However, normalizing may be understood as disqualification if the client is *convinced* that he has a problem that must be addressed. Thus caution needs to be used in pushing a normalizing position that runs the risk of making

clients feel invalidated or seemingly trivializing the problem or making them feel blamed for their distress or their actions.
- Used well, normalizing validates clients and places their problem in a context that is normal given the constraints of their situation. It may also set the stage for an implied change in that parents may actually stop their attempts to initiate change in their child for behavior they now see as normal given their stage of development.

The Use of Questions as an Intervention Procedure

The next type of intervention on the least intrusive intervention continuum involves asking questions. Asking questions is not just for gathering information, as we might have traditionally viewed it. When we interact with people for the first time we tend to ask them questions to confirm our initial opinion (Nickerson, 1998). In addition, we tend to answer questions they ask in ways that conform to the expectations they have of us (Nickerson, 1998). However, asking questions is an intervention in itself, as it can introduce new perspectives, alternative possibilities, and new views and frames that facilitate the process of change in treatment (Goldberg, 1998; McGee, Del Vento, & Bavelas, 2005). Research in non–mental health settings has found that merely asking questions can lead to behavior change in those asked the questions; this is called the *mere measurement effect* (Godin, Sheeran, Conner, & Germain, 2008; Fitzsimmons & Williams, 2000; Levav & Fitzsimmons, 2006; McCambridge & Kypri, 2011). Asking questions has also been found to be an essential part of the change process in mental health treatment situations (Adams, 1997; De Jong & Berg, 2008; Feldman, 1994; Goldberg, 1998; McGee et al., 2005; Selvini-Palazzoli, Boscolo, & Cecchin, & Prata, 1980; Tomm, 1987). In this section we address the use of questions as an intervention procedure to change frames, to change interactions and behavior, and to initiate a process of self-evaluation.

The Power of Questions

Microanalysis is the close examination of moment-by-moment utterance-by-utterance communicative actions in conversations, with an emphasis on how these sequences function in the interaction (Bavelas, McGee, Phillips, & Routledge, 2000). Two fundamental assumptions around communication is that communication as constructive and communication as directive (Bavelas et al., 2000). From a constructivist perspective practitioners' presuppositions are embedded in the questions they ask clients. These presuppositions invite clients to co-construct a particular version of their experience. Consequently, asking questions is a procedure that allows the practitioner and the family to co-construct frames or reframes for beneficial change. When communication is viewed as a directive, asking question becomes an indirect procedure to suggest new behavior (Bavelas et al., 2000; Eiser, 2000).

Just the act of asking question also changes the frame regarding who is the expert in the change process. Asking questions operates from the stance of curiosity and conveys the message that we believe that the client has the answers and we do not. It initiates a self-evaluative process in which clients are facilitated in carefully evaluating and thinking about their situation and come up with ideas and perceptions of their own. People are more likely to take ownership of their perceptions because these are not externally imposed and these perceptions are more likely to be viable and appropriate in their own context (Lee, Uken, & Sebold, 2003, 2007). In other words, *constructing useful questions is an important skill set. Asking questions allows clients to develop new frames and possibilities, engage in new behaviors, and take ownership of their change process.*

THE USE OF QUESTIONS TO CHANGE FRAMES

Clients may isolate themselves in their homes and avoid close relationships because they frame the world and relationships as unsafe. This belief influences their choice to withdraw. Perhaps they wish to go to the library but cannot because they fear it is unsafe. As discussed, questions embed a practitioner's presupposition of reality and change. Research has shown that a practitioner's expectancy that the client can positively change can affect treatment outcome (Coppock, Owen, Zagarskas, & Schmidt, 2010; Kirsch, 1990; Weinberger & Eig, 1999). In addition, the presuppositions embedded in questions can set up a self-fulfilling prophecy whereby the client's beliefs and behaviors actually change to conform to the expectations of the practitioner (Eiser, 2000; Semin & De Poot, 1997; Snyder, 1984; Snyder & Thomsen, 1988).

- For instance, *cognitive behavioral* approaches emphasize cognitive primacy and that people can make a rational decision about their experience. A cognitive-behavioral practitioner might ask:

    "What evidence do you have that the public library is unsafe?"

    The question presupposes that evidence is important to evaluate a situation, that is, evaluation of experience should be based on rationality. This question is an intervention attempting to help the client reframe the library as safe. The purpose of the question is not only to obtain information but also to encourage the client to begin to think differently, to reframe her view of public places.

- A Mental Research Institute (*MRI*) *strategic* practitioner might ask a client who is depressed and speaking very negatively about himself and his life:

    "Your situation is terrible; how come you are not doing worse than you are?"

    While validating the client's view, this type of question presupposes that the client could do worse and that the client is doing something positive to keep the situation from getting worse. Asking this question will direct the client in exploring and explaining some positive quality of themselves or his life to explain how it is he is not doing worse. The question shifts him into a more positive frame. Again the question is not simply an attempt to gain information but also to promote a shift in frames.

- A mother who describes the problem as her son's poor self-esteem can be asked:

    "What does your son do that is a sign of poor self-esteem?"

    This question presupposes that there should be observable behavioral indicators of poor self-esteem and is an attempt to shift the definition of the problem from something vague and global to something specific and behavioral. Again, a shift in frames is sought by the question.

- A *solution-focused* practitioner might ask a mother whose son does not go to school:

    "What is an example of your son getting to school?" This question presupposes that there are times that the son was able to go to school. Such a question is an attempt to shift the client's frame from focusing on the problems to begin noticing exceptions.

- A *narrative* practitioner might ask a client:

    "How have you fought off anxiety in the past?"

    This question presupposes that anxiety is something external to the client and that the client has done something positive to address the problem of anxiety. This is an example to shift the frame of anxiety from being internal to anxiety being external. In addition, the question also directs the client's focus from problems to solutions.

To note, the use of questions as an intervention procedure is a skill emphasized by numerous approaches such as *cognitive-behavior therapy* with the use of *Socratic questioning; solution-focused therapy* with the use of *exception-finding questions*; or *narrative therapies* with the use of *questions in externalizing the and mapping the effects of the problem, identifying unique outcomes*, and so on. In the preceding examples, representing numerous approaches, questions are offered not simply to obtain information but also to shift the frame. These questions embed different presuppositions that influence clients to revisit their experiences from a different frame. The skillful use of questions to shift frames can be utilized within I-FAST as long as the target of the intervention is a problem or goal the client has identified as something she wants to address in treatment.

THE USE OF QUESTIONS TO REINFORCE OR CHANGE BEHAVIOR AND INTERACTION

Questions can also be offered as an indirect way to reinforce or change interaction and behavior. Again, numerous approaches utilize questions for this purpose.

- When a client offers an example of successfully obtaining a goal, a practitioner might ask in an enthusiastic and approving tone: "How did you do that?" "How did you decide to do that?" Here, questions are being offered as an attempt to reinforce behavior.
- A client who has identified three specific methods he has used in the past to resist the influence of anxiety can be asked at the end of a session: "What type of week would you prefer, a week of anxiety or a week fighting off anxiety?"

    When this type of question is asked in the context described, it is clearly an indirect suggestion for the client to actively resist anxiety using the methods he identified earlier in the session. This is a question that indirectly promotes behavior change.
- In solution-focused therapy, scaling questions can be asked to identify small steps toward achieving a goal and indirectly to suggest taking those steps.

    "How will you know when you have moved up 1 point on the 0 to 10 scale from where you are now?"

    "When has there been a time when you were higher on the scale than you are now?"

    "What can you do to move up 1 point on the scale?"

In these examples, the client is not being directed to do anything. However, the identification of the next step is clearly an indirect method of suggesting she go ahead and take that next step. Again, in I-FAST, questions can be offered as an indirect method of suggesting new behavior or as a method of reinforcing successful behavior. This skill can be utilized in I-FAST as long as it is aimed at problems and goals the client and practitioner have agreed to focus on.

THE USE OF QUESTIONS TO INITIATE A SELF-EVALUATIVE PROCESS

People need feedback in the change process, as feedback provides indicators for progress and motivates change efforts. The act of asking questions assumes that the client and not the practitioner has the answer. Instead of the practitioner providing feedback or evaluation, asking questions serves to initiate a self-feedback process within the client. Questions allow clients to self-evaluate their situations in terms of their doing, thinking, and feeling. The practitioner abstains from making any interpretation of clients' situations or suggesting any ideas; he or she just asks good questions that help clients self-evaluate different aspects of their unique life situation (Greene & Lee, 2011; Lee et al., 2003). Asking self-evaluative questions sends a clear message that clients are the center of the change process. The list of self-evaluative questions is endless but the following are some useful examples (Lee et al., 2003):

- **Choice questions** "Are you going to continue doing the same thing next week, continue to say hi to people, or are you going to extend it to something else?"
- **Comparison questions** "So, how did you figure out when it's time for you to stand up for yourself and when it's time for you to walk away?"
- **Connection questions** "So, how did you do that, stay out of the fight instead of getting in the middle of it like you used to?"
- **Difference questions** "So what would you do differently to try to get along better with your dad?"
- **Effect questions** "What are you hoping will happen when you are friendlier to people?" "What thoughts do you have about what you're hoping will happen when you do this?"
- **Exception questions** "When was the last time you and your wife felt things were going well?"
- **Exploring questions** "What are you thinking about those possibilities?" "Would your mom have any ideas for you?"
- **Feasibility questions** "Where is it easy and where maybe is it not so easy?" "Are you feeling it's reasonable to do it?" "Have you ever done that in the past?" "How likely are you to be able to do that between now and the next session?"
- **Helpfulness questions** "Was it helpful that you were aware that you were angry?" "Do you think it would be helpful if other people knew that you are such a caring person?" "How do you think it would be helpful?"
- **Indicator questions** "How would you know that you have accomplished your goal (or work through the problem)?"
- **Meaning questions** "What does this crying mean about you as a person?"
- **Ownership questions** "When did you decide to do that?" "Where do you think it comes from for you, the commitment?"
- **Planning questions** "Is there something you'll need to do to make sure that you stay focused on your goal?" "So how are you going to do this (goal behavior)?"

- **Relationship questions** "Who will be the first person to notice the change if you were going to respect yourself more?"
- **Scaling questions** "On a scale of 0 to 10, 0 being that it doesn't matter that you get a job and 10 being it is the most important thing for you to accomplish, where are you at on that scale?"

THE PRACTITIONER'S RESPONSES TO CLIENTS' ANSWERS

A final note on the discussion on asking questions is around how we respond to what clients have said. Microanalysis uses the term "formulation" to denote the process in which the practitioner responds to what clients say (Bavelas et al., 2000; Garfinkel & Sacks, 1970). Microanalysis suggests that formulations serve three functions: They can (1) preserve, (2) delete, or (3) transform what the client has said (Heritage & Watson, 1979).

- In other words, we can *preserve* what the client said and by doing so we reinforce and expand the discussion. For example:

Client: School is very important to me.
Practitioner: In what ways is school very important to you?

- We can also respond to client's original statement by *deleting*, which represents our effort to block that line of discussion. For example,

Client: It really bothers me when my brother hassles me.
Practitioner: So, you don't wish to be bothered. Do you know at what point you need to walk away?

For a practitioner who does not see blaming talk as helpful, he or she can *delete* the focus on blaming and shift the conversation to what the client can do to avoid being bothered by his brother.

- Often, we **transform** clients' original statements to a different frame and level of understanding. For example,

Mother: My son is so rebellious.
Practitioner: What happens in your relationship with your son that allows him to be so rebellious?

In this example, the practitioner preserves the client's statement regarding "son is so rebellious," but *transforms* the focus from an individual focus on her son to an interactional focus between mother and son. How a practitioner preserves, deletes, or transforms clients' original statements has a clear influence on the direction and flow of the treatment dialogues that should be consistent with I-FAST's view of change.

PARAMETERS AND PRESUPPOSITION OF I-FAST

I-FAST, as a meta-model, has its presuppositions regarding the change process, which guide our way of asking questions or responding. The following are our parameters in constructing helpful questions that may bring beneficial changes in the family:

- Problems and solutions are viewed as interactional/relational as opposed to individual-focused.

- Strengths-based: Clients have the ability and resources to change and do something different as opposed to a deficits-based approach that may imply that clients do not have the ability to change.
- Problems are viewed as transient as opposed to being permanent, stable, and global.
- Clients take ownership of the change process as opposed to the change process being involuntary or external.
- Questions tend to be more open as opposed to closed.

Questions as an intervention procedure serve multiple purposes in the treatment process. In addition to the traditional use pertaining to seeking understanding, collecting information, and tracking interactions, I-FAST uses questions to change frames by expanding understanding or challenging existing understanding, indirectly suggesting new behaviors, and/or introducing a self-evaluative feedback process. I-FAST practitioners are welcome to embrace questioning techniques from different therapeutic traditions as long as these questions are consistent with the described parameters, which represent how I-FAST views the change process.

The Use of Tasks for Changing Interactional Patterns and Identifying Exceptions

Offering tasks is a common treatment tool utilized by a variety of family treatment approaches. The use of tasks has been generally utilized by approaches that focus on helping families directly change their habitual interactional patterns. Using tasks in family treatment involves requesting the family to attend to and notice something new, or to do something different than they have done prior to treatment. Tasks are used in family treatment as catalysts for the family to change habitual interactional patterns and/or increase interactional exceptions. Terms that appear in the literature that refer to what we are labeling "tasks" include directives, prescriptions, and homework.

Skills for Offering Tasks
THE PROPER ATTITUDE TOWARD TASKS

As noted earlier, it is not the task itself that has therapeutic value. It is how the family responds to the task or any other type of intervention that has value. When families improve it is because of their response, not the task itself. Practitioners therefore should not be married to their tasks. The most brilliant and creative task is meaningless unless the family does something with it. When a practitioner understands this, he can maintain a respectful and humble position toward the family. The practitioner understands that he does not know any better than anyone else how to live his life and tasks are not meant to suggest how to do so. Instead, they are offered in the spirit of experimentation. A task is offered and the practitioner then observes what the family does with it. This leads to either progress toward solving the problem or a deeper understanding of the family. A practitioner maintaining this stance is less likely to antagonize, insult, or pass judgment on a family.

Tasks, therefore, should never be offered unless the practitioner has an empathic and respected connection to the family. When a practitioner is frustrated with a family, tasks should never be offered. When the practitioner is frustrated, they have lost their alliance and the proper response to this is to regain that alliance, not offer interventions.

DEVISING TASKS

Beginning practitioners are often most concerned about devising tasks. Of all the skills involved in offering tasks, devising them may be the easiest. The main skill required for devising tasks is the skill of tracking interactional patterns and interactional exceptions. Understanding these interactions in detail and understanding what the contribution of all the participants is leads directly to the creation of tasks. To know what is "out of the box" for a particular family first requires a detailed understanding of what is "in the box." If a practitioner obtains a detailed understanding of what each pattern participant habitually does, he or she can then practice thinking of what would be "out of the box" for each individual participant. This is often a good exercise for beginning I-FAST practitioners. Each pattern participant's habitual response is described. Then a range of ideas for how each participant in the pattern could react differently is identified.

For example, a mother and son escalate, exchanging hostile verbal jabs. The father ignores the two. After the fight, the mother goes to complain about the son to the father. The father dismisses the mother's complaints. The pattern then repeats itself. Understanding this pattern can facilitate the design of interventions for each participant. When the son becomes disrespectful, the mother could become loving. When the father ignores the fight, the mother could request he deal with the son. When the mother complains to the father, he could be supportive. Each individual could produce a range of different responses. Practitioners who pay attention to the details of these patterns will have no difficulty devising tasks that deviate from them.

FRAMING TASKS SO THEY WILL BE ACCEPTED

Much attention has already been paid to this skill set in Chapter 6. How to frame tasks so they will be accepted is perhaps the most difficult skill to learn, yet it is one of the most important ones associated with offering tasks in treatment. *No task should ever be offered without a frame, or rationale offered first.* The rationale for assigning the task must make sense to the family and client. As has been noted, this requires detailed knowledge of how the family frames the problem, how they frame the solution, the language they use to describe the problem, and a clear agreement on what the goal of the task should be. Selecting frames that families will respond to requires an intimate understanding of that family, their values, their motives, and their beliefs about the problem and its solution. The more practitioners can immerse themselves in clients' thinking, the more they will be able to construct a frame that is accepted by the clients.

TRACKING RESPONSES TO TASKS

Tasks given to families are only as good as they are understood, accepted and acted upon by all parties involved. It is important, therefore, to observe or track how the family or individuals in systems respond to the tasks given and adjust appropriately to their response.

- **In-session responses to tasks.** When a task is offered during a session, parents can respond in a number of ways. They could agree and be pleased they have something to try. When they express reluctance or reject the task, the practitioner should use this as an opportunity to learn more about the client. What are they concerned about? What do they think the roadblocks might be? When clients express reluctance about a task offered, this should produce a discussion between practitioner and client that deepens the practitioner's understanding of the situation, not resistance and tension between practitioner and client. Once a more detailed understanding is obtained, the practitioner will understand better either how to frame the task so it is accepted, or if a new task is required.

- **Out-of-session responses to tasks.** Once a task is offered and accepted it must be followed up on. Often beginning practitioners offer task after task, session after session, without ever following up. When viewing tasks as experiments and avenues to understanding the family more deeply, the follow-up discussion is more important than the task itself. Following up on tasks, therefore, is a key part of the skill set surrounding the use of tasks. When following up, practitioners should be curious about a wide range of issues. What did they end up trying? What did each person actually do differently? How did they do that? Why that particular response? What happened when they tried whatever they ended up trying? Did anything improve? How did everyone else respond? If they did not do the task, what did they do instead? How did they decide to that? Note that following up on tasks is essentially interviewing for *exceptions*. The line of questions is basically the same. The skill at interviewing for exceptions can enhance following up on tasks.

At the very least, a proper follow-up discussion should deepen the practitioner's understanding of the family, their beliefs about the problem, and the patterns that support them. The best case scenario is that, however the family responded, their response set a change process in motion. Changes can be either incremental or discontinuous. In either case, the practitioner must then shift to a mode that reinforces and supports any changes that may have occurred.

STRENGTHS AND THE USE OF TASKS

Making Use of Whatever Response the Client Gives to a Task

There is no failure, just data. When this attitude is adopted, tasks become experiments, not assignments. I-FAST practitioners then become more interested in how clients respond than in the task itself. When this view is adopted, the client's response, not the task, is what is useful. The client's response to the task is in essence their expression of their strengths. The point of the task is not the task. It is what the family decides to do with the task that counts. The task can become a tool to elicit strengths.

Making the Task the Client's, not the Practitioner's

When a task is received and either modified or inspires a novel response by the family, the task becomes the family's. The task allows the family to utilize their strengths in the unique ways they adopt the task. The family strengths are in fact their responses to being given a task.

TYPES OF TASKS

What follows is a list of types of tasks that represent the range of ways to offer tasks in treatment available within I-FAST. I-FAST practitioners are free to choose any or all types on a given case. The type of task chosen should match the client's readiness for change. How clients respond to whatever type of task offered should be tracked and modified with the eventual goal of finding an approach that facilitates both a resolution of the identified complaints and a shift in the interactions that support those complaints.

- **In-session tasks**
  - Offering tasks to families in session that request deviations from their interactional patterns is permissible within I-FAST as long as the request also focuses on resolving the presenting problem. The in-session task is a request for families to change how they interact in the session. This tradition is best illustrated with the structural family therapy approach (Minuchin, 1974; Minuchin & Fishman, 1981). The in-home practitioner has both an opportunity to observe the family's interactional response to the problem, and if properly aligned, request deviations from that pattern. When families successfully respond to the problem differently while in conjunction with the direct participation of a practitioner they are much more likely to continue that change between sessions. A successful in-session task can then be followed up with requesting that the family repeat the task between sessions.
  - The changes in interactions requested during in-sessions should have an obvious connection to the problem the family is requesting help with. For example, in the case of a youth with conduct disorder, parents who are in conflict over how to respond to the youth's behavior can be asked to talk to each other in the session and try to reach a compromise on how to deal with the youth's most recent or most frequent infraction. The practitioner may then observe that the father dominates the discussion and the mother acquiesces to his demands. Their interaction pattern is being directly

---

A CASE EXAMPLE

Who habitually deals with a problem youth can also be changed within a session. A single mother and her six-year-old daughter moved in with the mother's mother shortly after the girl's parents divorced. The girl was very hyperactive and impossible in school. The mother, the grandmother, and the girl attended a session together and during the session the girl was very hyperactive. She climbed on the furniture, crawled under the furniture, and opened every drawer of the practitioner's desk. While this was occurring, the mother participated in the discussion as if nothing was happening.

The grandmother, however, was all over the girl, constantly correcting her. When asked how the two women dealt with the girl at home, the grandmother insisted she did not want to interfere. She then reported that when her grandchild was being a problem, she often intervened because she feared her daughter would lose her temper and hit the girl. There was obvious tension between the grandmother and the mother regarding how to respond to the girl.

This tension and the interaction pattern of grandmother just taking over for mother were thought to be contributing to maintaining the girl's difficulties. This pattern prevented both the tension between the two women from being

(continued)

> resolved and relegated the mother to the sidelines with the girl. It left mother and six-year-old daughter disengaged from each other.
>
> An in-session task was offered. While the girl was busy crawling under furniture, the grandmother was asked to advise her daughter right then on what she should do with the girl. This was a deviation from their pattern. The grandmother's first response was to instruct the little girl herself, not to advise the mother. The practitioner interrupted the grandmother and repeated the request that she advise her daughter what to do. The grandmother then suggested that her daughter get up, gather up the girl, sit next to her, and hold her. The mother followed the advice and the girl settled down.

observed. The practitioner can then ask the father to give the mother a turn and the mother's thoughts can be drawn out. Once both parents have stated their ideas, something that their typical interactions do not allow for, the practitioner can encourage them to meet each other half way.

This example follows the typical pattern of how families often respond to in-session tasks. When asked to deviate from their pattern, their first response is to follow it, not deviate from it. The grandmother initially wanted to deal with the girl herself. This illustrates the power of these patterns. Even when asked to change them, the first response is to stick to them. The practitioner then must push for the initial request of deviating from the pattern to be followed. With this family, after successfully dealing with the girl in the session, the grandmother agreed for her daughter to take more charge of the girl during the week. The daughter agreed to follow her mother's advice if difficulties with the girl arose. The mother was moved to a central role with the girl, and the grandmother was made an advisor. The girl completely settled down both at home and at school.

- **Between-session tasks: New action or attention**
    - In using between-session tasks the practitioner asks the family to do new things or direct their attention in new ways.
    - The first and most obvious task is when the practitioner asks clients to do new things or direct their attention in new ways.
    - These tasks might include reading something, or going to some new place, or talking with someone who might share their plight, or directing their attention to when things are happening, or even directing their attention to the times when they resist the temptation to fall into the same old habits, and so on. With at-risk youth new parenting behavior may include offering clear expectations for behavior and following through on consequences.
    - Such tasks require that the clients are in clear agreement with the intervener on frames, rationales, goals, and related tasks. These tasks assume the clients will agree to the new action and try it out; thus it must both make sense to them and fit with their motivation and values.
    - Between-session tasks should have an obvious connection to resolving the problems the parent(s) is (are) identifying and require deviations from the interactional patterns that support those problems.

- Parents can be asked to change how they are interacting with the identified client or they can be asked to change how they are interacting with each other about the identified client.
- Who is habitually involved and who is habitually not involved can be switched.
- Extended family members who are not involved can be recruited.
- Extended family members who are overly and directly involved can be asked to become advisors.

Examples include:

- The practitioner can ask parents to discuss privately for ten minutes each day how the identified client did that day and what to do about it.
- The practitioner can offer ideas for how a parent can respond to provocative statements by the identified client without becoming hostile or defensive in return.
- The practitioner can ask parents to switch who is directly dealing with the identified client.
- The practitioner can ask parents to negotiate and compromise with each other on how to respond to the identified client.
- When relatives are chronically involved and phone calls between relatives and either a parent or the identified client are part of the pattern, who calls whom and who talks to whom about what on the calls can be changed.

A CASE EXAMPLE

An 11-year-old boy was brought to treatment by his mother. He lived with his father, mother, and 14-year-old sister. The mother defined the problem as the boy being defiant. He and the mother engaged in terrible arguments every evening. The arguments occurred if the boy did not get his way or if he was asked to do a chore or his homework. The arguments were dominating the household. The father and daughter withdrew when they occurred. The mother felt unsupported. The mother was offered the frame that the boy was in charge of the mood of the house. His fits dominated the house. They also controlled the mother's mood. When he became hostile, she followed his lead. This all made sense to the mother. She agreed to the goal of taking back control of the mood of the house. This would require her to not respond with anger to her son's provocations and fits. The goal was for her to remain calm during the heat of battle. She was given two tasks: (1) Enlist the father's help for her to stay calm when the son becomes provocative. She was coached on how to approach him on this. The father was to rescue the mother if she became angry. He was to take her for a walk or to the bedroom to help her regain her composure. (2) Practice "brain dead" responses when the boy becomes provocative. For example, when the boy complains about a task, the mother can respond with, "Life is not always fair."

- **Tasks for amplifying interactional exceptions.** Tasks for amplifying interactional exceptions fall into two main categories: observation tasks and behavioral tasks. In an observation task, the practitioner suggests—on the basis of information gathered in the interview—that the client pay attention to a particular aspect of his or her life that is likely to prove useful in solution building. Behavioral tasks require the client to actually do something—to take certain actions that the practitioner believes will be useful to the client in constructing a solution. As with observation tasks, behavioral tasks are based on information gathered during the interview and should therefore make sense to the client within his or her frame of reference.
- **Formula first session task.** Often families have the feeling that nothing is going right for them and they are losing control of their lives. This task helps refocus the family's attention to something they are doing *well* rather than problems or failures. By asking families to notice what goes well in their lives, they are encouraged to "discover" things that are going well for them. This change of focus can lead to the family having a feeling that there still is something working in their lives (Berg, 1994). For example, a practitioner might say:
    - "Between now and next the time we meet, we[I] would like you to observe, so that you can describe to us[me] next time, what happens in your [*pick one*: family, life, marriage, relationship] that you want to continue to have happen" (de Shazer, 1985, p. 137).

    The name of this task comes from its successful use at the end of the first session with a wide variety of clients regardless of the presenting problem (de Shazer et al., 1986). The formula first session task is especially useful with clients who present vaguely defined problems and are not responsive to attempts to get them to define it more concretely and specifically.
- **Keep track of current successes.** The purpose of this task is to help families focus on identifying the skills and abilities they have and how they use them to make their situation better. The more specific and detailed the family is in providing these descriptions the more likely they are in anchoring such behaviors into their frames.

    "Identify the ways you are able to keep doing_____"
    (behaviors that are exceptions to the problem behavior) (Molnar & de Shazer, 1987, p. 356).

    Or

    "Pay attention to and keep track of what you do to overcome the temptation or urge to. . .." (perform the symptom or some behavior associated with the problem) (Berg & Gallagher, 1991, p. 101; Molnar & de Shazer, 1987, p. 356).

    Or

    "Pay attention and notice when you have moved up 1 point on the 0 to 10 scale and notice what you did to get that to happen."
- **Prediction task.** Often the client is able to identify exceptions but reports that they just seem to happen randomly. In the prediction task the client is asked to predict the likelihood of the exception occurring, "First thing each morning rate, the possibility of _____ (an exception behavior) happening before noon" (Molnar & de Shazer, 1987, p. 356). The

purpose of the prediction task is to help families discover that the exception behaviors may be much more within their control than they think. By asking the family to keep a careful record of what they predicted and how the day actually turned out can produce important insights into the client's ability to make what appears to be a random or spontaneous exception into a deliberate one (Berg, 1994).

- **Paradoxical tasks.** Paradoxical tasks, or prescribing the symptom, is defined as asking a youth or parent to engage in or direct another to engage in the problematic behavior he or she is requesting help to change.
    - A common rationale for such tasks is to gain further knowledge or understanding of the problem or sequence of things involved in the escalating problem.
    - The other prominent goal of such tasks is to help clients take control of interactions they formerly felt were out of control; or alternatively to change the nature of the interaction around the typically escalating battles.
    - When a parent in effect asks her child to have a tantrum, or notes the start of a meltdown and calmly guides the child to his "meltdown" place so he can have his tantrum, the dynamics of such escalating battles are altered and tantrums often dissipate or are altered.
    - Paradoxical tasks are often helpful when the problem brought to treatment is defined as involuntary behavior. Examples include specific or generalized anxiety; depression; obsessive or ritualistic behavior; or trauma symptoms such as nightmares, flashbacks, intrusive thoughts, or avoidant behavior.
    - Asking clients who are experiencing such symptoms as involuntary to produce the symptoms on purpose often helps them regain voluntary control of that symptom. When a child is the client exhibiting such a symptom, the *parent* is coached to deliver the paradoxical task. The parent, not the practitioner, delivers the task to the child. As with all I-FAST interventions, one goal is most often for the parent to be the change agent with the child. This is so with all types of tasks given, including paradox.
    - Offering paradoxical tasks require skill and should be avoided by inexperienced practitioners unless under the direct supervision of a skilled supervisor. The procedure follows clear steps.
- **Think in opposites.** A useful concept that can help in the devising of tasks comes from the MRI tradition (Weakland Fisch, Watzlawick, & Bodin., 1974). Problems can be formed when clients take a path that is opposite from the path that is needed to solve the problem. It is like a football player who on receiving the ball is hit and turns in the direction of the opponent's goal. Because problems can form in opposites, solutions can involve opposites as well. In effect, the practitioner must help the problem solvers to move in the opposite direction of the direction that they are pursuing. More simply, the problem solvers must stop their advance or retreat and go the other way. When thinking of tasks, think what would be the opposite of what is already being attempted.

Positioning in relation to the positions of others. One way to implement the use of opposites is for the practitioner to take a position with involved parties that *differs from others and often is the opposite of what others might be stating or pushing for.* This is most often done to keep the practitioner from falling into the same problem-escalating stances of the rest of the systems involved. In other words, if everyone is pressing for change and the clients are reluctant or pushing back, then the practitioner will do best to agree with the clients that things may need to slow down or even be redirected. Two variations of this are "soft" and "hard" restraints.

- **Soft restraints from change**
    - Soft restraints are defined as cautions offered from the practitioner about the dangers of moving too quickly on change, bringing up real or perceived potential hurdles for change or potential dangers or reactions of an all-out press of action.
    - Soft restraints are a second-order shift for practitioners when involved parties expect them to push for change. The practitioner is taking the opposite position of what involved parties are expecting from him.
    - Soft restraints are often either met with relief by parties worried about their abilities to take the actions needed or concern about the potential consequences of creating more strife or other problems.
    - Soft restraints are also often received as respectful concern for the clients and their ambivalence, frustration, and uncertainty about how to resolve the problem at hand.
    - Soft restraints may also serve to engage clients in the enviable position of arguing for a greater press for change, in which they are more clearly committing to an action stage. With this, the practitioner can agree to collaborate while still bring up potential obstacles and pitfalls that they can all anticipate, rehearse, and be ready for.
- **Hard restraints from change**
    - Hard restraints from change are defined more as challenges to clients or other parties regarding change. They are often attributed to the perceived opinion of a third party such as an external authority, an agency, or even an alternate theory or rationale.
    - Hard restraints usually are designed to enlist the motivation or reactance of specific involved parties, often the youth, in the service of defying or proving the third party's skepticism wrong!
    - Though high reactivity of youth, parents, or others involved is most often seen as an obstacle, the skillful positioning of the practitioner in putting forward hard restraints to change can turn such client reactivity to their credit and in service of achieving their goals.
    - It is most often important for the practitioner to remain neutral and aligned with the client when delivering these hard restraint messages. This allows for the practitioner to remain supportive and aligned with clients' strengths and resilience while still acknowledging the strong skepticism of others. Clients need to react to the message and not to the messenger, or in this case their practitioner!

It must be noted here that this list of tasks and their targets is certainly not complete. These, in fact, represent a sampling of those tasks most often used by the current authors according to their own individual strengths and perspectives. There are a wide range of tasks available to I-FAST practitioners. The only qualification for a task to fit into the I-FAST approach is that it fit the general meta-model premises and strategies of the overall I-FAST approach. It needs to interrupt or redirect the identified vicious cycle pattern of the problem and create or note a significant difference from that pattern. Once the difference is created or identified, then the task of all involved is to amplify and build upon it to create positive ripples in the involved systems. Using tasks that both fit a chosen treatment rationale and are those that fit the practitioner's expertise are well within the I-FAST model of work. In fact, they reflect the flexible core of the model itself.

THE ESSENTIAL ELEMENTS OF INITIATING CHANGE

- The practitioner articulates strategies that block or reverse patterns of interaction that maintains problems.
- There are tasks other than those discussed here that directly follow from several family treatment rationales. These tasks may certainly be used as long as they conform to the general meta-goals of the I-FAST approach and fit well into the treatment rationale agreed on between the practitioner and the clients and involved systems.
- The practitioner articulates strategies that amplify exceptions, for example:
  - Doing more of what works
  - Observation tasks
  - Pretending tasks
  - Prediction tasks
- The practitioner and the family/child mutually agree on tasks to be accomplished.
- The practitioner demonstrates competence in delivering, pacing, and timing of the task assignment.
- The practitioner is attuned to and respectful of the family's/child's stage of change (e.g., customer, complainant, or visitor).

8 BUILDING RESILIENCE AND TERMINATING/STEPPING DOWN

CONCEPTUALIZING

The process of treatment is essentially experimental. The practitioner's role is to trigger change processes either by directly helping families deviate from their interactional patterns or by amplifying exceptions that are already occurring. When changes occur, they can unfold in a multitude of ways. I-FAST practitioners must be prepared for many possibilities and have the skills to track and solidify all types of change. This means that the practitioner must continuously observe his or her impact on the family and the family's responses to his or her input. All responses provide information. It is the practitioner's job to use this information to alter his or her approach to the family. When assessing responsiveness to therapeutic procedures the practitioner has the following tasks:

- The practitioner carefully assesses the family's responses to procedures.
- If the family did not do the assignment or partially did the assignment and reports change, the practitioner will support the change.
- If the family did the assignment and reports that it didn't work the practitioner will take responsibility for the failure of the assignment.
- If the family did the assignment and it worked the practitioner will credit the success to the family.

When desired changes occur the practitioner will assist the family in processing their specific contributions. The practitioner will then negotiate with the family any needs for more changes. If desired results are not achieved the practitioner will conduct an assessment to determine what happened. The practitioner will operate from the premise that there must be a legitimate reason for the failure that needs to be understood. This is done without blaming the family.

STRATEGIZING

Types of Responses to Change
When change begins to occur we assume there are a multitude of possible responses by family members and or key professionals. Practitioners must be observant and inquisitive regarding how key participants are reacting to change and be prepared for a multitude of possibilities. I-FAST practitioners must be skilled in a range of strategies that are appropriate for the various ways family members and professionals can react to positive change. What strategy to employ will depend largely on the type of response the family makes when change occurs. There are a number of possible options.

THE CLIENT IMPROVES AND EVERYONE IS PLEASED

One possibility is that the client changes and everyone is pleased. The client improves, the changes are noticed and acknowledged as meaningful, everyone is happy, and the case can be closed. This reaction to change occurs in numerous cases. It should not be assumed that positive change will always be met with anxiety or not be noticed or anything else that could be negative. But there are other possibilities.

CHANGE IS NOT NOTICED

Change can occur and it is either not noticed or not responded to as if it has actually occurred. This can occur when change is incremental. Small changes may not actually be noticed, or they may be noticed but not considered meaningful, or they may be dismissed because they do not represent the ultimate desired outcome. First and foremost, the practitioner must notice. To do so, careful tracking must be done to how families are responding to interventions. When the change is dismissed as not coming up to expectations, an affirmation can be sought to weather the small change that is acknowledged is a step in the right direction. If so, an inquiry can be made as to what the next step would be and what everyone should do to achieve it.

THE CLIENT IMPROVES BUT IS NOT TREATED AS SUCH

One possible response to improvement is that although positive change is noticed and acknowledged, the client is not treated as if he or she has made a change. Either family members or professionals can respond to improvement this way. A child can improve significantly in school, for example, but not be removed from the special class for behavior problem children. Or, a child can improve at home but not receive privileges back. In all of these cases, important participants may be acknowledging change, but there is not a corresponding response appropriate for improvement. If responses that logically go with improvement are not obtained, a relapse is very likely. In this situation, the practitioner must support the individual who has changed and hold him or her to that change while encouraging the rest of the system to come around and respond appropriately.

ANXIETY IS A RESPONSE TO CHANGE

One common reaction to change is anxiety. The client can improve but the client, family members, or powerful professionals can become anxious that the problem will return. This is a human response to positive change, especially if the problems involved serious and unsafe behaviors. If a teen has been using drugs, or becoming violent, or sneaking out of the house and being gone for days, it is a human response to be anxious that these types of behaviors will occur again even if there are clear signs that the client has changed. Who has the anxiety when change occurs can vary from case to case. It could be one of the parents, or it could be a professional. The parents may be pleased if their child has improved and confident in the changes, but the probation officer (PO) is worried. When change does occur, the practitioner must track the responses of everyone involved. The anxiety if unchecked can then bring about a relapse. One common method for dealing with this reaction is to *predict a relapse* and define it as a desired part of the change process (Fisch, Weakland, & Segal, 1982). In this way, anxiety or other unfortunate responses can be bypassed and changes can be amplified.

A CHILD IMPROVES BUT INTERACTION BETWEEN PARENTS DOES NOT CHANGE

Parents can be coached to change how they habitually respond to their child's problem and the child then may improve. Both the practitioner and the parents may acknowledge the parents have changed how they are dealing with their child and the child has improved. The practitioner can then give the parents credit. All this can occur but the parents may continue to minimize the child's improvement and/or their own contribution to that improvement. Sometimes when this scenario is present, the problem is that although the parents and child are interacting differently, *the two parents* have not changed how they are interacting *with each other about the child's problem.*

A common example can involve a biological parent and a stepparent. A typical interactional pattern can be: one parent is critical of the child and interacts negatively about the child with the other parent. Only one parent interacts with the child about the problems. The other parent complains only to the parent who is dealing directly with the child, not the child herself. When the uninvolved parent complains to the involved parent about the child, that parent then deals with the child's problem that is upsetting the other parent. In this scenario, even if the child improves, the uninvolved parent may not cease complaining about the child to the involved parent. The involved parent then may continue to describe the child with the practitioner as unimproved, minimizing, or not acknowledging the child's improvement. How the two adults habitually interact and the fact that it has not changed must be on the practitioner's radar screen. If not, the involved parent's continued complaints to the practitioner about the child, despite the child's improvement, will not make sense to the practitioner. Once it is realized that the problem is no longer the child, *but how the parents interact about the child,* interventions can then be designed to deal directly with these interactions.

CHANGE OCCURS AND FAMILY MEMBERS BRING UP WORSE PROBLEMS

One classic response reported by several authors when a client improves is that someone else in the family becomes worse, or a worse problem emerges (Jackson, 1957; Haffner, 1983; Haffner & Ross, 1983; Haley, 1997; Stanton & Todd, 1982). In I-FAST we do not have a theory that when a client improves the underlying family problems emerge. It is simply an observation that occasionally when a client with serious problems improves dramatically, the adults can become unstable. For example, when the client improves, one of the parents may threaten divorce. If this happens, the divorce threat is not viewed as the underlying cause of the presenting problem, but as adjustment and reaction to change. Another possibility is that a change can occur and the functioning of one of the adults can dramatically deteriorate. When this type of reaction occurs, the client must be persuaded to continue to improve despite the adults' difficulties. Practitioners will be tempted to be drawn in to successive problems and begin what may seem to be interminable treatment. I-FAST operates on an episode of care model. If a new treatment contract is to be made, the true gains of the current treatment need to be acknowledged and solidified. Then all may consider addressing another problem or not.

IMPLEMENTING

Skills for Building Resilience

TRACKING CHANGE

The main skill for tracking change is tracking responses to treatment procedures. Who did what in response to interventions? How did the client respond? How did each individual involved in the case, including other professionals, respond? If positive change occurred, what did each person do to contribute to it? How did they do that? How did they decide to do whatever they did? What do they each think is the next step? Tracking these responses will make it clear exactly what changes occurred, how the changes were brought about, and *define the changes as a result of the family's actions*. To do all of this, practitioners must learn how to follow up on their interventions. Practitioners must learn to restrain themselves from offering additional interventions until a full understanding has been obtained regarding what interventions have already been given.

GIVING THE PARENTS CREDIT FOR CHANGE

In I-FAST a basic goal is to help the adults to help their own children. Interventions are designed to arrange for this to happen. Once changes occur, the adults must be given credit and must accept that credit. If an out-of-control teenager improves, it cannot be framed as due to medication or fear of court consequences. Sometimes parents will not see themselves as the main instigators of change and will give credit to something else. When this happens, they must be reminded of everything they did to help their child and asked to share their own observations regarding how their child responded to the parents' specific efforts to help.

RESTRAINING CLIENTS FROM CHANGE

One classic approach to amplifying changes once they begin to occur is to restrain clients from changing too fast (Watzlawick, Weakland, & Fisch, 1974). For example, once a mother agreed her school phobic son would have to be exposed to school a little bit at a time to help him with his problem, she was given a laboriously slow and meticulous procedure for reintroducing her son back to school. First she would have to take him to school every day and just sit with him in the car until he could do that without having a knot in his stomach. After that, they could get out of the car and take one step toward the school building and do that every day until the boy did not have a knot in his stomach. Because his anxiety was so intense, months might pass before he could actually enter the building.

After a few days of this, the mother called and reported that she thought we were underestimating her son. She thought he was ready to go back to school part time and if that went OK, in two weeks he could go back full time. We cautioned the mother that he had a very serious anxiety problem and we wanted to make sure she did not push him too hard and produce a relapse. She insisted she knew her boy better than we did and that she was confident he could start back part time right away. After six months of her son not going to school at all, the mother had him back in school full time in two weeks.

PREDICTING RELAPSES

One way to manage anxiety when change occurs and to amplify those changes is to predict a relapse. If a relapse does occur, it has been predicted and the family does not have to feel all is lost. On the other hand, organizing the family in response to a possible relapse can further amplify changes that are occurring. For example, a 16-year-old boy had moved from the home of his mother and her boyfriend to that of his maternal grandmother and her boyfriend. The boy had a history of manipulating both households and causing all of the adults to argue and blame each other when he did not get his way. Several interventions were offered to both the mother and grandmother and this pattern was changed. To support this change, it was predicted that the boy would revert to acting out when he did not get his way. The adults were asked to watch for this. Ways were talked over for them to respond in a more coordinated manner. They were also told that the boy would be instructed to purposely test them so they could practice observing and being coordinated. When the boy did attempt to manipulate his mother and grandmother again, the women were ready for him and did not react like everything had failed and they were back to square one. It was then noted how the boy had used similar tactics with adults at school and with his PO. The mother and grandmother were instructed to look out for this also and respond similarly.

ADJUSTING TO CHANGE THAT HAPPENS QUICKLY

When change occurs rapidly and a client improves dramatically the family may bring up a new and serious problem. For example, the functioning of one of the adults in the family can seriously and rapidly deteriorate, or a threat of divorce may be made by one of the parents. When such reactions occur several methods can be employed in response:

- The new problem can be dismissed and framed as a temporary response to improvement. For example, if a parent threatens divorce and the client informs the practitioner, the divorce threat can be framed as something that happens sometimes when major family changes occur and that it will most likely subside. The client need not worry. In fact, with both Haley's schizophrenia (Haley, 1997) project and Stanton and Todd's (Stanton & Todd, 1982 heroin addict project, when parents did bring up divorce after the clients improved, it was just a temporary threat and was ultimately not followed through with. If the client accepts this, the treatment can continue to focus on solidifying the client's improvement.
- Another option if parents threaten divorce after the client improves is to frame the client as too unstable for the couple to be discussing divorce. In this option, the parents are asked to put the divorce on the back burner in the interest of making sure the client can continue his or her improvement. The parents can revisit the issue once their child is on more stable footing. Often, if the parents agree, the client will continue to improve, and divorce is not brought up again.
- A third option if the client improves and a parent threatens divorce, or one of the parents falls apart, is to switch the focus of treatment to the new problem. At the beginning or in the middle of treatment it is an error to switch the focus directly to adult problems when the treatment initially focused on a child problem. However, once the child has clearly improved, it is not necessarily an error to switch the focus at this stage of treatment. If done, it should be thought of as freeing the child from having to deal with the

problem. The practitioner may be framed as replacing the child as the one who helps the parent or focuses on the divorce threat. In this scenario, this may be viewed as a tactical move to help the child continue to improve without being involved in the adults' difficulties. The practitioner may or may not help with the adult problem, but by freeing the child from having to worry about the adult, the child can then change and a potential relapse can be avoided. When this works out, even if the adult problem is not solved, the child's attitude about it changes. The child has moved on and is no longer overly worried about adult problems.

CONCEPTUALIZING

A chronic problem with numerous home-based models is that families experience serious relapses after intensive in-home involvement is terminated. With the support of an intensive in-home practitioner, many families make successful changes. During the in-home intervention, safety is maintained and out-of-home placement is avoided. Evaluations across numerous programs indicate these gains are not maintained or significantly diminished within six months after in-home treatment has terminated (Little, 1997; Little & Schuerman, 1995; Unru, 1997; Wells & Whittington, 1993). There is some indication, however, that an important factor in preventing relapse after intensive in-home treatment is the linkage of families to natural support systems, as opposed to linking families to stepped-down mental health treatment.

One useful way of examining the problem is to take a larger systems perspective. The majority of families who typically receive in-home treatment are involved with numerous systems simultaneously. In addition to their in-home practitioner, they are typically also involved with POs, Children's Services case workers, individual practitioners for perhaps a multitude of family members, and psychiatrists who may continue to medicate the identified client. One way to attempt to understand relapses after termination from in-home treatment is to examine how these various professionals respond after home base is terminated and to compare these responses to how families and particularly parents are treated by most in-home practitioners.

Common elements in home treatment models include:

- A parent-friendly approach in which parents are respected and joined with
- A strengths-based approach in which the best is assumed of families instead of the worst
- An episode of care model in which specific problems are the focus of treatment
- An understanding of problems from an interactional perspective

However, this way of working with families concerning any remaining problems may not continue with professionals who remain on the case. POs continuing to dictate rules and consequences for clients do not represent a strengths-based approach nor does such treatment represent a parent empowerment model. Individual practitioners who see children alone may end up antagonizing parents at worst, and disempowering them at best. One possible cause for relapses after termination of in-home treatment can be that the multitude of professionals who remain on the case do not operate in a similar way to the home-based practitioner and the results gained from home-based intervention end up being undone.

Faced with these possibilities, merely providing home-based intervention within a larger context of services that do not operate from the philosophies that organize in-home treatment may not be sufficient to sustain the changes obtained with the in-home treatment. To minimize or avoid relapses after in-home termination, a strategy must be employed to influence professionals and agencies that will remain on the case after termination. This can be done both on a case-by-case basis and by design regarding how an agency implements its home-based services. In this chapter we examine the larger system factors required to sustain improvements gained with in-home intervention on case-by-case basis. Chapter 11 addresses programmatic methods of sustaining improvements gained with in-home intervention.

STRATEGIZING

All good things must finally come to an end, so it is said, and so it goes with intervention. Successful termination of treatment is always everyone's goal. The question is, how do we define successful intervention? If we see success as the elimination of all problems or the achievement of some ideal state for the family and children, or the end of future problems as we know them, treatment is likely to be interminable. For I-FAST, successful termination usually means successfully accomplishing the goals the parents initially set forth. To quote a venerable system thinker and mentor, John Weakland, it is better to see life as ". . . just one damned thing after another. . . but the only game in town." There will always be new challenges, and the idea is to learn by mastering the past ones, anticipate the new ones, and do the best we can, if not truly enjoy the better times in between. Another metaphor for this view is that "life is a roller coaster" with plenty of ups and downs. The trick of it is to learn to enjoy the ride, anticipate the dips, and maybe learn to master them enough to be able to hold our hands in the air and laugh and scream as we go down, anticipating the next rise.

The idea of ending treatment is to focus on goal achievement, congratulate clients on their strength in the face of adversity and their successes, anticipate the next hurdles, and assure everyone that "the door is always open" if they need to check in again. I-FAST assumes an "episodes of care" approach to treatment, similar to that of a family physician or pediatrician. The goal of intervention is:

- To address the family and system as it is struggling right now
- To treat the dilemma and the reasons for it escalating
- To build knowledge of the causes of the problem and support the way it has been resolved
- To discuss prevention and how to address recurrences as they arise again
- To welcome the clients' return when the next difficulty arises

Because the I-FAST practitioners know the family from past consultations, trust and alliances tend to be carried over to future visits, and new episodes tend to be more "booster shots" or more efficient variations of what worked in the past, now applied to the next phase in the life cycle or the next challenge.

Achieving the originally agreed on goals is the main signal for ending this set of visits. By setting clearly defined goals as discussed in previous chapters, these goals can be regularly visited, and progress measured all along the way. With goal achievement as a major part of each session or visit, the idea of ending this episode of care will not be a surprise. All involved will have been noting and even celebrating successes all along. Also, ending intensive intervention with a highly distressed family does not always mean fully terminating them from services in general. Often clients and families are linked with other needed yet less intensive case management services within the agency or community, and further linked with other positive and helpful community groups and organizations to continue to reinforce their change. We return to this ending process in more detail in chapter eleven. For now, it is important to remember the three key elements of termination.

Termination as a Special Issue for Home-Based Treatment
In the ideal treatment world, termination occurs when the presenting concerns of the client are successfully resolved. The question is whether this simple rule applies to intensive in-home treatment when the removal of a child is at stake. As noted, traditionally, relapses after in-home treatment has successfully terminated have been a chronic and widespread problem. This suggests the issues of termination are more complex than just resolving the presenting client concerns. Assuming improvement on a given case has been obtained and the family is satisfied with the results, the practitioner needs to address what additional issues might be looked at to ensure the continuation of the client's improvement.

IS IMPROVEMENT ACKNOWLEDGED BY OTHER PROFESSIONALS?
In-home treatment cases inevitably involve child welfare case workers, juvenile court POs, and in most instances, psychiatrists prescribing medication. All of these professionals have power. POs and case workers have the power to place children out of the home involuntarily. Psychiatrists have great influence over parents, POs, and case workers.

When a family improves, serious problems can return if any of these powerful professionals do not acknowledge improvement or become overactive once the in-home practitioner is gone. An out-of-control adolescent can improve from his parents' perspective, but still be involved with a PO. It is common with in-home treatment for probation officers to recede to the background while home-based treatment is in place. In fact, several of the major in-home treatment models require POs to step aside at this time. Once in-home treatment has terminated, however, many POs return and can become overactive, intervening in ways that produce a relapse. The teen can be placed in detention by a PO for violating terms of probation, such as coming home after the deadline the PO sets. This outcome can easily occur if a teen improves but the PO continues to have serious concerns about the case. At a minimum, termination should not occur unless the PO agrees the case has improved. The same idea goes with other involved agents and systems. I-FAST involves all parties and systems into the treatment plan to help ensure that everyone is taking the same position with the youth and family. Once this is done, then it is less likely that other agents will disrupt the gains made.

In some cases, even after treatment goals have been met, it may be wise to stay involved until the court case is closed. Many families attribute change in their teen to the teen's fear of the court. Despite all efforts to help the parents take credit for their child's improvement, many may continue to harbor doubts about how much influence fear of the court contributed to positive changes. This can easily be assessed by asking the PO to begin talking of terminating the court case and observing the parents' response. Even in the best cases where the teen has improved due to obvious efforts of the parents and the parents agree they have helped their child improve, these same parents can exhibit serious anxiety at the first sign of court departure. This alone can possibly account for many relapses after in-home treatment has terminated. Parents and PO might both be pleased at the time of in-home treatment's termination but the court and PO remain involved. When the PO begins to terminate, the parents become anxious and the teen relapses. Staying involved until the court is clear can help avoid this outcome.

Psychiatrists and medications must also be considered at termination. A child can improve significantly but remain on a high dosage of multiple medications. The fact that no medication changes are made despite the child's improvement sends a conflicting message to the family. The child has changed, but that change is implicitly not acknowledged because the child continues to be heavily medicated. Change has occurred, but a key professional on the case is not behaving as such. This can also account for relapses. At a minimum, if significant changes do occur, this should be reflected in some sort of adjustment to the child's medication. Medications do not necessarily have to be eliminated, but a reduction often helps to validate that the changes made are significant and that they are a result of the changes that the youth, family, and involved others have made.

IS THE CLIENT'S FUNCTIONING DEVELOPMENTALLY APPROPRIATE?

Problem behaviors can be eliminated, symptoms can be successfully resolved, parents can be pleased with improvements, but a client can continue to have no social life. When the resolution of specific problems does not result in a shift to developmentally appropriate activities, relapses can occur. Should treatment be terminated when an oppositional teen calms down with his or her parents, but continues to isolate socially? The parents may be pleased by the teen's improved way of dealing with them. They may not be upset about the teen's isolation. They do not have to worry about their child getting into trouble if he or she stays home all of the time. How should in-home treatment professionals respond to this situation? A case will probably have to be terminated if the parents cannot be persuaded to focus on a new goal of helping the teen associate with peers. However, there is no rule against attempting to persuade the parents. It can be pointed out that as long as their teen is either uninterested or unable to associate with appropriate peers, they are not out of trouble. Pressing for developmentally appropriate behaviors once goals are met or including developmentally appropriate behaviors as part of the goals at the outset of treatment can often help to sustain change.

DISENGAGING FROM FAMILIES

When successful, in-home treatment professionals become very powerfully connected to families. Typical professional boundaries are stretched when professionals go into homes. Many families become reliant on the in-home professional in ways that are not necessarily apparent. When termination is looming, parents can become very anxious about the in-home professional's departure. Perhaps they feel protected by the in-home professional from other powerful professionals such as child welfare workers. Perhaps they lack confidence that they can continue to exhibit competence with their child without the support of the in-home professional. Perhaps the only person they think really understands their situation is the in-home professional and losing this support is anxiety provoking. One key to terminating in-home treatment without a relapse is finding support for the family once the in-home treatment is over. Ideally, that support should come from the family's natural environment. An extended family member or a friend can be connected to a parent or parents as a "teammate" helping them think through how to respond to future difficulties that may arise with their child. Church or other community organizations can also provide support. If support is found from other less intensive mental health professionals, it is crucial that the help be parent friendly. A new practitioner who focuses on diagnoses and works with the child individually can be a problem. In this situation parents can lose support previously offered by the in-home professional, or at worst, be antagonized by an individually focused practitioner. Relapses can then occur. To avoid this, in I-FAST, we hope that by training clinic supervisors, I-FAST treatment philosophies are shared by other clinic professionals, making transfers to other clinic services more congruent with the in-home services being terminated.

Implementing Summary

As a final review, the following points need to be remembered when approaching successful termination:

- **Review what worked.** Attribute the change to the clients and systems involved. They are the ones who have achieved this success and their strengths and resilience should be celebrated.
- **Emphasize the strengths and resilience of all involved.** Lasting change is change that clients own as their own achievements and not necessarily the result of good work by the practitioner.
- **Emphasize episodes of care.** Part of termination is predicting future challenges and inoculating family members and related systems against future dilemmas. Clients are encouraged to "be in the world" and not necessarily to be in treatment. Clients are assured that they can always check back in as needed. "The door is always open."
- **Link the family to resources in their natural environment.** As noted earlier, linkage to natural supports can reduce relapses after in-home treatment. Natural resources could be Boy Scouts, the school chess team, the local gym, engagement of uninvolved extended family members, or changing how involved extended family members are engaged. There are several advantages of linkage to natural supports. First, it promotes participation in normal activities. This then reinforces more normal behavior. Second, linkage to natural supports reinforces the idea that no more treatment is necessary and does not require the client to continue to be seen as abnormal. Two variations of linkage to natural supports are finding a godparent for abused children and finding a teammate for single parents.
    - **Find a godparent for abused children.** When serious abuse or neglect has been the problem, finding an adult, preferably an extended family member, to engage in an ongoing relationship with the abuse victim can support family changes and continued safety of the victim. The strategy

was fully developed by Madanes (1990). Finding an adult who lives outside the home to help take responsibility for the safety of the abused child can reassure Children's Services and the court, resulting in allowing the abuse victim to remain in the home. The idea can be framed to the family as finding a "godparent" for the child. Finding an extended family member to remain involved with abuse victims is one way to break a common interactional pattern associated with abuse: secrecy and rigid boundaries around the household in which the abuse took place. Having an aunt or uncle become regularly involved with the child creates a permanent boundary breaker. This also can help satisfy the court and protective services who may continue to fear further abuse if they close their cases.

- **Find a teammate for a single parent.** One view is that a parent learns new parenting behaviors and then goes forth and forevermore produces them. Another option is that new behavior results from a new social organization. A single mother with an in-home practitioner, for example, has a teammate to validate her position of authority, strategize with, and report to. This social function of the in-home practitioner is especially profound owing to the intensity of involvement of in-home treatment. In this social organization, the single mother can function at a higher level. But what happens when treatment is over and the mother's teammate departs? For single parents it is especially important to find someone in their natural support system who can replace the in-home practitioner as their teammate. This strategy was developed by Price (1999). The teammate can be a sister, a best friend, or a boyfriend or girlfriend. The teammate's job is not to take over parenting, but to function as a sounding board, an aid to develop parenting strategies when needed, and to validate the parent's position of authority. They can be called on a Wednesday night when the mother is at her wits' end and just does not know what to do. She has someone she can vent to and help pull herself together before deciding how to approach the latest parenting challenge.

Though there are numerous other options available for building resilience and moving toward termination, the main goal is to consolidate gains while empowering the family and helping all involved others stay on the same page as the successful treatment process.

TIPS FOR BUILDING RESILIENCE

Once the family has made sufficient change the family will either be terminated or moved to a lesser level of care. Because families may return to baseline behaviors under stress the main task of this process is to develop a relapse prevention strategy. This may be done in a number of ways depending on the family.

- **Use scaling questions to amplify incremental changes.** When small changes are occurring, the use of scaling questions can be offered to amplify those changes. If a child is depressed, for example, practitioner can ask a parent to rank on a scale of 0 to 10 where the depression before treatment and where is it now. Once the parent has rated the improvement, he or she can be asked what each person did to help obtain that improvement and what the sign would be that showed improvement has gone up another notch. A discussion can follow regarding what everyone can now do to help that next small step to occur.

- **Predict a relapse and develop a prevention plan ("Life is a roller coaster!").** Quite often, when clients and other systems have experienced positive and rather rapid change, they either come to expect it to always be that way, or feel that it is fragile and one false step will bring things all back to the way they were before. The metaphor of "life as a roller coaster" is often used to point out that recurrences of the past problem will likely arise again, and that new difficulties will invariably come up. Moving through the life cycle alone will always present new challenges. The point of this position is to spend time coming up with what things are likely to happen next and decide whether they simply need to be accepted, or if not, then how the currently successful game plan may be reapplied. Predicting is most always done at termination, but may also be done at several points along the way.

- **Prescribe a relapse to test the plan ("fire drills").** Prescribing a "relapse" may sound illogical to most clients. Why should they try to bring on the thing they have apparently mastered and left behind? Also, some clients may also feel that they are unsure if they have really mastered the past difficulty, and are unsure if they do have the skills to handle it on their own. Others may be afraid that any hint of the past problem behaviors or negative feelings will be a sign that the apparent "house of cards" they have built with their successes is about to come tumbling down. Of course, the more clients try to rigidly hold on to that they have created, or again rigidly try to prevent what they most fear, the more likely that fear of relapse is to come true.

  - The technique of prescribing a relapse is most often used when successful change has been achieved and all involved are concerned about it being robust and sustainable. Most often change is seen as potentially fragile and susceptible to erosion given new challenges and old familiar ways of responding.
  - The purpose of prescribing a relapse is to help bring the old symptomatic or problematic behaviors under voluntary control. Prescribing that the clients revisit the old challenges to see how they do with them offers many advantages. Not the least of these advantages is the apparently paradoxical effect that, trying to bring on old problems, fights, and related distress puts the clients in control or in change of these past problems. Thus the old problems may be difficult to recreate, or they just don't happen, or everyone decides not to do that old stuff again, or if they do manage to create the old difficulty, it is handled with relative ease. If it isn't handled easily, then everyone has the advantage of reviewing how things got off track and how things can go better the next time. No real problem.
  - Once seen as out-of-control fights, resections or behaviors, once clients actively and deliberately attempt to reengage in them they usually find

it either hard to do so or they learn that they can actually control them quite well.
- Relapse prescription is always done well before termination so that clients can return to meet with the practitioner and process their success and frame their responses and even their potential for a few more skills or more practice.
- A variation of this stance is *predicting a relapse*. This is done to alert all clients to future transitions and challenges and predict potential reactions and rehearse new responses. This comes under the heading of "forewarned is forearmed." The more clients can anticipate and prepare for stressors the better they can respond to them and the less likely they will be to view new challenges as simply relapse or reoccurrence of the former problems.
- One more of a number of other useful predicting options comes under a behavioral rationale. This is the idea of predicting what behaviorists call an "extinction burst." When parents start setting limits or start using time outs and other shifts in their parenting, children will invariably escalate their efforts to get their way before they give up and start changing in new directions. Reframing these escalations as proof that their efforts are working and not that they are making things worse will help parents weather the short storm and stay consistent in their new parenting routine.

Prescribing relapses is always done before final termination. This is because there is always the need to have all involved return and review what happened. Successes may be celebrated. If the relapse just didn't occur or everyone decided they didn't want it to, then this can be framed positively for everyone as a sign of their progress and their choice to move ahead. If there were challenges in dealing with the re-created problems, then everyone can track the process and see how things got off track, and what needs attention in the future. Doing "fire drills" is an easy rationale to use to help everyone understand the value of this and to go along with it.

- **Normalize relapse and make it part of the prevention plan ("stuff happens!").** Without needing to say much more on this intervention, needless to say, it is very important for clients to get the idea that being in life or in families, or being a kid is not always a bowl of cherries. It is important that all clients learn that their future successes will be a process with new challenges. New problems are just new problems, not backsliding or sign of weakness, or the recurrence of the same old thing. As mentioned previously, the main idea is to emphasize that, "Life is one damned thing after another. . . but it's the only game in town!" A plan of action is likely to inoculate all involved family members and systems against being overly alarmed, labeling the next challenge as the same old thing, and returning to the same old solutions. An ounce of prevention really is worth a pound of cure.
- **Develop a comprehensive list of what worked in the treatment process ("How the heck have you all done this? Look what you've done. You're amazing!").** This process amounts to not only reviewing all clients' and involved systems' achievements, but also attributing these successes to their

own strength and hard work. Positioning with clients and involved others at this time and asking questions like, "Really... how have you done this?" "I wish all parents were as strongly committed to the welfare of their kids as you... how did you manage to hang in there?" Clients need to be put in the position of doing a positive scan to inventory their strengths in the face of adversity. Even if clients can't answer these questions, they are left with the strong sense that they have done it themselves. Owning change is critical to lasting change for clients.

9 SOME FINAL THOUGHTS ON PRACTICE

RUSSELL BARKLEY (1997) AND ROSS GREENE (2001) are preeminent scholars in the treatment of disruptive behavior disorders. Each has developed a framework for working with disruptive kids and their families that is highly effective. Research has shown that when compared head to head, the rate of effectiveness is about the same (Greene et al., 2004). At the same time, when examining the frameworks there are differences in both frames and procedures that are used to bring about change. That each framework is effective yet conceptually different is not surprising. This is consistent with predictions that might be made from the perspective of I-FAST. In essence we propose that it is not a model per se that brings about change. Instead it is the practitioner's skill at connecting with families that is most important as he or she works within a given, coherent approach. The connection occurs on multiple levels and includes the strategic use of various models. In the end, therapy models are useful when they serve the purpose of providing a hopeful framework for families and practitioners in organizing problems and solutions.

With many treatment approaches, emphasis is placed on adherence to the model. In I-FAST there is also a need for adherence; however, this occurs at a different level. Practitioners are required to adhere to meta-level constructs that fall within the process of change theory. In this chapter we present the larger level concepts that frame I-FAST clinical skills. In the strategy section we describe specific skills that I-FAST practitioners need in order to provide effective treatment. In the implementation section we offer some thoughts that clarify the integrative nature of I-FAST.

CONCEPTUALIZING

Bruce Wampold (2001) indicates that fidelity to a treatment model includes two dimensions, adherence and allegiance. Adherence refers to treatment protocol and the extent to which the practitioner follows the protocol as has been put forth. Allegiance refers to the practitioner's belief that the protocol works.

Adherence

Most fidelity measurement protocols exclusively target adherence to specific treatment methods. Yet there are limitations to adherence as a one dimensional construct. Taking these limitations into account, and including allegiance changes our understanding of adherence in an important way. The following list of findings illustrates this point.

- Mazzucchelli and Sanders (2010) reporting on Barlow (1981) indicate that most practitioners deliver interventions comprising an eclectic mixture of goals and methods fashioned from their own previous training and clinical experience.

- They report further that practitioners often express concerns about the relevance of empirically supported treatments for their clients.
- Mazzucchelli and Sanders (2010) indicate that there is evidence that overemphasis on technical procedures can result in the therapeutic relationship suffering, which may in turn hamper change (Castonguay, Goldfried, Wiser, Raue, & Hayes, 1996; Najavits, & Strupp, 1994).
- However, flexibility within fidelity may be easier said than done.

Allegiance

- Allegiance is more difficult to study and so has often been neglected as a dimension of fidelity.
- Wampold (2001) included measures of allegiance in his meta-analysis of psychotherapy outcome.
- Wampold found that allegiance effects were consistently present and notably large. Surprisingly, close adherence to treatment protocols was generally not associated with positive outcomes, but for a few notable exceptions. In these exceptions it was the organizing or structuring aspect of adherence that was found to be important versus the protocol or treatment model itself.

What Matters

Given that allegiance is more important to outcome than adherence to a specific treatment protocol the question of what matters becomes important. In other words, can a practitioner pull together any set of techniques and ideas and throw them at a family with the expectation of facilitating change? Of course, the answer is no. There is a form that effective practitioners knowingly or unknowingly follow. This form is summarized by the following points.

- The practitioner listens to problems and hears points of view from all concerned parties, empathizing with all sides, even though differing views may be in conflict or seem contradictory.
- The practitioner provides a rationale or conceptual scheme that explains the symptoms of the youth in a way that validates all persons involved in the case situation.
- The rationale is worded in a manner that implies a pathway for change and that enhances hope that something can be done behaviorally to alleviate the families' concerns.
- The practitioner then offers a procedure or ritual that is designed to change how the family is attempting to solve the problem.
- The practitioner focuses on changing the way that a family is trying to change. This is pattern shift or second-order change.
- The practitioner observes the family's response to procedures and adjusts them as needed.
- The practitioner does not blame the family if they do not follow the procedure or change it in some way but uses this as information to adjust his or her position with the family.
- The practitioner identifies and empowers change, finally building resilience and relapse prevention.

STRATEGIZING

I-FAST treatment skills are centered on not judging clients (acceptance) and conceptual flexibility. I-FAST practitioners bring knowledge of multiple behavioral treatment frameworks to the treatment setting or are prepared to learn different treatment protocols to best serve clients. The ability to present novel ideas in a genuine, sincere manner is also an important skill.

Because I-FAST is inherently flexible, previous knowledge about various treatment modalities is welcomed. Practitioners are warned that because I-FAST is based in the common factors and the general process of change, rationales that have been learned for why a particular treatment works may be different from what they have learned. For example, a practitioner experienced with Eye Movement Desensitization and Reprocessing (EMDR) may believe that the treatment works because of the fixation on the practitioner's finger movement while recovering a painful memory. However, from the perspective of I-FAST, EMDR does work but not for that reason. Instead it works because it fulfills the requirements in the preceding section. Moreover, independent research has not been able to verify that eye movement is involved in the underlying change mechanism. In the following sections we more specifically identify the skill set that is possessed by effective I-FAST practitioners.

Becoming Nonjudgmental

Acceptance of clients who are different and who have a worldview counter to the clinician can be a formidable challenge in providing effective treatment. The following summarizes the emphasis that I-FAST places on acceptance.

- I-FAST practitioners are able to be accepting of interpersonal differences and variable parenting styles.
- The I-FAST practitioner understands that clients, community partners, and others involved in the case are more likely to engage in change when they are first validated. This means that the practitioner must be prepared to actively seek information that allows him or her to validate parties who may be at odds or represent values that differ from those of the practitioner.
- I-FAST practitioners understand that parents have usually been blamed by professionals and others for the behavior or their child. They often easily put on the defensive by interaction that comes across as critical. At the same time it is the parents who we are seeking to empower. I-FAST practitioners go to great lengths to show acceptance for parents in such a way that they feel affirmed and not blamed.

The I-FAST practitioner focuses on change and believes this is possible no matter how problematic the family situation may be. Focus on change requires that the clinician maintain conceptual flexibility. The following assumptions underlie conceptual flexibility.

Conceptual Flexibility
- I-FAST practitioners understand that various treatment models carry both possibilities and limitations.

- There are no models that have rationales and treatment approaches that are "true" in all senses of the word. For example, in working with families it is currently popular to use frames from brain science. It is important to remember that brain science is in an early stage of development. This means that rationales from brain science will change as the science evolves.
- There is no one treatment model that works for all clients.
- The judgment about what treatment model to use in a specific case is based on how it fits for the family. If the fit is not there, the I-FAST practitioner either modifies the model to fit the family or finds another model that best fits with the needs of the family.
- The key to fit is that the family (as well as the practitioner and others involved) believes in the proposed rationales and procedures; and that the rationales and procedures lead to interventions that promote pattern shift.

Rationales

For interventions to be effective it is important for clinicians to provide a conceptual framework that enables clients to understand the nature and purpose of treatment. The following assumptions are critical to developing effective treatment rationales.

- I-FAST practitioners understand that human beings are meaning makers and as such have a need to understand the nature of problems and how potential solutions are logically connected.
- I-FAST practitioners understand that the power of behavioral therapy is in language. The words used by the practitioner make a difference.
- The I-FAST practitioner understands that the purpose of framing, reframing, and deframing is to introduce novel ideas that carry hope for change.
  - In the process of framing, reframing, and deframing, the practitioner attempts to validate the client or match his or her presentation while introducing a "twist."
  - For example, the practitioner may tell parents who yell a great deal at their child that the yelling is a sign of their caring–protective natures. The practitioner may then ask if the parents are willing to turn up the heat by letting go of the yelling and allowing the youth to endure the natural consequences of his or her behavior.
- The I-FAST practitioner understands that with regard to treatment rationales, believability trumps scientific truth or fidelity to a particular treatment model.
- Effective rationales are framed in language that makes sense to the family and all others involved.

Listening

I-Fast stresses the importance of rationales that fit within the language of the family. To work within the family's language system listening becomes crucial. The following are key points related to listening.

- I-FAST practitioners listen with empathy to different parties and their views of problems.

- All parties' perspectives need to be included in the treatment planning process.
- At another level the practitioner listens to learn the language of the family and other parties involved in the case. The objective here is to pick up the manners of speech, metaphors, and analogies used in the family.
- The I-FAST practitioner uses the language of the family when introducing rationales and procedures.
  - For example, Greene's perspective negates the view that youth with disruptive behaviors are motivated by a need or desire to engage in power struggles while Haley endorses this as a potential motivation.
  - The I-FAST practitioner listens to determine the family's view on this matter and will develop and use language that is consistent with how the family views the child.

Mutual Goals

I-FAST clinicians are aware that mutually agreed upon goals are vital to effective treatment. Yet, when multiple parties are involved with differing interests complications arise. The following guidelines are useful for establishing mutual goals.

- The I-FAST practitioner is prepared for the idea that various parties may have different goals that may appear to conflict with one another.
- There may be a need to organize interviews so that various factions and persons who represent differing views can be validated without losing rapport with other family members or constituent groups.
  - For example, this allows for the practitioner to work with a youth on getting space from parents while working with parents on obtaining more compliance from the youth. Because compliance leads to space these goals are not incompatible.
  - The language that the youth and parents are using to accomplish their goals may be so conflictual that talking to the youth and parents separately is the only feasible way of getting the work done.
- It is important to take into account all persons who have power within and outside of the family when establishing goals, noting and aligning with each powerful agent.

Procedures

Procedures are used to directly interrupt problem patterns or amplify exceptions. I-FAST clinicians use the following guidelines for developing procedures.

- The I-FAST practitioner understands procedures must be tailored to fit the unique needs of the family.
- Procedures are designed to produce a change in the way that a family is trying to bring about change; the target is to interrupt and/or redirect solution patterns that are making problems worse.
- Procedures are directly linked to the problems identified and the mutual goals that have been established.

- Procedures are designed in a manner that they can be delivered with empathy to the family and other involved parties.
- Procedures are understood as an extension of the therapeutic relationship.

Responsiveness

I-FAST clinicians are aware that human behavior is very complex. Consequently, even the most carefully constructed procedures may achieve different effects than were intended. The following guidelines are useful for observing and responding to procedures.

- The practitioner is continuously observing how family members respond to his or her rationales, efforts at conveying empathy, and procedures.
- The objective is to use information to adjust the approach.
- The practitioner takes responsibility for resistance exhibited by the family and shifts his or her stance to obtain cooperation.
- The I-FAST practitioner continuously looks for small signs that desired change is occurring.
- The I-FAST practitioner notices signs of change and empowers it by focusing attention on who is doing what to make it happen among all involved.
- The I-FAST practitioner assigns credit for wanted change to family members and involved others, and does not accept credit personally.
- The I-FAST practitioner looks for ways that family members have contributed to change even when medication is involved.
- The I-FAST practitioner also looks for ways to assign credit for desired changes to significant others such as probation officers, teachers, and children's services workers.

Genuineness

At the end of the day, the clinician's ability to be an effective agent of change hinges on her credibility with the family. Credibility in turn is earned through a process where the clinician demonstrates that she genuinely cares for all members of the family. The following tools are useful to maintaining genuineness.

- The I-FAST practitioner realizes that the skills of conceptual flexibility are important to being nonjudgmental. Multiple frames, different rationales, and language must make sense to the practitioner so he or she can deliver them authentically and genuinely.
- The I-FAST practitioner uses social constructivism or other philosophical frameworks to further support a nonjudgmental approach. Clients are not blamed for their actions or motives.
- The I-FAST practitioner uses supervision to challenge his or her own beliefs and theories that get in the way of a genuine nonjudgmental stance.

IMPLEMENTING

When training practitioners we are often asked about the integrative nature of I-FAST and how it differs from other frameworks such as Collaborative Problem Solving (Greene, 2001) or Parent Management Training (Barkley, 1997). Our response is that

I-FAST is like a conceptual umbrella. Frameworks such as Barkley's or Greene's fit under the umbrella. Each framework calls the practitioner to a nonjudgmental point of view through rationales that explain how children become oppositional and defiant. The rationales free both children and parents from blame. Although the rationales are different, a nonjudgmental perspective is the common thread. The rationales lead to different processes for establishing goals. Though the processes are different they both lead to goal consensus and a scheme for determining priorities for working on goals. Though both frameworks offer different procedures for achieving goals, they have important common elements. Procedures are logically linked to rationales and are directed at changing the way the parents are attempting to change their child. In addition, the frameworks establish parents as the agents of change. Finally, genuineness is built into the frameworks through research that assists practitioners with believing that they are providing an evidence-based approach.

In I-FAST we give much credit and respect to model developers such as Greene and Barkley. An I-FAST practitioner with previous training in any of the evidence-based approaches is free to use the approach that they have learned. I-FAST requires that the practitioner understand that his or her chosen approach fits under the larger conceptual umbrella. It is also necessary that the I-FAST practitioner can relate his or her work in this manner. For example, if the practitioner uses the three-basket approach that is in Greene's work it is important for the practitioner to see that the baskets represent a rationale and a procedure. The value of the rationale and procedure is that when followed they change the way that the parents are trying to change their child. It is also critical for the practitioner to understand that how he or she implements the three-basket approach makes a difference. For it to work, it must fit the world view of the parents and be presented in a manner that demonstrates genuineness and responsiveness.

Because of the larger umbrella, the practitioner is also aware that the rationale for a particular framework may not fit the world view of the family. Greene's axiom is that children do what they can; he does not view defiant children as engaging in a power struggle. Some parents may not be convinced that this is the case and insist that their child is into power struggles. When this occurs, I-FAST calls for the practitioner to change his or her rationale to fit the family. This might mean adopting Haley or Barkley's rationale or creating one that better fits. This may not preclude using Greene's three baskets. However, the use of the baskets would be to gain control of the child versus teaching him or her to be more flexible.

In essence, I-FAST is about expanding the flexibility of practitioners so that their creativity can come to play when simply following a manual doesn't work. Though maximum flexibility is the objective, this does not mean that anything goes. Different approaches may be cobbled together or a new approach may be invented for a particular case. The integrity of the treatment is maintained by adherence to the broader principles that we call I-FAST.

Implementing Through Matching

In the following few chapters we address the process of matching or fitting the practitioner's approach to that which personally fits him or her best and, as importantly, that fits the values, world views, language, and goals of the families and agencies involved in each case. This becomes quite a unique and creative, case-by-case process. It calls for the I-FAST practitioner to be well grounded in the basic concepts underlying I-FAST as a meta-framework. This includes the idea that clients and involved others are likely to be doing the best they can at trying to resolve the problems with their youth in the ways they understand them. It directs the I-FAST practitioner to become acutely sensitive to the values, frames, and language used by youth, family members, and other agency practitioners. This sensitivity not only helps the I-FAST practitioner understand how the lens of those world views shapes the problem-generating system, but it also enables the practitioner to enter those worldviews and use those values and goals to fit frames and rationales to the family and involved others. At times, the treatment rationale most favored by the I-FAST practitioner will fit well with a given family and other providers, and yet just as often, the practitioner will need to creatively shift his or her language and frames to fit the perspectives of the clients and those of other involved providers.

The importance of this creative flexibility within the general guidelines of I-FAST cannot be overstated. Yet it is also a process that evolves with practice. To use a metaphor, just as those learning to dance need to learn different styles and types of dance along with the unique steps of those different dances, so too must the practitioner learn the general rationales and intervention techniques of a number of different approaches to treatment. Yet there are also basic steps and turns common across most all forms of dance. Those common steps are simply adapted to different rhythms and styles. So too are there general types of positions and intervention common across different approaches. The foxtrot or the waltz will not always fit the rhythms of samba or salsa music, even though the waltz and foxtrot may be the dancer's favorites. General steps and styles must be learned and yet fit to the style and tempo of different music. I-FAST basic skills represent a range of basic interventions and strategies common across a wide variety of approaches. Each family and involved schools or agencies represent different music and tempos and practitioners need to recognize this to fit the dance and their approach to the music of these systems. Furthermore, learning to dance well is a process, just as is learning the skill of becoming an expert practitioner. It's important to become comfortable with one's partners and become attentive and sensitive to their ways of leading and following in the give and take of the dance. For the best dancers and the most effective practitioners, this looks like an effortless process. However, it comes from continual practice and the guidance of teachers, coaches, and supervisors. Experts at the dance fit their style to the music played, are familiar with different styles, and have become skilled at both leading and following different partners.

So too is the evolution of strong I-FAST practitioners. They become sensitive to the style of different systems; become familiar with different options for describing problems and rationales for treatment; they fit their style to the systems involved and are willing to be led by their goals and approach to resolving their dilemmas to collaborate well with them; and ultimately they match their approach to that of those involved in each case and through that matching help all involved shift their patterns to a collaboratively achieved new pattern or resolution.

We have chosen this metaphor to drive home the idea that the process of implementing the general I-FAST skills is based on its flexible basic concepts. Refining and fitting these I-FAST skills becomes a unique process of fitting the general meta-concepts and general skills to the different values, frames, and approaches of each new system encountered. If we could teach this in this final section on implementing the general I-FAST skills we would. However, such a structured approach to teaching would likely begin to violate the basic value of flexibility and matching of practitioner, agency, family, and larger systems that is at the heart of the I-FAST approach. Becoming an expert I-FAST practitioner is like becoming an expert dancer. It is a process of rigor in adhering to the basic premises of the approach, learning to dance to the time of the music, and being willing to flex to different styles and tempos; of learning the general skills that tend to be common across treatments and learning the steps and how they are done differently in different approaches; and finally, it is a process of creatively and imaginatively fitting these to each unique case. After that, it is a matter of practicing with supportive teachers, coaches, and supervisors who fit well with you and who have your best interests and those of each case as their highest value.

I-FAST SUPERVISION, AGENCY CONSIDERATIONS, AND SUSTAINABILITY

3

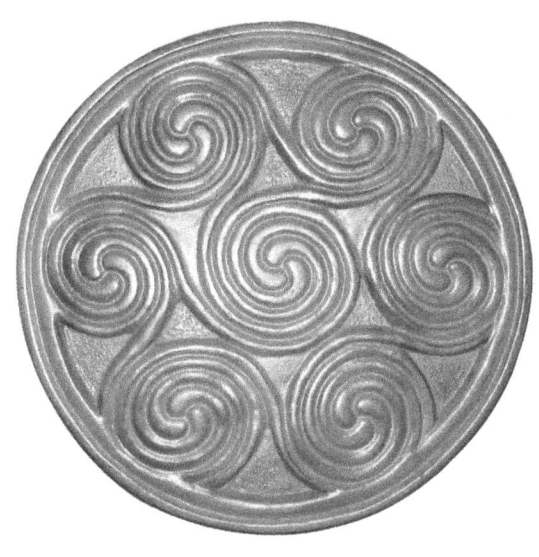

TEACHING AND SUPERVISING I-FAST

10

SUPERVISION OF SPECIFIC EVIDENCE-BASED MODELS EMPHASIZES ADHERENCE to the model by the supervisees. Obtaining strict adherence to steps and procedures outlined in manuals is a primary goal of supervision. In this model of supervision, supervisors and consultants assume roles of teachers of the models they support. The model itself is the customer in this supervision process, as an ultimate goal is to obtain data in support of the model by ensuring fidelity by its supervisees.

Should the goal of supervision emphasize practitioner adherence to a model? Or should the goal of supervision emphasize the successful resolution of problems families want help with? Clearly both can be a focus, but which should be emphasized? Should the role of a supervisor emphasize teaching a specific treatment model? Or should the role of a supervisor emphasize consulting and collaborating on resolving problems with cases? Should the customer of supervision be the model a supervisor represents and is promoting or should the customer be the practitioner who wishes clinical support and help on a case?

These are complex questions. Where an I-FAST supervisor should place his or her emphasis on each of these issues should be carefully thought through. Considering the concepts of parallel processes, adherence versus allegiance and a view of the setting in which I-FAST is being implemented can offer guidance into how an I-FAST supervisor should deal with these issues.

CONCEPTUALIZING

Parallel Processes

Supervision and treatment are isomorphic processes (Liddle & Saba, 1984). What a supervisor does with a practitioner can then be paralleled by what a practitioner does with a family. If the supervisor is supportive and strengths-based with the practitioner, the practitioner will be so with the client. If the supervisor is critical of the practitioner, the practitioner will be so with the client. If the supervisor loses empathy and does not validate the practitioner, the practitioner may treat the family in a similar fashion. Treatment parallels supervision. In view of this, when supervising I-FAST the philosophy and principles emphasized in the model must also be paralleled in supervision. Some of these key principles and their relevance for supervision are presented in the sections that follow.

FLEXIBILITY AND EMPOWERMENT

I-FAST emphasizes flexibility and empowerment. As a model, a multitude of ways of working can be incorporated into any given treatment. This allows supervisors to empower practitioners. A given practitioner can utilize many of his or her existing skills and beliefs within I-FAST. I-FAST supervisors can support existing skills and beliefs. A supervisor who is responsible for a staff that may represent a multitude of beliefs and skill levels is not required to push a rigid model on the group that may ask practitioners to forgo their existing skills. Instead, supervisors can empower staff to utilize their existing therapeutic repertoire within the larger, flexible I-FAST frames.

Navigating issues of supervisor power and hierarchy are identified as keys to the supervisor/practitioner relationship (Fine & Turner, 2002; Lee & Everett, 2004). Managing a collaborative supervisor/practitioner relationship within the context of a clinic in which the supervisor has power as both a clinical expert and possibly a manager can become very sticky. In such settings, it may be more crucial for I-FAST supervisors to emphasize practitioner strengths and expertise rather than impose an additional power-based approach of focusing on adherence to I-FAST.

STRENGTHS-BASED SUPERVISION

Just as I-FAST is a strengths-based approach with clients, it is also a strengths-based supervision model. This does not merely mean supervisors should be positive with practitioners and pointing out strengths. It means truly collaborating with practitioners, respecting their judgments on cases whenever possible, and utilizing their preexisting skills.

Collaborative supervision is stressed by Fine and Turner (2002). They identify mindfulness of the impact of supervisor power, creating a practitioner/supervisor alliance, and collaborating on goals of supervision as key components to collaborative supervision. Creating a sense of teamwork is stressed by Henderson, Cawyer, and Watkins (1999). Developing a working alliance can enhance greater satisfaction with supervision (Ladenay, Elliks, & Friedlander, 1999), ability to work through conflicts (Ladenay & Friedlander, 1995), and allegiance to the treatment model (Patton & Kivilghan, 1997), which have also been found to be core elements of effective supervision across models.

LISTENING TO THE PRACTITIONER

Just as I-FAST emphasizes listening to clients and empathizing and validating families, supervisors are encouraged to listen to, empathize with, and validate their supervisees. Falender and Shafranske (2004) emphasize the importance of warmth and genuineness by supervisors, as well as developing a supportive relationship with supervisees. They emphasize empathy and validating as major components of effective supervision. This means allowing practitioners to vent about difficult cases without judging them, hearing them out about their views on the case regardless of whether these views fit with I-FAST or not, and validating their struggles on their cases. When practitioners feel listened to, they are then more receptive to new ideas on their cases.

TRUSTING THE PRACTITIONER'S JUDGMENT

Trusting a practitioner's judgment on cases goes along with strengths-based supervision. Knowing when a practitioner's judgment can and cannot be trusted is a skill for any supervisor. In I-FAST supervision, it is assumed that practitioners' judgment can be trusted under certain conditions: first, when their own personal biases are not dominating their thinking, and second, when they have an empathic connection with the family and client. If they are clearly biased, or if they have not gained or have lost their empathy for a family, in these instances, the supervisor's job is to help practitioners regain empathy, or recognize their biases are clouding their own judgment.

On the other hand, when a practitioner does have an empathic connection with the family and is relatively objective, the practitioner's judgment can be trusted and in fact should be relied on regarding a multitude of therapeutic issues. What goal or specific problem does the practitioner think the family might buy into? What frames would they like? What tasks might make sense to them? When a practitioner is properly connected to the family, the supervisor can trust the practitioner's judgment on these issues and may also rely more heavily on him or her to come up with ideas the family is likely to respond positively to.

It could be argued, especially for beginning I-FAST practitioners, that they inherently miss important aspects of interviews and so trusting their judgment is questionable. They do not know what they do not know, so to speak. Feist (1999) notes the limitations of practitioner descriptions due to limited conceptual and observational abilities by the practitioner. Although the limitations for trusting practitioners' judgments have been noted, regarding when the practitioner's judgment can be trusted, the literature appears to be amazingly silent. It may often be true that beginning practitioners may not be aware enough of important aspects of their family interviews to be able to verbalize certain issues or ask certain questions. It is suggested here that if they are empathically connected to the family and unencumbered by serious biases, when asked questions by the supervisor regarding what goals, frames, or tasks a family might like, their connection to the family will inform their responses and those responses can be trusted. Practitioners may not know what they do not know, but if they are connected to the families, they will know it when they hear it.

UTILIZING PRACTITIONER RESPONSES TO SUPERVISOR IDEAS

Just as the practitioner skill of observing and utilizing client responses in treatment is emphasized in I-FAST, it is also a major skill in I-FAST supervision. In I-FAST, a major emphasis is placed on observing responses and being responsive to them. If the practitioner is empathically connected to the family, what the practitioner accepts or rejects as ideas appropriate for a given case should be a guide to supervisors. In this process, supervision is a give and take with feedback going in both directions. It is a collaborative process, not a top-down communication. Just as in treatment, when a family rejects an idea, this should be received as data and information about the family, in supervision when a practitioner rejects an idea this should be taken as information about the family and further inform the supervisor about what the family will ultimately accept and respond to.

As stated previously, research on model fidelity suggests that allegiance to the model is more important than strict adherence to it (Wampold, 2001). The issue is winning the hearts and minds of participants rather than obsessively forcing them to adhere to something. If the goal is winning their allegiance, then an approach to supervision must be adopted that is different from one intended to monitor and maintain adherence to fidelity measures. How does one get someone to change his or her belief system? One way is to adapt to and utilize his or her existing belief system. To do this, one must become interested in what the practitioner already believes and has skill in doing. One must think how these existing beliefs and skills can be retained and utilized in the model. The supervisor must approach the practitioner with respect and in the spirit of collaboration. This is a different approach to supervision than what might be expected when the goal of supervision is to obtain and monitor adherence to something. It also parallels the core beliefs of the I-FAST model when working with families and larger systems. The same ideas go for respecting the strengths and perspectives of the supervisee and building on them.

The Setting

Community mental health centers and other agency settings can be very demanding places to work, requiring heavy case loads, with overwhelming amounts of paperwork, and at low pay. When agencies require their staff to work from specific models the staff themselves did not choose to learn, with strict fidelity guidelines the staff must be constantly monitored on, adherence to that model can easily become one more burden placed on an already overloaded plate. Staff morale in these settings is typically not good, as evidenced by high staff turnover in many of these clinics. How to fit a model in this setting that improves rather than further diminishes staff morale becomes a crucial question regarding both sustaining the model in the setting and obtaining positive outcomes on cases. Perhaps the demands of these settings and how to fit a model into them provides the best guideline for how to best address the above raised issues with respect to supervision of I-FAST.

It is assumed that practitioners will be more likely to develop an allegiance to a model if their existing skill set is respected and incorporated into the new model as much as possible. If at all possible, they are not asked to give up cherished beliefs and skills. It is also assumed that practitioners will buy into a model if they have choices on how to work within the model and those choices are made in a collaborative supervision process as opposed to a top-down approach in which the supervisor is primarily a teacher. Finally, buy-in is intensified if what the practitioner is doing is working. Nothing helps morale and model buy-in more than successfully helping a family.

If these assumptions are correct, then I-FAST supervisors would be wise to place a greater emphasis on helping the practitioner succeed on their cases than on rigidly adhering to fidelity. They would be wise to view supervision as collaborative and respect what the practitioner already knows and believes and to seek out and utilize the practitioner's feedback on cases. This makes supervision a two-way collaboration rather than a top-down communication. In this way of approaching supervision, the practitioner is the customer, not the model. Although the ultimate goal is allegiance to I-FAST, on a case-by-case basis the goal is for the practitioner to find the encounter helpful and useful. The practitioner should be the customer the supervisor is attempting to satisfy.

STRATEGIZING

Expanding the Practitioner's Skills

One emphasis in I-FAST is to utilize practitioner's existing skills and incorporate them into I-FAST as much as possible. If a practitioner is skilled at solution-focused or structural family treatment, most of their skill set can easily be included in I-FAST. At the same time, the flexibility and integrative nature of I-FAST affords practitioners with a wide range of ways of learning new methods to do treatment. In supervision, learning opportunities frequently arise regarding decisions and choices that must be made on cases. As noted in chapter two in I-FAST, treatment choices must be made on each case regarding a range of therapeutic issues that in other models are dictated by the approach. In I-FAST, frames can be constructed on each case, rather than provided by the model. Constructing frames can become a new skill to learn for practitioners accustomed to being given the frames by the model they are familiar with. In many models, unit of analysis and decisions on whom to work with directly are also choices that are dictated by the approach. Learning to think in different units and work with different subgroups of the family can also become a new skill for many practitioners.

In teaching flexibility to groups of practitioners, the list that follows has often proven useful. Different approaches emphasize different skills listed below.

Evaluating I-FAST Skills

Practitioners and supervisors can utilize the following list to see what skills the practitioner already has that fit into I-FAST and what additional skills they can learn that also fit into I-FAST.

Skill	Strength	Growth
• Establishing alliances		
• Constructing frames		
• Identifying clear problem/goals		
• Thinking in different units		
• Flexibility on who to work with		
• Identifying patterns/exceptions		
• Use of frames as an intervention procedure		
• Use of questions as an intervention procedure		
• Use of tasks as an intervention procedure		
• Tracking change/following up on interventions		

As a given case unfolds and these issues arise in supervision, dealing with these decisions in supervision becomes a tool for expanding the practitioner's knowledge and skill base. In I-FAST, much of a given practitioner's skill set can be utilized on a given case. However, if the family does not respond, in I-FAST there are numerous ways to adjust and find a way of working that the family will respond to. These are the times when practitioners can learn new skills as they attempt to match the family and find a way to work with them that they will respond to. In addition, when stuck on a case, practitioners may be more open and receptive to learning a new approach. They are not forced to give up their own beliefs and skills at the outset of a case. They are asked to consider something new when they themselves see the necessity of doing something different. This is a more respectful and collaborative approach to supervision in which a model does not have to be force fed to a resistant practitioner but can be offered in smaller doses when the practitioner is most receptive to learning something new.

The Minimum Elements Needed to Be Practicing I-FAST

Although I-FAST supervision emphasizes flexibility and utilizing existing practitioner skills and beliefs, ultimately these skills and beliefs must fit within the larger I-FAST frames to be faithful to the model. The following is the minimum requirement for a practitioner to be faithful to I-FAST:

1. **Collaboration with colleagues.** In numerous evidence-based in-home treatment models, the approach to colleagues on the case is to either insist they are off the case, or take a back seat on the case while in-home treatment is occurring. In I-FAST, listening to, collaborating with, and reaching agreements with other colleagues who share the case is emphasized. How to share the case and work together is the goal.
2. **Parent friendly.** I-FAST practitioners must be parent-friendly. They must be willing to view parents in a positive light despite the potentially unfortunate ways a parent may be dealing with their child. The practitioner who is out to save a child from the "damaging" influence of a parent is not operating within the frame of I-FAST.
3. **Focus on something specific that the parents agree to focus on.** It should be clear what problem the practitioner is helping a family to solve, or what goal they are trying to achieve and this represents something the parents' desire to focus on.
4. **The problem is understood in an *interactional* context.** Ideally I-FAST practitioners understand specific problems and specific goals interactionally. They are either able to track habitual interactions that support the problem or are able to track interactions that represent exceptions to these habitual interactions or both.
5. **Flexibility in choosing whom to work with.** Whom to work with is a strategic decision made on each case. I-FAST offers flexibility on this decision. The decision is based on the practitioner's skill, what the family will cooperate with, and on what patterns are being focused on for change.
6. **Offering frames the parents agree with that set a treatment direction.** I-FAST practitioner and supervisor construct overarching treatment rationales that the family will accept and allow treatment to be organized around.
7. **Offering frames the parents agree with that set up interventions.** The rule is no intervention is offered without a frame and that frame must first be accepted by the family before the accompanying intervention is given.
8. **Offering interventions that promote deviations from patterns.** The I-FAST practitioner and supervisor devise interventions that have an obvious connection to resolving the problem the family is requesting help on while simultaneously requiring the family to either deviate from the interactional patterns that support the problem or amplify exceptions to those patterns.
9. **Following up with interventions.** When interventions are offered, they are followed up with in detail. Detailed information is obtained about what was done, what was not done, how it was decided to do or not do something new, how everyone else responded, and most importantly if whatever was done produced any kind of change.

IMPLEMENTING

Case Consultation

Case consultation involves verbal case presentations and discussions between practitioner and supervisor. Although over the years, family treatment has emphasized live supervision and demonstration interviews as a way of teaching and supervising, within community mental health and similar agency settings, by far the most frequent opportunity for supervisor and practitioner to interact is within the format of case consultation. Case consultation is the most widely used form of supervision (Goodyear & Nelson, 1997). Advantages of this form of supervision include:

- It is time efficient and thus allows for discussion of multiple cases (Lee & Everett, 2004).
- As opposed to live-supervision, or tape review, it is more conducive to focusing on the broader picture of a particular case (Lee & Everett, 2004).
- It allows for more focus on merging theory and practice (Lee & Everett, 2004).
- It promotes practitioner autonomy and development (Nichols, 1988).

Disadvantages include:

- It is an inaccurate way of presenting the raw data of the treatment process (Campbell, 2000).
- It is limited by the conceptual and observational abilities of the practitioner (Feist, 1999).

I-FAST Recommends Weekly, One-Hour Contact with Each Staff Member

Although this can be expensive, if successful, staff morale and productivity can be enhanced, allowing the time devoted to consultation to pay for itself. When staff members are successful and excited, their attitude carries over to their work with families. They are more likely to develop positive connections with their families and this can lead to less no-shows in treatment and thus increased productivity and less staff turnover.

GOALS OF CONSULTATION

It is important to begin a consultation with an understanding of what the practitioner wants to accomplish during his or her time with the supervisor. There are a number of possibilities.

- **Allowing a practitioner to vent.** Just as it is important to validate the family's difficulties and struggles, it is equally important to validate the practitioner's struggles. They may have lost his empathy for a family and just need to vent his complaints and struggles on the case. It is important to allow for this. The supervisor must allow for the practitioner to express his struggles on the case before attempting to shift the practitioner's view of someone.
- **Validating.** Sometimes a practitioner has an idea about where she wants to go with a case and is simply seeking reassurance that what she has in mind is OK. She is not stuck on the case and is not requesting help to change anything she is doing. They want validation that what she is doing is alright. As long as what she has in mind fits within the broader frames of I-FAST, her ideas should be validated.
- **Celebrating success.** Sometimes a practitioner just wants to share and celebrate a success. He may be excited about a positive outcome and want to

share this with his supervisor. It is important to include success stories in supervision. Just as it is important for practitioners to follow up on interventions with families, it is important for supervisors to follow up about families who have been the focus of past supervision, particularly if the case is going well. Supervisors need to hear about success cases to assess fully the skill level of their supervisees and to avoid supervision focusing only on problem cases. This allows for a positive tone of supervision and facilitates a positive supervisor/practitioner relationship.

- **Helping the practitioner past an impasse.** This is the most common goal of consultation, but it is important for the supervisor not to assume every case presented is a request for help getting unstuck. Before offering suggestions, it is helpful to ascertain the practitioner's idea for where and how she is stuck and what specifically she needs in the consultation. If the practitioner is viewed as the customer, and helping the family is viewed as the primary purpose of the consultation, an overemphasis on adherence to I-FAST should be avoided.
    - An important consultation goal is to obtain an affirmation from the practitioner that consulting has provided something that makes sense to him that he can do to help get unstuck. The practitioner deciding to write something down is one sign that the consultation is useful to him. The goal should be for an idea or ideas to be generated from the discussion that the practitioner has some confidence will help. It is not important whose idea it is, or even that the idea is overtly stated. What is important is that the consultation end with the practitioner receiving something of value that he believes he can implement in the treatment. The supervisor or the practitioner or the interchange between the two can generate that idea.

ASSESSING WHERE THE CASE IS IN THE TREATMENT PROCESS

An early step in a consultation, especially when help is needed to get unstuck, is for the supervisor to assess where the case is in the treatment process. Is the practitioner stuck engaging important participants? Does she have an interactional understanding of the problem? Is she stuck with formulating a useful goal, or at initiating change, or at following up on interventions and supporting change? If the practitioner is ahead of the family, pushing goals that the family is not interested in focusing on, or if she is behind the family and not aware that positive change is already occurring, then the practitioner herself will not have an accurate understanding of where the case is in the treatment process. For a supervisor to understand where the case is in the treatment process, therefore, she must ascertain if the practitioner is in synch with, ahead of, or behind the family.

ASSESSING IF THE FAMILY AND PRACTITIONER ARE IN SYNCH, AHEAD, OR BEHIND EACH OTHER

Practitioners can be in synch with, ahead of, or behind families at any point as treatment unfolds. This continuum refers to how well the practitioner is matching the family's attitude toward change.

- **Ahead of families.** Being ahead of the family refers to situations in which the practitioner is pushing for change or focuses on goals that the family

has not agreed require change. The family may not feel change is needed, or they may feel change is needed regarding a different problem than what the practitioner is pushing for.
- This error can be common when practitioners become over-joined with probation officers (POs) or child protection case workers who have referred the family for treatment. The PO may be very involved with the family and pushing a court-ordered agenda on the family. To satisfy the referral source and or the court, the practitioner adopts the referral source agenda and pushes it on the family as well. The practitioner may then describe the family as noncompliant or unmotivated to change. In these cases, the supervisor must refocus the practitioner on what the clients say they want and on how the family is viewing the necessity or non-necessity of change.
- **Behind families.** Practitioners are behind a family when change is occurring but the practitioner either does not realize the changes are happening or responds as if they are not happening. This problem can arise in several ways.
  - It can occur when practitioners push for changes other than what may already be occurring. The practitioner is focusing only on whether change is happening regarding his goals.
  - It can also occur when change is happening incrementally and/or outside the practitioner's observations. When change occurs incrementally, the changes may be off of the practitioner's radar.
  - Also, as noted earlier, change can be initiated simply by validating and empathizing with clients, and/or when clear goals are agreed on. Change can be initiated when practitioners are not expecting it to be and so they do not inquire about it.
  - Perhaps the most common way practitioners get behind a family occurs when they do not follow up properly or in enough detail with interventions they have already given. A common error for beginners is not following up with interventions that are intended to promote change. Tasks may be given and accepted in one session, and in the next session additional tasks are given without inquiring about the outcome of the previous tasks or without obtaining detailed descriptions of how everyone responded to the earlier task given. Continuing to give tasks implies change is still required or not happening at all. When changes are occurring, the proper response is not to continue to give new tasks, but to understand exactly what changes have been initiated and then supporting them. In these situations, supervisors should focus the practitioner on following up in detail on previous tasks given.
  - Practitioners can also miss change if they view tasks as assignments and not experiments. As noted, offering tasks can inspire families to come up with their own solutions. They may not do the task, but receiving it gives them their own idea for how to produce improvement. If practitioners are operating from a model that requires homework to be completed, they can get too focused on what the family did not do and miss what they did do. By getting over-focused on the roadblocks of doing the homework, the practitioner fails to inquire what the family did do instead and if this produced change.

- A final way a practitioner can be behind the family also relates to matching the family's position on change and on what they want from a treatment provider. Though much emphasis is placed on restraining practitioners from pushing goals and treatment on families who are not ready for it, the opposite problem can also occur. The family can be desperate for help, in crisis, and wanting direct intervention and advice from their treatment provider and the provider can be busy just validating, looking for strengths, and asking about exceptions. There are families who want help and want to be told what to do. They want their practitioners to be experts. For these families, restraint is not meeting their needs.

Struggles with Colleagues

Cases can become stuck when professionals who are concurrently on the case develop impasses with each other. Outpatient practitioners working individually with the child, POs, and case workers are the most common participants that family focused in-home treatment practitioners may butt heads with. An impasse with colleagues can occur at any point in the treatment process. There are three common scenarios. First, goals are not agreed on. Second, safety is an issue. One constituency believes the situation is unsafe, or has imposed safety interventions that another constituency believes are not necessary. Third, change is not acknowledged by one constituency that is acknowledged by another. One response to such disagreements is for the practitioner to over-join with the family and become hostile to professionals who are seen as unfairly imposing their professional power on the family. The most common scenario occurs when an in-home practitioner successfully helps a family make changes but a probation officer or child welfare worker does not acknowledge those changes and continues to impose safety measures on the family. The in-home practitioner's response is then to become hostile to the PO or case worker. In this scenario, the in-home worker is over-joined with the family and too detached from the case worker or PO. He must intensify or regain his alliance with the PO or case worker before attempting to persuade them that change has occurred.

When a supervisee is in a struggle with a colleague, the supervisor must first direct the practitioner to hear her colleagues out and make sure the colleagues feel listened to, understood, and that their concerns are valid. Not doing any of these can be the primary cause of the impasse. Second, when disagreements occur among professionals the disagreements are often *ideologically* driven, not *case driven*. The fight is over theory, not fact. One way out of this is to focus the practitioner on the facts of the case. What, specifically, have her colleagues observed that is of concern to her colleagues? Case workers and POs also go into homes and they may have observed something directly that is of legitimate concern. When the facts of these concerns are tracked down it is easier to obtain agreements on how to deal with them. Inquiring into the facts alone is one way of being respectful to the colleague. It is being assumed that they have important knowledge about the case. Also, once the facts are shared, the opposing colleague now may feel heard and understood and therefore become more receptive to reaching an agreement. Once alerted to new facts, the in-home practitioner may agree that there are indeed safety issues or that more change is still needed.

Therapeutic Alliance

One of the most common causes of a therapeutic impasse is a problem with the therapeutic alliance. An important participant, in I-FAST usually a parent, is not engaged or the practitioner has a hostile attitude toward the parent and has lost empathy for him or her. If a practitioner is not joined with an important participant it is first necessary to obtain an agreement from the practitioner that this is indeed where they are stuck. The practitioner must accept the goal of going out and obtaining an alliance, or re-obtaining one.

Assessing a relationship without the benefit of direct observation is a special problem. In case consultation the supervisor has only the description to go on.

- When a practitioner describes a parent as noncompliant, or preferring crises, or some other derogatory descriptor this typically indicates the practitioner has lost his empathy for the parent. This is a general rule but is not always the case. When offering live supervision, for example, a supervisor may be given a negative description of a parent by the practitioner, and then directly observe an interview in which the practitioner is obviously joined with the parent.
- Another sign that a practitioner may not be joined with a parent is that the practitioner knows very little background information about the parent, or is aware only of the presenting problems in the family. The family has not opened up to the practitioner. This may be an indication that the family does not trust the practitioner.
- On the other hand, when a client or family member decides to open up and tell about their own background, or tell about other serious problems in the family, this could be a sign to practitioner and supervisor that the family member has decided to trust the practitioner.
- Sometimes practitioners can assume that a family member's disclosure of additional family problems is an invitation to offer help on those problems. When practitioners do assume these disclosures are invitations to focus on additional problems, the practitioner can become overwhelmed and unfocused.
- Instead, when families open up about additional problems it should first be taken as a sign that the family trusts the practitioner. This is a sign that a therapeutic relationship is established, not an invitation to focus on additional problems.
- When a trusting relationship has not been established, a useful task to give the practitioner is for them to learn the family history and life story of the parent. When given this task, the practitioner must think about how she is going to win the trust of the parent so the parent is comfortable telling about their own background. The practitioner is not oriented toward what task to give or what goal to focus on, which is inappropriate if the family members do not yet trust the practitioner. Also, by learning more about the life story of a parent, the practitioner is more likely to develop empathy for that parent, and this then will produce the proper conditions for a therapeutic relationship. When a practitioner comes back to supervision after being given such a task, if successful, the supervisor will usually note a changed and more compassionate attitude toward the client.
- A second common problem for therapeutic relationships occurs when the family is patronizing the practitioner. During the sessions, the family agrees

on goals and agrees to try different ways to solve the problem, but then never follows through on anything. This will typically produce a frustrated practitioner who describes the family as noncompliant. Families may have learned from past experience that professionals, particularly ones who come into the home, have power and cannot be trusted. For them, the most intelligent way to deal with such professionals is to tell them what they want to hear and hope they go away sooner.

- Typically, when a practitioner is being patronized, he will become frustrated with the family and perhaps upset that the family does not appreciate that they are trying to help. They might even have the attitude that the family owes them their trust and respect as a professional. Sometimes, the higher the degree of the professional and the more the professional has invested in obtaining their expertise, the more the professional has the attitude that the family owes them their trust and respect.
- The problem when being patronized, however, is that the family does not trust the practitioner. We all must remember that trust is not owed to us; it must be earned. It is on the practitioner to earn that trust and demonstrate to the family that they can be trusted. When being patronized, the practitioner must earn the family's trust before any goal can be truly established and certainly before any interventions can be offered. Once it is recognized that a family is patronizing, the practitioner must essentially start the treatment process over and focus on obtaining an alliance. Goals the practitioner may have thought the family agreed to must be put aside. The practitioner must demonstrate she is going to be different than previous interveners. Once it is recognized that the client is patronizing the practitioner, the practitioner must reassess what the client's position on change is and then match whatever that is.

Goal Consensus

A second common problem that produces a treatment impasse relates to goal consensus. Either there are no clear goals, or the goals the practitioner is focusing on are not the goals of the family. Families with multiple problems can produce an unfocused treatment. Every session the focus is on a different problem. The practitioner goes around in circles, focusing on one problem one week and another problem the next with no progress on any. In this scenario, there are no priority goals. One way out of this problem is simply to have the practitioner ask the family what problem is the most upsetting to them. They may not have asked this. Another possibility is to find a central problem that if solved will simultaneously help on other problems the family is bringing up. Sometimes this will help a family get focused. A third possible solution is to engage other family members in the goal-setting process. If only the mother has been worked with, the father or a grandmother or another adult in the home can be included in the discussion about what specific problem or goal to focus on. Often, when more than one adult in the family can agree on this, the treatment will then focus on the goal that has obtained a larger consensus.

Perhaps the more common goal problem is a practitioner focusing on a goal or goals that the family is not motivated to work on. This can easily occur when too much emphasis is put on what stakeholders and referral sources want, confusing the idea that stakeholders and referral sources, not the family, are the customers.

The rule is you work for who pays you. If it is the medical card, the court does not possess it—the family does. Though collaborating with and satisfying stakeholders and referral sources is very important, the reality is, the focus of treatment must ultimately be on what the family themselves want. Stakeholders and referral sources are more likely to be satisfied if a practitioner can focus a family on solving some problem, even if not the exact ones the referral source wants solved. Often, when successful, a domino effect can occur and in the end, everyone's goals can show improvement.

Useful questions for supervisors helping practitioners focus on family goals include: What problem are you trying to solve? Who is upset about that problem? Who wants what from you? When you first met with the family, what did they say they wanted help with? How did they describe the problem? What word or words did they use to describe it? When they no longer have the problem what will that look like? The practitioner who is not focusing on the family's goals will have difficulty answering these questions and should be sent to find out what the answers to them are.

Identifying Interactions

Once an alliance has been obtained, and specific problems have been identified that the family wishes help on, treatment is now entering a middle phase where interventions are needed. A major goal of an I-FAST supervisor is obtaining an interactional understanding of the problem being focused on and the goal being pushed for. Can the practitioner describe an interactional pattern associated with the problem? Can they identify exceptions and who does what differently when those exceptions occur? There are two common errors.

- One is that the practitioner can describe what the problem person does only when he has the problem. She cannot describe what everyone else does in response, or the interactions about the problem among secondary participants. She has not inquired into how the family habitually attempts to solve the problem.
- A second common error is that the practitioner gives interventions without any awareness of the patterns involved with the problem. A strict focus on behavioral interventions can sometimes produce this error. Offering interventions without knowing the patterns associated with the problem allows for the possibility that the interventions can be reinforcing the very problems they are intended to resolve.

When problems are being described by a single family member, that family member will typically not offer an interactional description. She may offer her theory about why the person with the problem has the problem, or may offer a detailed description of what only the problem person does, leaving out how everyone else is responding when the problem person exhibits the problem. In this instance, I-FAST practitioners must be coached to inquire about and closely track how everyone involved responds when the problem occurs and how they all talk to each other about the problem.

When observing families directly, beginning practitioners will err most often by interrupting the interactions before they have reached their habitual conclusion.

Typically, the practitioner's internal limit to conflict, or their belief in what is proper parenting, or their observation of boundaries either being violated or not existing will motivate them to interrupt the process. This is a difficult error to detect in a case consultation setting and will most likely be apparent on videotapes or during live supervision.

A supervisor can habitually ask the practitioner questions regarding interactions in the hope that the practitioner will eventually internalize them. What does everyone else do when the problem occurs? How does each person respond when the problem happened, or when he heard about the problem? Who offers advice, what is the advice, and does the recipient agree with it? Who talks to whom about the problem and what do each of them say about it? This will produce a practitioner who wants to be able to answer those habitually asked questions in supervision. The supervisor will be in his mind when he is interviewing the family and will then more likely make sure he obtains the information. At some point, practitioners themselves will learn the value of having an interactional understanding of the problem and they will be able to obtain one on their own.

Identifying Interactional Exceptions

There are two common mistakes when working from a perspective of finding and amplifying interactional exceptions. First, the family is not given enough of a chance to tell about and commiserate over their problem. The practitioner is so busy being positive and looking for strengths that the client does not feel heard or understood. The client may feel like the practitioner does not appreciate the severity of the problem. When this problem occurs, the client does not feel validated. The practitioner has too quickly pushed his frame on the client before the client is ready to receive anything.

When a client does not feel the magnitude or severity of their problem is appreciated by the practitioner, the client will not only not improve but may also become worse. A pattern between practitioner and client can emerge in which the more the practitioner attempts to find strengths, normalize, or be positive, the more the client feels compelled to prove to the practitioner that the problem is worse than the practitioner realizes. This pattern can emerge with any way of working with clients, not just with an approach that emphasizes exceptions. When this pattern occurs with practitioners attempting to identify exceptions, the client will not cooperate with finding exceptions until she feels the practitioner understands the severity of her problems.

A second mistake that can arise from working primarily with identifying exceptions has already been noted. Some families are ready for change and desire direct interventions from professionals. They expect the practitioner to be an expert and give them advice. In this instance, the family may feel let down by the practitioner, and lose their faith and hope that the practitioner can help.

Unit of Analysis and Getting Unstuck

Sometimes changing the unit of analysis in which the case is being conceptualized can solve an impasse. There are two possibilities. Sometimes when treatment is unfocused and/or the practitioner is confused and unable to focus, it is due to information overload. The practitioner has too many problems and too many people in mind when conceptualizing the case. In this case, the practitioner is over-thinking the case and the supervisor can help by helping the practitioner simplify the way she views the family and problem. If the supervisor can help focus the practitioner on a smaller unit a doable plan can then be devised.

On the other hand, cases can also become stuck when the practitioner is oversimplifying how she conceptualizes the case and over-focusing on particular goals. One way this problem presents itself is when specific goals are being reached but the family is reporting no improvement. This can occur for two reasons. First, the problem being focused on is not the main problem the family wants help on. Treatment may be focused on getting a child to school and this goal may be in the process of being reached, but the problem in the family is that the single mother is ill and requires the child who has been truant to stay home and help look after his younger siblings. In this example, the larger picture has not been grasped by the practitioner and she has put a focus on a problem that does not make sense given that larger picture. She is oversimplifying the case.

A second way families will report no improvement when change has obviously occurred happens when the client improves but someone in the family has not recognized it and this person's participation in the pattern is not on the practitioner's radar. For example, a teenage boy was truant from school, belligerent at home with his mother, and failing academically. With help, the mother changed how she dealt with the boy and his attendance and grades improved. He and his mother began to get along better. Despite these obvious and verifiable improvements, the mother complained that nothing was better. The practitioner was baffled. Enlarging the unit from mother and son to include mother, stepfather, and son made the situation comprehensible. The stepfather was angry over numerous complaints of his own. He constantly nagged the mother about the boy. Even though the boy's behavior improved, the stepfather's nagging the mother did not. The mother then reported "things" had not improved. She was indirectly referring to the stepfather's nagging. Once the unit of analysis was enlarged to include the stepfather, the case made sense to the practitioner. Cases can be oversimplified or overcomplicated. When one or the other of these occurs, supervisors can help to expand or contract the unit of analysis to break an impasse.

Constructing Frames

Constructing frames is typically one of the more difficult skills to learn. Practitioners trained in other models typically have been supplied with pat frames from those models and so have not had to learn the skill of devising frames for each case. There are two types of frames that need to be devised on any given case, overarching frames, or treatment rationales that set a direction for treatment, and frames that set up tasks. Many practitioners have received training in models that provide overarching frames and pat frames used to set up interventions. They have not learned the skill of constructing frames to fit each unique case.

When a treatment is in trouble regarding frames it is either because the client does not buy the overarching treatment rationale, or does not buy the specific frame offered to set up interventions. In either case, the practitioner is not tuned in to the client's belief system and must be oriented to what that is to ensure frames are offered that will make sense to him.

If possible it is often wise to allow practitioners to begin a case offering the frames they are accustomed to using. This is OK as long as offering the frame is not in itself going to lose the case. If the practitioner offers the frames she does know and the family does not respond, the practitioner will then be more open and motivated to learn how to construct a frame that the family will respond too. If the practitioner is empathically connected to the family, she can be asked what she thinks the family would buy into. If she cannot come up with her own ideas, the supervisor can offer suggestions until a frame has been found that the practitioner affirms the family will like. This is a collaborative supervision process in which the practitioner's feedback is trusted and relied on.

Using Questions and Responses
A common error for practitioners is that they use questions or responses based on the theoretical orientation of the selected approaches without noticing the inherent nature of communication as constructive and directive, and are thereby not able to utilize fully the power of language in the process of change. Consequently, I-FAST supervision aims to develop BOTH the sensitivity and skills in practitioners regarding the use of questions and responses as an intervention procedure. In I-FAST supervision, we help practitioners to comprehend clearly that questions are not just for acquiring information for understanding or assessment purposes. Instead, I-FAST supervisors help practitioners to recognize fully the importance of and develop the skills to construct and ask useful questions for the following purposes: (1) to help clients develop or change frames, (2) to reinforce or change behavior and interaction, and (3) to initiate a self-evaluative process so that families take ownership of their change process.

In addition to constructing useful questions, the second set of skills is for the practitioners to formulate consciously and appropriately their responses to preserve, delete, or transform clients' dialogues for change purposes. Though most practitioners have a broad sense of how to respond to their clients usually based on a particular approach or therapeutic style, practitioners might not pay close attention to the moment-to-moment communication, despite the fact that these interactions convey important messages to clients. Preserving clients' language will reinforce a particular view or direction. Deleting any part of client's description will distract the therapeutic conversation from that end, while transforming clients' description will lead to a new perspective or viewing of the phenomenon. Because therapeutic communication is dynamic and fluid, practitioners will need to know clearly and explicitly the parameters as to what types of questions or responses will be helpful and consistent with I-FAST assumptions and values. Consequently, an important task in I-FAST supervision is for supervisors to clearly help practitioners to embrace I-FAST assumptions of change that include (1) problems and solutions are viewed as interactional as opposed to individual-focused; (2) a strengths-based perspective that clients have the ability and resources to change and do something different as opposed to a deficits-based one that may imply that clients do not have the ability to change; (3) problems are viewed as transient as opposed to being permanent, stable, and global; (4) clients take ownership of the change process as opposed to the change process being involuntary or external; and (5) it is more helpful for questions and responses to be open as opposed to closed.

Devising and Offering Tasks
Practitioners often request help devising tasks. The first requirement is a detailed understanding of the interactional patterns associated with the problem. Tasks can be devised to interrupt any part of the pattern whether it involves those directly engaged

with the problem person, or those who interact with each other about the problem. It is best if the task comes from the practitioner. One way to elicit a task from the practitioner is to ask: "If the family would do anything you asked to solve the problem, what would you ask them to do?" Often when asked this, practitioners can come up with a task. If not, the supervisor and practitioner can list multiple ways each pattern participant could deviate from the pattern if he or she chose to. This is often a useful exercise for beginning practitioners. Once a task or tasks are identified, the practitioner should be asked how to frame the task so it will make sense to the family. How does one sell it to them?

There are several common errors related to giving tasks that will generally result in clients not doing the task or initiating changes on their own. The errors will most generally present themselves to a supervisor as a practitioner who is frustrated with the client and/or describing the client as noncompliant or unmotivated.

- **Offering tasks when the client is not ready for change.** If the client is not at a stage of the change process at which she is receptive to actively changing something and the practitioner is offering tasks, the practitioner is ahead of the client and the client will most likely not be responsive. In this situation, the supervisor must help the practitioner match the stage of change the client is in and this will most likely mean not offering tasks.
- **Not having the proper attitude about tasks.** If a practitioner is of the view that his tasks must be completed, if he views the task as a trick to try to get the client to do something, or if he thinks his task is brilliant and will work if the client would just do it, the practitioner has an improper attitude about tasks. If he truly believes his task must be followed, or if he is trying to be manipulative, he lacks a respectful position toward the client. When this happens, the task either will not be followed, or if it is, the client will not be given credit for the improvement. When tasks are truly viewed as experiments, not merely framed as them, the practitioner truly does not know what will happen and is truly curious about what will happen. This attitude maintains the practitioner in a genuine, humble position and the client in a respected position.
- **Offering tasks while frustrated with the client.** When practitioners become frustrated with clients, regardless of this, they often do intervene. When this happens and the client still does not follow through on the task, the practitioner will usually become even more frustrated. When a practitioner is frustrated with a client, she has lost their empathy for that client. When this happens, the proper response by the practitioner is to regain her empathy and this means not intervening. In this instance, the supervisor must restrain the practitioner from intervening and help her regain her empathy for the client.
- **Offering tasks that do not relate to the client's goals.** Offering tasks that are not related to the goals or problems the client wishes to focus on is a very common error. When this happens, the supervisor must orient the practitioner to what the client wants and make sure interventions offered relate directly to that.
- **Offering tasks without offering a frame.** Offering tasks without offering any frame to set them up is also a common error, especially with new

practitioners. When this happens, the supervisor must orient the practitioner to the motives, values, goals, and language of the client to help him come up with frames the client might like.
- **Framing the task in a way the client does not buy.** Sometimes a practitioner will offer a frame for the task, but the frame does not make sense to the client. She is not buying it. Despite this, the practitioner pushes forward with the task anyway. When this happens, the supervisor must again orient the practitioner to the client's motives, values, goals, and language to help him construct frames the client might buy.

Following Up on Interventions

A common error with beginning practitioners is failure to follow up on interventions. A typical scenario involves a practitioner continuing to give tasks week after week without following up with previously given tasks. When this happens, practitioners can often be unaware of changes that have been instigated by previous interventions. They can fall behind the family. Besides being unaware of improvements, by continuing to give new interventions, the practitioner is behaving as if no changes have occurred when in fact they may have.

One of the major skills in intervening is following up in detail on exactly what has happened since the last session. Has anything improved? If so, what has improved and how? Who did what? How did they do that? How did they decide to do what they did? How did everyone else react? When supervisors grill practitioners with these types of follow-up questions, practitioners are more likely to follow up with interventions on their own.

Another error that can occur if the practitioner is not strengths-based is being skeptical when families do report positive change. Instead of inquiring in detail what they did and how they did it and celebrating improvement, the practitioner pushes for changes in other areas or dismisses the improvement being reported. Supervisors should always inquire if the family is reporting improvement and what those improvements are.

Changing Whom to Work with

When a treatment is stuck for reasons other than lack of alliance and goal consensus, often a powerful variable to change that can resolve the impasse is whom the practitioner is working with. There is an old family treatment guideline that says "when stuck add people." The larger conceptual issue involves changing who is being worked with. This could mean either expanding or contracting the group. If one parent and child are the primary participants in interviews, the other parent could be recruited. If the entire family is regularly participating, a smaller subgroup could be chosen as the focus. Perhaps one individual can be chosen to work with. In some instances, recruiting extended family can produce a big change. Changing who participates is a powerful intervention by both practitioner and supervisor. It is perhaps a more powerful aspect of treatment to change than changing frames, goals, or interventions offered. Often this can be the difference maker if a treatment is really entrenched. It requires skill at how to frame the change to the family so no one feels blamed or singled out and it makes sense to the family to change who will participate in treatment. If the change involves recruiting someone new, skills are required for how to engage them successfully in a process that has already been underway and how to conduct the first interview they participate in so something positive comes from their addition.

Termination Problems

Cases can become stuck at the end when termination is near. The most common problems include:

- The family does not take credit or notice significant change.
- Powerful colleagues on the case do not acknowledge change.
- The family has anxiety about termination and continues to ask for help on new problems.
- The family is having difficulty adjusting to change.

Termination problems typically present in supervision as one in which either relapses continue to be reported as termination is discussed or the practitioner is drawn into new problem after new problem as termination is approaching. The supervisor must then assess why the family is having difficulty terminating.

Techniques for helping families take credit for change have already been presented. Sometimes, despite the use of these techniques, the family continues to give credit for change elsewhere. Sometimes this is understandable. If a teen has been on probation, even when the family changes how they deal with the teen and these changes clearly helped, there still may be belief by the family that fear of the court was a major factor in helping their teen settle down. The family then fears what will happen when the court goes away.

Another problem occurs when a PO or case worker who has remained in the background during in-home treatment is now prepared to get seriously involved again if treatment terminates. The PO may believe that change has not really occurred or the changes that have occurred are not sufficient. The family may then be anxious about this. When colleagues cannot be persuaded that significant change has occurred, the decision for the supervisor is either to keep the case open until the court is finished or the PO is truly satisfied that change has occurred, or to step the case down to less intensive clinic services. Any of these options may prevent the PO from becoming re-involved in a way that may produce a relapse. When the in-home supervisor is also responsible for supervising other clinic programs stepping the case down can be an ideal solution. The supervisor will continue with the case and ensure continuity.

When practitioners present cases in which the presenting problems are solved and the family is bringing up new additional problems they wish help on, there are two possibilities:

- The most common possibility is that the family and practitioner are having difficulty disengaging from each other. Going into homes can produce powerful connections between practitioner and family. It then can become difficult to part ways when the time comes. The most typical sign of this is the family relapsing or bringing up new problems when termination is near.
- A second possibility is that the family is having difficulty adjusting to change. This is most common when treatment produces changes that are rapid and require major reorganization of the family. The most common

signs of this are: an adult in the family deteriorates, or there is a threat of divorce by one of the parents.

A family having difficulty adjusting to change and a family having difficulty letting go of an in-home practitioner are two separate issues and must be dealt with differently. If the family is having difficulty adjusting to change, it is often wise to remain on the case and focus directly or indirectly on those difficulties. Tips for doing this have been offered elsewhere. On the other hand, if the family is having difficulty letting go of the practitioner, it is an error to offer new interventions.

- When the problem is a family and practitioner having difficulty disengaging from each other, this problem will emerge in obvious connection to termination. The practitioner can be drawn into a pattern of the family continuing to bring up new concerns and the practitioner responding by offering new interventions as termination is imminent. In this situation, the act of offering new interventions indirectly suggests the family does indeed continue to need professional help, when the problem is convincing them they no longer need such help.
- One way out of this is to instruct practitioners to stop offering interventions. They can empathize and be curious how the family will solve the new problem, but not offer help or ideas for how to do so. This is a way of disengaging gradually by first ceasing to offer help but remaining involved anyway. If this is effective, the family will solve the new problems they bring up without help from the practitioner, demonstrating that they no longer require advice and then the practitioner can completely disengage.
- When a family is struggling to adjust to major changes, their reaction to the change is typically swift and acute. The two most common reactions are the acute deterioration of another family member, usually an adult, or the threat of divorce by the client's parents, either of which occurs in obvious connection to the positive changes. In these instances, the practitioner must stay involved and ensure the original client does not relapse in the face of new family problems.

Helping Practitioners Get Unstuck

To summarize, I-FAST practitioners can become stuck on a case at any point in the treatment process. One can divide the process up into beginning, middle, and end of treatment problems. Beginning treatment problems occur when the practitioner is unable to engage a parent, or agree on a specific problem or goal, or focus a family on something specific. Middle treatment problems occur when the practitioner is not able to identify interactional patterns or exceptions to them, or is unable to construct frames the family responds to, or is unable to construct tasks that focus on the problem and require pattern deviations. End of treatment problems include not following up on interventions, not tracking and supporting changes that are occurring and, especially with in-home treatment, not able to terminate without relapses.

Because I-FAST offers a wide range of choices at each step of the treatment process, supervisors have a multitude of ways to help practitioners get unstuck. Goals can be changed, frames can be changed, unit of analysis can be changed, whom to work with can be changed, and what intervention approach to offer can be changed.

The variety of these choices increases the possibility that some approach can be devised that the family will respond to; which choice to change depends largely on the stage the treatment.

BEGINNING TREATMENT ERRORS

Following is a summary of types of errors and the stages of treatment in which they typically occur:

- The practitioner is not strengths-based. He or she does not believe the family is changeable or has the resources to solve the problem.
- The practitioner does not use pre-suppositional language that fosters hope and possibilities of change in participants.
- The practitioner continues paying attention to repetitive negative, blaming, or self-defeating descriptions and thus reinforces these conversations when those descriptions no longer provide useful information to the practitioner in tracking interactions.
- The practitioner is frustrated and not aligned with the parent(s).
- The practitioner is ahead of the family and pushing for goals the family has not identified they want help on.
- The practitioner and family do not have something specific to focus on. They both go back and forth on different problems and cannot maintain a focus.

MIDDLE TREATMENT ERRORS

Often there are errors that occur in mid-treatment such as:

- The practitioner is pushing an overarching frame the family does not buy.
- The practitioner has insufficient information to identify a pattern or an exception.
- The practitioner's unit of analysis is too large and he or she is confused or unfocused.
- The practitioner's unit of analysis is too small and he or she is over-focused on a problem that does not make sense to focus on, or the family is complaining that change is not occurring even though progress is made on the goal being focused on.
- The practitioner is offering interventions without frames that make sense to the family.
- The practitioner is unable to construct tasks and interventions that require deviations from patterns, or amplify deviations.
- The practitioner is offering tasks but the family is not responding.
- The practitioner does not have key participants engaged in the process who are needed to produce change.
- The practitioner is unable to recruit key participants into treatment who are needed to produce change.
- The practitioner misses opportunities to use questions in helping clients develop or change frames, or reinforce/change behavior and interaction.
- When a family is describing positive changes, the practitioner does not recognize and reinforce the change, thus missing the opportunity to reinforce positive change efforts.

- When a family is engaging in repetitive blaming- and negative-talk, the practitioner does not redirect the conversation in a more helpful direction.

 END STAGE TREATMENT ERRORS

The list below notes a number of errors common to the end stage of treatment.

- The practitioner continues to offer new interventions without following up on previous interventions.
- The practitioner is behind the family. They are unaware of change.
- Significant change has occurred but key participants do not acknowledge the changes.
- Goals have been met and acknowledged but when the practitioner begins to terminate, relapses are reported or additional new problems are brought up.
- The practitioner continues to offer interventions at a point in treatment when practitioner and family must disengage from each other.
- The family does not take credit for change.
- The practitioner did not use language that reinforces family's ownership of the positive changes.
- Important and powerful colleagues do not acknowledge change.

The Use of Video in Supervision

The use of videotapes in supervision can be an intensive learning tool for practitioners and a reliable method of informing the supervisor about crucial aspects of treatment. I-FAST recommends using this method in conjunction with case consultation and live interviews. This form of supervision has been rated as the most valued by both supervisors and practitioners (Goodyear & Nelson, 1997). It is valued as both a teaching tool and an effective form of modeling when it includes supervisors showing tapes of their own work (Larson et al., 1999). By viewing tapes of sessions the supervisor can observe directly how the practitioner is interacting and connecting with the family, how the family is interacting with each other regarding the problem, and how the family is responding to the practitioner's attempts to empathize, offer goals, and offer interventions. The use of videotapes in supervision can be utilized in group and individual supervision but is perhaps best suited to individual supervision. Without knowing what is on the tape, a supervisor allowing the practitioner to show it to a group of colleagues, sight unseen, can produce unanticipated dilemmas. When viewed individually the supervisor is freer to comment without having to consider the politics of the group.

- Advantages of this form of supervision include:
    - Sections of tape can be replayed to stress important concepts (Protinsky, 1997).
    - Alliances are more obvious (Protinsky, 1997).
    - Replaying segments allows for identification of interactions and provision of role play opportunities (Haynes, Corey, & Moulton, 2003).
    - Viewing tapes across time can show how the practitioner is developing (Haynes et al., 2003).
    - Enhances understanding of how all parties are actually interacting (Whiffin, 1982).

- Can allow for the identification of the practitioner's personal biases (Lee & Everett, 2004).
- Disadvantages include:
  - Practitioner anxiety of being videotaped (Lee & Everett, 2004).
  - Can produce too much focus on a single session rather than the larger clinical picture of a case (Nichols & Lee, 1999) or overall case planning (McCollum & Wetchler, 1995).

It is often not possible to view an entire tape in the space of the typical one-hour supervision, especially if the tape generates intense discussion. It is therefore wise to ask the practitioner to make sure a priority is given to seeing the parts of the interview the practitioner most wants the supervisor to review. Doing this will ensure the supervision meets the needs of the practitioner. The goals for the supervisor can include obtaining a good sense of the relationship between family and practitioner, making direct observations for how family members interact with each other, and getting a sense of what interventions the family is responding positively to or might respond positively to. Ideally, viewing the tape will intensify the supervisor's grasp of the practitioner's skill level as well as his or her understanding of the particular family. This intensified grasp of the family can then become useful in future supervisions regarding the case. Viewing the tape can generate intense case discussions and enhance learning for the practitioner. Tips for the use of videotape review include (Lee & Everett, 2004):

- To reduce practitioner anxiety, collaboratively decide on specific questions to focus on during tape review.
- Have the practitioner prepare segments important to him or her to review.
- Process what the practitioner has learned at the end of the tape review.

Team Day

I-FAST recommends setting aside at minimum one half day per month for staff to meet as a team to discuss cases and do live demonstration interviews and/or live supervision. Staff can take turns bringing families and presenting cases. The ideal group should consist of staff from across departments, not just limited to in-home treatment staff. This is especially ideal if cases are shared or referred across departments. Conducting teams this way ensures continuity of care and a shared view of the case among staff from different departments. It can help to ensure I-FAST is not just done in a remote corner of the agency, but has influence with outpatient, case management, and other staff who may share cases with the in-home treatment team.

Team day can serve multiple purposes. First and foremost it should be a fun, engaging, stimulating, and useful day for staff. Promoting this type of atmosphere enhances creativity, learning, and especially staff morale. It should be a day staff looks forward to. Offering this type of time can help retain staff as well as provide a regularly scheduled time to continue to teach and reinforce I-FAST within the agency. If the time is organized properly and staff look forward to team day, it can produce an effective atmosphere for learning I-FAST concepts, increasing staff receptivity as well as demonstrating directly both how I-FAST is implemented on actual cases and its effectiveness in treatment.

Live Supervision

Live supervision, in which the supervisor participates directly by observing interviews behind a one-way mirror or from another room viewing a monitor, is an effective way to both train new staff (Saltzburg, Greene, & Drew, 2010) and help experienced staff past a therapeutic impasse. In addition, live supervision can be employed on a clinic "team day," in which a group of practitioners also participates behind the mirror or in an observation room. In this format, supervisors can observe directly the interactions of family members and family and practitioner and can intervene directly if the situation requires. Montalvo (1973) offers guidelines for carrying out live supervision, especially when it also involved a training group observing.

- Advantages of live supervision include:
    - It provides the opportunity to observe family interactions directly and to modify those interactions (Montalvo & Storm, 2002).
    - It provides first-hand knowledge about both family and practitioner skills (Lee & Everett, 2004).
    - It can provide immediate help for practitioners in over their heads (Lee & Everett, 2004).
    - It can change the direction of a case that is stuck or in crisis (Lee & Everett, 2004).
    - A team of observers can also learn and participate (Lee & Everett, 2004).
- Disadvantages include:
    - It produces serious practitioner anxiety (Haynes et al., 2003).
    - It can become a hindrance to the development of practitioner autonomy (Lee & Everett, 2004).
    - It can dilute the practitioner's authority with the family (Lee & Everett, 2004).

STEPS OF LIVE SUPERVISION

Live supervision with concurrent training groups can be broken down into steps, with goals and protocols identified for each segment.

- **Planning the interview.** Before beginning the interview, the supervisor and practitioner must organize a plan for conducting it. By the end of the planning session it should be clear to the supervisor and practitioner what the goal of the session will be. The goal might be gaining an alliance with a particular family member, establishing a clear goal for treatment, identifying patterns, or constructing frames and tasks. The practitioner should have a clear direction agreed on with the supervisor for how to conduct the session. The plan should include how the practitioner will frame the beginning of the session to set a direction and gain family cooperation. From the supervisor's standpoint, the plan should allow for an interview in which the supervisor can observe the family and have flexibility regarding different directions in which the session might go. This allows the supervisor and practitioner to be responsive to how the family responds during the interview. A generic plan might include having the family summarize what the treatment has been about, what the goals have been, and what has helped so far. From this discussion, a direction for the session that fits in with where the treatment is in the treatment process can be generated.

- **Introducing the set up to the family.** The practitioner should obtain an agreement from the family for conducting and taping a team interview before the session. The team and supervisor should be described as added consultants. The family should be informed about possible phone calls and a consult with the team at the end of the session. If the family does not want to do the session this way, their wishes should be respected. Generally, if the practitioner is comfortable working this way, the majority of families will be also. On the other hand, if the practitioner is reluctant to work this way, the family is most likely to be hesitant also. Families can be given the option of meeting the team before the session and seeing the observation room if they desire.
- **Phone calls.** During the interview, the supervisor is free to call in suggestions and interventions. Phone calls should be brief and include one or two concrete instructions. The general rule is to limit the number of phone calls to three per session; however, this should not be taken as a rigid rule. If a serious error that could jeopardize the case is being committed, the supervisor should call regardless of how many calls may have preceded. If the family and practitioner are responding positively to calls and not seeing them as interruptions, additional calls can be made. What should be avoided is creating a situation in which the practitioner is awaiting the next instructions from the supervisor and not asserting himself in the interview. Too many calls can sometimes produce this phenomenon. Generally speaking, over-intervening by the supervisor can result in the practitioner losing credibility with the family (Lee & Everett, 2004).
  - When considering if a call is warranted, Liddle and Schwartz (1983) suggest:
  - Consider the urgency and necessity of the call.
  - Consider the possibility that the practitioner may do what the supervisor has in mind on her own.
  - Consider whether the practitioner can implement the suggestion.
  - Consider whether the call may impede the practitioner's authority with the family and/or their autonomy.
  - The interview should be conducted with the idea that the family and practitioner will go on meeting on their own, and so a direction must be set that the practitioner can carry out with his or her relationship with the family improved or at least intact. What is called in should be considered optional, with the practitioner's judgment respected as to how exactly to phrase something and even if it should be done or not. If the supervisor thinks an error is clearly being committed and the case could be in trouble, they should specify that these particular instructions are not optional. If the practitioner is not in agreement, he or she can politely dismiss themselves from the interview and come to the observation room to discuss the situation (Montalvo, 1973).
- **Behind the mirror etiquette.** The tone of the discussion behind the mirror should reflect a positive, strengths-based approach by the supervisor. This tone is crucial for several reasons including reducing participants'

anxiety about taking turns in front of the mirror. Discussion behind the mirror should be respectful, positive, and constructive if mistakes are made in the interview. The supervisor should set the tone by how they talk about the interview and how they respond to what the practitioner is doing in the interview. Both practitioner and family should be framed positively by both the supervisor and team behind the mirror.

- **The session-break and team feedback.** When the practitioner comes behind the mirror for a break, he or she should be given final questions and interventions for the family to end the session. Goals the family has identified during the session should be central. How the family has framed problems and words the family has used should be incorporated into the questions or interventions offered. The supervisor should have an idea of interactional patterns based on what was said during the interview and how the family interacted with each other. When the practitioner enters the observation room, there should be only one spokesperson for the group, usually the supervisor. The practitioner cannot be bombarded with numerous suggestions from numerous participants. The supervisor can obtain feedback from the group before the practitioner comes into the observation room. Before offering interventions the supervisor should inquire if the practitioner has his or her own ideas for how to end the session and what to offer the family. During the break, the practitioner should write down suggestions and so suggestions can be more numerous and accurate in communicating them to the family. It is often a good idea to have the practitioner repeat back how she intends to end the session so it is clear she has thought through what she wants to offer and how she wants to frame it.
- **Processing the interview.** Processing the interview with the team affords excellent teaching opportunities as well as a forum for sustaining I-FAST in the agency. It is important to obtain the interviewer's perspective on what he viewed as key moments in the interview, what he felt was helpful input from the supervisor and the team, and what he thinks the next step in the treatment process should be. Besides eliciting important feedback, this keeps the practitioner in a respected position, allows him to think through his own case, and establishes a precedent in the group that encourages others to volunteer to bring in a case.
  - Also important in the post-session discussion is the supervisor describing how she arrived at interventions, what patterns she observed, how she constructed frames, what the family said during the interview that inspired her ideas, and how she devised tasks. These discussions should be lively, positive, and promote a learning environment that practitioners look forward to as opposed to one more task they must complete at their clinics.

The use of live supervision with practitioners and teams can be thought of as a high-risk/high-reward method. If used properly, staff morale, practitioner development, and learning and an intensified therapeutic modality for families can be offered. To achieve this, the supervisor's attitude and manner with their teams, not just their skill in the use of live supervision, is paramount. Producing a climate conducive to openness, willingness to take risks, and a spirit of fun is vital. Lee and

Everett (2004) listed being personable, open, genuine, and willing to acknowledge their own mistakes as important attributes of supervisors when using this form of supervision.

Demonstration Interviews

A variation of live supervision is the demonstration interview. It holds most of the same advantages and drawbacks of live supervision with an added benefit of giving the supervisor or trainer a chance to demonstrate the model in real time with the team of practitioners involved.

Demonstration interviews can be a valuable learning tool. In a demonstration interview, the supervisor or trainer solicits a case from the group that presents particular difficulties. The case can then be discussed with the entire group on a team day using the I-FAST perspective. The idea is for the team to come up with an approach or a set of questions that may lead to a new direction. Then the supervisor or trainer has the practitioner gain permission from the family for the supervisor to join in a session with the team as a part of the process through either closed circuit video or through one-way mirror observation. Assurances of confidentiality are offered and the family is invited into an agency setting to accommodate the interview and observation. As the session begins, the practitioner introduces the supervisor as a colleague from his team who would like to take the lead in asking some more questions and maybe help with some new directions. Often the practitioner sits directly beside the supervisor or just off his shoulder to offer easy line-of-sight for all members interviewed with both interveners. These demonstration interviews typically follow the following format:

- **Planning the interview**. As discussed previously, the entire team is invited into discussing the dilemma around the case and they jointly develop a strategy they feel will be helpful for the session. They also discuss how the family may best be made comfortable with the consultation process and decide on what the team may need to look for to help with the demonstration.
- **The first interview break**: Soliciting questions from the team. Usually a longer time is set aside for these sessions. Most often these demonstrations are scheduled for from an hour and a half to two hours. This allows for the supervisor and practitioner leading the interview to conduct an initial interview segment of around 30 to 45 minutes and then take a brief break to consult with the team. The clients are given a break as well. Then the supervisor and practitioner share their views of how the planned strategy has gone in their view and they request input and ideas from the team observing. A next step plan of action is then devised and the session is reconvened. This break usually lasts from 10 to 15 minutes.
- **Processing the interview**. The interview then is brought to a conclusion and the supervisor and practitioner reconvene with the observing team. The supervisor offers ideas and input on what she felt she was able to do, pointing out particular tactics or frames or interventions and noting their response. Questions and feedback are invited from the group in a way that makes this kind of training and supervision a very real and engaging process. Real-time learning with live cases is energizing and offers real credibility to the model and brings life to the interventions.

SUMMARY

I-FAST supervision is strengths-based, focusing on utilizing existing practitioner skills within the context of the I-FAST model as much as possible. Obtaining practitioner allegiance to I-FAST is a primary goal. To help obtain this, supervision is viewed as collaboration between the supervisor and practitioner with an emphasis on resolving cases. Teaching opportunities arise when a practitioner is stuck and his or her usual methods of treatment are not working. Although I-FAST supervision emphasizes flexibility and permission for practitioners to work in the ways they are most familiar, I-FAST practitioners must operate within the major concepts and treatment steps of I-FAST. The most common errors associated with each I-FAST step have been reviewed. I-FAST supervision can be offered in the form of case consultation, review of videotapes or live supervision, and supervisor demonstration interviews. When teaching I-FAST and helping to sustain it within a community mental health setting, hands-on learning methods such as live supervision, review of videotapes, and observation of supervisor-demonstrated interviews are highly recommended.

FITTING I-FAST AND AGENCY TOGETHER

11

CREATING SUSTAINABILITY

CONCEPTUALIZING

The difficulties of successfully implementing and sustaining evidence-based (EB) in-home treatment models that have been devised and researched under controlled settings in the more diverse, uncontrolled, and "messy" settings of community mental health clinics and other public agencies has been noted throughout the EB literature (Hoagwood et al., 1995; Rowe & Liddle, 2003; Sexton & Alexander, 2002). Henggeler, Schoenwald, Rowland, & Cunningham (2002) found that when implemented in community settings multisystemic treatment was half as effective as when used in a laboratory setting. Despite these findings, Goldman et al. (2001) reports there are no standardized methods for how to implement these models in community mental health settings.

Families at risk for having a child removed from the home present many challenges to mental health agencies. These families often have multiple and longstanding problems. To qualify for services it is necessary for the child with the presenting problem to receive a formal diagnosis based on the *Diagnostic and Statistical Manual of Mental Disorders (DSM)*. In addition, the child is often prescribed psychotropic medication to treat the diagnostically related symptoms. A frequent effect of receiving the diagnosis and medication is that the primary method of treatment is individual treatment with the child, with the involvement of the parents being ancillary to the treatment process. Treatment such as this usually is long term with a high rate of dropout. Even when the child and family remain in treatment it is not very effective. In recent years several EB family treatment approaches have been developed to address these issues. These EB family treatment approaches have been found to be effective but many mental health agencies that originally embraced them found that they could not be sustained over the long term and consequently "de-adopted" them for a variety of reasons such as costs; difficulty hiring and retaining qualified staff; and poor match with the agency's philosophy, culture, and climate (Massatti, Sweeney, Panzano, & Roth, 2008). Given these realities we have developed methods of implementing I-FAST in agency settings that we think address these issues and enhances sustainability of I-FAST in agency settings.

Evidence-based Family Treatment Models
Recall from the beginning chapter of this workbook/manual that there are four well-established EB approaches to family treatment: Brief Strategic Family Therapy (BSFT; Horigan et al., 2005; Szapocznik et al., 2002), Multisystemic Therapy (MST; Henggeler, Schoenwold, Rowland, & Cunningham, 2002; Schoenwald & Henggeler, 2005), Multidimensional Family Therapy (MDFT;

Hogue, Liddle, & Becker, 2002; Hogue, Liddle, Becker, & Johnson-Leckrone, 2002; Liddle, Rodriguez, Dakof, Kanzki, & Marvel, 2005), and Functional Family Therapy (FFT; Sexton & Alexander, 2005). An EB approach that is not as well established is Ecosystemic Structural Family Therapy (ESFT; Lindblad-Goldberg, Dore, & Stern, 1998). For the most part, these current family treatment approaches were initially developed outside mental health agencies. This often creates problems of agency/model fit when community mental health and other related agencies adopt home-based EB models.

Community Agencies: "Messy" Environments

Despite difficulties with fit, many community mental health systems and public agencies have made efforts to adopt home-based EBPs. The main challenge posed in the EB literature for sustaining fidelity of their models is how to control treatment in a mental health clinic and community environment. Contrary to the controlled environment of research programs, community agency delivery of services is very "messy." The typical family referred for intensive in-home treatment may have multiple mental health professionals and other community professionals all working with them simultaneously. They all may be working with different family members, and/or with the same family members but focusing on different goals. Powerful court appointed professionals such as case workers or probation officers can also share the case, but not share the goals or treatment philosophies of the mental health professionals working the case. How to offer a focused, singular treatment within this environment presents a real challenge.

> **A CASE EXAMPLE**
>
> A 14-year-old girl who is very sexually active, using drugs, failing in school, and running away from home at night is already in treatment at a mental health clinic. The clinic has diagnosed her as bipolar. She has a psychiatrist who is giving her medication to treat her bipolar disorder. The diagnosis defines her as having a biological illness and calls into question what she has voluntary control over. She also has an individual practitioner. The practitioner is employing cognitive-behavioral therapy, viewing the problem as the girl distorting events and becoming emotionally reactive to them. The practitioner has also become sympathetic to the girl's complaints about her mother and stepfather. The mother and girl also have a case manager who is working with the two of them together. The case manager goes into the home and is trying to help the mother parent the girl differently. This is contrary to how the individual practitioner is working with the girl and also contrary to the idea that the girl's behaviors are involuntary. The girl is also in group treatment focusing on making better choices.
>
> At some point, the school files truancy on the girl and the court gets involved. A probation officer is assigned. The probation officer sets the rules for the girl at home and expects the mother to enforce those rules. This is contrary to how the case manager is working with the mother. The probation officer also orders the girl into drug court and adds a drug treatment component to the case. In addition to all of the previous practitioners, she now also has a drug treatment practitioner.

> The girl's younger brother and sister are also receiving services from the mental health clinic. One is diagnosed with attention-deficit/hyperactivity disorder and the other with oppositional defiant disorder. They both receive medications and also have individual practitioners. One is also in group treatment focusing on social skills. The mother describes herself as depressed and is also receiving medications and is in treatment. The majority of all of the services that the family is receiving is from one community mental health clinic. In all, four family members are receiving services from a total of eight professionals focusing on at least seven different problems.

If this family is assigned to an MST or FFT or I-FAST program, one problem is how to measure the effects of this additional service in the context of a multitude of services. Solving this problem has been the main focus of how to implement EB treatments in a community mental health setting. How to offer an EB model that is not interfered with by other professionals on the case and how to sustain fidelity to the model within this diverse setting has been the focus.

Clearly, looking at this case example, how to maintain fidelity and offer an EB model that is not contaminated by all of these additional services is problematic. But equally clear is that this is not the only problem that must be addressed regarding successful, long-term implementation of EB models in this setting. If an EB model is offered to this family, what happens to all of the other professionals? Even if they agree to step aside while the EB model is offered, what happens when the EB model is finished? It is very unlikely that this family will go forth and not have any services after in-home treatment is complete. What will happen to the outcomes obtained by the EB model once a symphony of professionals re-enter the case who are not family systems oriented or strengths-based? As previously noted, families having a relapse after intensive in-home treatment has been successfully completed has been a serious problem.

SUSTAINABILITY OF EFFECTIVE TREATMENTS

Within the EB literature, three factors have been identified as crucial for sustaining fidelity within community mental health agencies:

- Implementation of the program within the setting (Sexton, 2011; U.S. Public Health Service, Office of the Surgeon General, 2001)
- Organizational support (Beidas & Kendall, 2010)
- How other professionals are involved on the case

Successful implementation of an EB model within an agency requires attending to how implementers interact with various agency programs, the culture of the agency, the background and training of the staff, and the type of clients served (Sexton, 2011). Attention must be paid to how the agency and model fit together. Although this is identified as a very important factor for successfully sustaining EB models, little attention has been paid to this issue. The major in-home models implement their programs within community agency settings by setting up their own staffs, sometimes supported by trained internal supervisors and ongoing periodic contact with model consultants. The main focus is to devise a support system within the clinic whose sole goal is to maintain fidelity to the model from the front line staff who are delivering it. These staffs and their supervisors function separately and independently from other clinic services. They are not truly integrated into the array of other clinic services.

Organizational support has been defined as pre-training support from the agency employing the trainee and a commitment from the agency to pay for ongoing supervision in the EB model for those agency personnel trained in that model. If EB models are to be widely disseminated and sustained it is argued that organizational support from within the clinic settings in which EB-trained practitioners operate must be obtained. This is described as a *systems-contextual* perspective (Beidas & Kendall, 2010).

How other professionals who share cases with EB models are dealt with has gained considerable attention regarding the potential to contaminate fidelity to the model. How probation officers, children's services case workers, or other mental health professionals who may share the case with the EB practitioner can potentially interfere with or undermine EB treatment has been noted by the major in-home models. The traditional and most common method of dealing with this problem has been to insist to other professionals who share the case that they must recess their involvement on the case while in-home treatment is being delivered. This practice was begun by the Homebuilders model, the first intensive in-home model (Kinney, Booth, & Booth, 1991), and later adopted by both MST and FFT. Becoming the exclusive treatment provider ensures fidelity to the model. Only staff members trained in the model have direct dealings with the family. Henceforth, we shall refer to the setting up of separately functioning EB home-based staffs within mental health clinics and the exclusive dealings with cases as the standard model for sustaining fidelity within community clinic settings.

THREE LEVELS OF SUSTAINABILITY

Considering the de-adoption studies that show the struggle to sustain EB models long- term and the studies that point to relapses after termination of intensive in-home services, we define sustainability more broadly than simply maintaining fidelity within community agency settings. When considering sustaining I-FAST we consider three levels of sustainability:

- Maintaining faithfulness to the model
- Sustaining the use of I-FAST within the agency on a long-term basis
- Maintaining I-FAST outcomes once the case is terminated and stepped down to less intensive treatment

The standard model for sustaining fidelity does not address the problem of sustaining outcomes once a case has terminated treatment or stepped-down nor does it address the long-term difficulties of sustaining expensive EB models within publicly funded mental health settings.

STRATEGIZING

Agency/Model Fit

When viewing sustainability more broadly to include the agency's capacity to sustain I-FAST long term and sustaining outcomes obtained by I-FAST practitioners as well as sustaining fidelity to I-FAST, agency/model fit must be examined in detail. An extensive analysis of the agency context and how EB services fit within that context must be obtained. Several questions must be addressed with respect to sustainability:

- How does a particular EB model fit into and operate within the larger array of services of a given agency?
- If a client completes EB treatment but requires further treatment, how is continuity of care sustained when a client moves from EB services to other agency services?
- How do EB and other agency staff collaborate if there are multiple clinic staff assigned to the same case?
- How does the theoretical orientation of a given EB model fit with treatment as usual in community mental health? If there are incongruities, how are they dealt with to ensure the EB model is sustained in a larger agency environment that operates differently?
- What is the impact of training specific agency staff in an EB model with the larger staff of the agency?

These questions must be adequately addressed to successfully implement and sustain I-FAST within a given agency. We propose a five-step process to help address these issues:

1. Assess how training and implementation impacts the agency.
2. Assess agency functions and how services are delivered.
3. Enhance agency/model fit.
4. Strategically design a training package to fit with a given agency's staff and services.
5. Design ongoing agency procedures that will reinforce adoption of the model and help to ensure its sustainability after the training is over.

Long-Term Sustainability: How EB Training and Implementation Impacts the Agency

Understanding how EB training and implementation within a community agency setting impacts the agency is crucial to ensuring long-term adoption of the model within the agency. Three factors that impact long-term adoption of these models within an agency setting are cost, staff turnover, and how well received the model is by other professionals who work with client families. We will look at each of these factors in detail.

COSTS

Cost must first be addressed as a major factor in the dissemination and sustainability of I-FAST. The emphasis on EBPs in general denotes a major trend in the field toward more and more specialization. Taking the EBP trend to its logical conclusion suggests that in the future each diagnosis will require an EB approach. For example, to satisfy stakeholders, community mental health clinics will be pressed to purchase EB models for traumatized children, school phobic children, depressed adults, substance abusing adolescents, conduct disordered youth, and so on. This trend is on a collision course with the reality of funding for social services in general. Many have experienced and continue to experience draconian budget cuts for social services, and mental health will not escape these funding realities.

Specific EB models can also be cost prohibitive by design. Initial training alone can be costly. In addition to initial training costs, many EB models require ongoing consultation. These requirements create a dependency on EB consultants to sustain the model, incurring never-ending consultation costs.

Hidden (Uncompensated) Costs

Besides overt costs of initial training and ongoing consultation, many EB models impose hidden uncompensated costs to agencies. Some approaches vastly increase paper work requirements for practicing practitioners. This requires significant time commitments that cannot be devoted to direct, billable service with clients. Practitioners' caseloads and productivity requirements must be reduced to accommodate the additional paper work demands. Producing less billable hours costs the agency dollars that cannot be billed for. Finally, data collection can also result in additional hidden costs to agencies. Time spent by support staff and practitioners at data collection is a real cost.

Currently EB models are often funded by grants or by pooling community resources. This type of funding cannot support EB model after EB model, particularly considering all the costs of each model. With funding cuts many clinics may be hard pressed just to pay the salaries of line staff. Paying for multiple costly EB models in addition to normal operating costs can be severely prohibitive for many if not most agencies, threatening the long-term sustainability of EB models.

TRAINING AND STAFF PRODUCTIVITY

Sensitivity to how EB training will affect staff productivity is essential when considering how EB training can impact a given clinic. A balance must be struck between offering sufficient training as to allow minimum competency in the EB model, and how much staff time will be tied up being trained and not producing billable hours.

STAFF RETENTION

In addition to the costs of the EB program, retaining staff is also an important factor influencing the long-term sustainability of the model within a community setting. Staff retention indirectly relates to cost and overall effectiveness of the program. Constantly replacing staff costs money. New staff must be trained and their caseloads must be brought up to full levels; both of these cost money. In addition, every time one person leaves and a new practitioner comes on board, the continuity of the staff group is disrupted. Working relationships are severed and new ones created. There is no chance to develop a well-oiled high-functioning team in this environment. Someone is always coming or going.

Staff retention has been a chronic problem for several intensive, in-home models (Glisson, Schoenwald, Kelleher, Landsverk, Hoagwood, Mayberg, & Greene, 2008). The difficulty of the cases taken by intensive in-home programs, the pressure to produce good outcomes, and the pressure to stay faithful to the model are all factors that contribute to staff departures. Models that stress strict adherence to fidelity tend to offer a top-down approach to supervision. Feedback from the practitioner is minimized. Opportunities for practitioners to utilize what they have learned from other approaches and/or being creative are limited. Practitioners can become disgruntled and feel unheard and unsupported in this model of supervision. This can then also contribute to staff departures.

HOW THE MODEL IS RECEIVED BY OTHER PROFESSIONALS ON THE CASE

Stakeholders are typically very sold on these models as they represent cost-effective, EB methods of working with difficult cases. But how do other professionals who work concurrently on the cases receive these models? As stated, the standard approach to achieving fidelity while in-home models are actively on the case is to insist that all other professionals recess while in-home treatment is involved. This is not a negotiated agreement. It is typically a requirement for the in-home model to take the case. Clinic treatment providers must be out. Probation officers are asked to take a back seat. It is clear why this is done. As noted on the example case, a multitude of providers concurrently offering services can at a minimum contaminate fidelity and at worst cause the case to fail. The issue is how this decision is arrived at. If other professionals are simply instructed to remove themselves from the case, as opposed to the decision as to who is in and who is out being made collaboratively, it can be assumed that the EB model will be negatively received by other professionals. Our own study on de-adoption indicated this. One complaint of community professionals about EB models is their insistence on exclusivity on the case and that this decision is not negotiated but forced on everyone. When some of these professionals work within the clinic itself in which the EB model is being implemented, this can exacerbate the problem.

How the model is received within the clinic itself may also be affected by the decision on whom and whom not to train. The status of those who receive EB training is elevated among their clinic colleagues by virtue of having received special training. The question becomes, whose status can be elevated without disrupting the clinical hierarchy? Giving outpatient practitioners special training that is not given to clinical supervisors, for example, can depower the supervisor's ability to supervise the newly trained staff.

Some EB models require ongoing consultation from EB trainers. This essentially amounts to clinical supervision. When this is done, clinic supervisors are depowered and replaced by consultants who are experts in the EB model. Deciding whom and whom not to train in a given clinic is a strategic decision that should be made by being mindful of how receiving special training will affect the working relationships of clinic staff that operate from differing hierarchical positions within the clinic.

To summarize, long-term sustainability must address three issues:

- Affordable costs
- Staff retention
- The model must be positively received by other professionals who share the cases and especially from those who work in the same clinic.

Sustaining Outcomes

ASSESS AGENCY FUNCTIONS, SERVICES, AND HOW
SERVICES ARE DELIVERED

The difficulties of working from a family-oriented, problem-solving model within a community mental health setting have been well documented (Grove, 2009). Agency procedures are most strongly influenced by how services are billed for and by demands of accrediting agencies. Typically services are paid for by Medicaid. Medicaid dictates that services are organized around an individual and are diagnosis driven. A formal "diagnostic assessment" is typically done when a client first accesses services. This is a broad-based assessment that seeks to analyze the totality of clients' functioning and their social environment. These two procedures have profound impact on what services are offered and how they are delivered.

Specific problems are viewed as symptoms of a larger diagnosis. Problems are defined as ongoing illnesses as opposed to episodes. Parents may or may not be sufficiently engaged. Parents' goals may or may not be attended to. Parents may or may not be empowered to be the change agents regarding their child's problems. As the case described earlier illustrates, treatment as usual is diagnosis driven, defines problems as illnesses requiring ongoing contact with professionals, and is multifaceted and unfocused. Numerous professionals can and will be assigned to any given case, and those professionals will not represent a consistent treatment philosophy to the family. Problems will simultaneously be defined as medical, psychological, and interactional. Hence, there will be no focused approach. This can be described as "treatment as usual."

How does one fit in this environment an intensive in-home EB treatment, which operates as an episode of care model, is parent friendly, focuses on specific problems, is driven by what parents want help on, and conceptualizes problems primarily as interactional and individual and medical? What happens if an EB practitioner is attempting to empower a parent and focus a family on a particular problem, while other clinic colleagues who are concurrently on the case are unwittingly depowering the parents and focusing the family on completely different problems, or are defining the problem in a way that is contrary to how the EB practitioner is working? Clearly, understanding how the larger clinic operates and how EB treatment fits in this process is essential to maintaining EB outcomes after the EB treatment has been completed.

As noted, the standard method of sustaining fidelity solves the problem of doing EB treatment in the "messy" environment of community agencies but does not address problems of sustaining EB outcomes or sustaining the long-term adoption of EB models in community settings.

EB Treatment and Continuity of Care
How continuity of care will be maintained on a given case is an important consideration regarding sustaining outcomes obtained by EB treatments. Continuity of care can be affected by two issues. First, how well do professionals who share the case collaborate? Do they agree on goals? Do they agree who should be the focus of treatment? Do they share a similar way of conceptualizing the case? Do they share ways of framing the problems that are presented to the family? Continuity of care will suffer when families are exposed to numerous professionals who differ on one or several of these issues.

The second issue affecting continuity of care, as noted in earlier chapters, concerns who will work with the family once intensive in-home EB treatment is complete. Once the family has become accustomed to working with one treatment provider who works from a single model, how will they respond when they return to the treatment as usual model described previously? Once a family has received EB treatment that is parent friendly and empowering, is focused on goals parents choose, is nonmedical and non-blaming, how do these families respond if they are then stepped down to treatment as usual that is very different? We suggest that the vast differences between the ways the in-home intensive EB models approach families and particularly parents, and the ways families and parents are worked with in the treatment as usual approach impact both continuity of care and treatment outcomes. As noted earlier, relapse after intensive in-home treatment is an ongoing problem for many client families.

The standard method of sustaining fidelity solves the first problem. When no other professionals share the cases, families cannot become confused by differing approaches. However, this method does not address the problem of continuity of care once the case is referred back to other clinic services.

IMPLEMENTING

Enhancing Agency/I-FAST Fit

If intensive EB models are to be successfully disseminated and sustained on a large scale within community mental health, not only fidelity to the model must be sustained, but outcomes obtained by the EB treatments also must be maintained after termination, and the long-term use of the model within the clinic must be sustained. How to fit the model to the setting and the setting to the model becomes a major consideration. Although these problems have been identified in the EB literature, only sustaining fidelity has been addressed adequately.

Key Principles

How I-FAST fits into the agency setting is organized around four key principles:

- **Flexibility.** As a model, I-FAST is designed to be flexible enough to have wide applicability. It can be applied to the full range of child mental health problems. With wide applicability comes the possibility of wider influence with clinic services. This type of wide influence is not possible from models that focus on a narrower range of child problems.
- **Empowerment.** I-FAST is a clinic empowerment model. I-FAST certifies whole agencies, not individuals within agencies. Once certified, the agency owns the model. To ensure fidelity, certification must then be reviewed every two years by I-FAST trainers. However, at recertification time, each agency will likely have developed its own unique adaptation of the broad I-FAST model, if the model is working well. Agency recertification looks only at how the major core elements of the I-FAST approach are being sustained. We do not discourage adaptations of I-FAST unique to each agency culture, staff, and clients. In fact adaptations of I-FAST are celebrated at times of recertification. We aim to empower clinic staff to sustain fidelity to the model with minimal consultation with I-FAST trainers once training is complete.
- **Collaboration.** I-FAST emphasizes collaboration among professionals sharing cases. We do not insist on working cases exclusively. We teach and emphasize collaboration as a major component of our model.
- **Cost friendly.** I-FAST seeks to provide effective training and a model that can be sustained long term for costs that can be absorbed within the normal funding streams of community agencies.

These principles of flexibility, empowerment, collaboration, and cost friendliness are embedded in the I-FAST treatment model and are incorporated in numerous ways at all levels of clinic service delivery, from I-FAST training to supervision of I-FAST staff, to how other professionals are treated and finally to how families are treated. These principles are implemented to create a user-friendly EB model for mental health clinics and represent our attempt to be sensitive to the issues faced by mental health clinics from both a fiscal standpoint and the need to satisfy stakeholders.

Goals of Fitting I-FAST with Agencies

We pursue two goals when attempting to fit I-FAST with agencies:

- A true integration of I-FAST services within the larger array of services offered by the agency
- Influencing the treatment philosophy and procedures of the larger array of agency child treatment services

GOAL ONE

To fit I-FAST and agency together, we are suggesting a different approach from the exclusive EB treatment delivery approach. Instead of operating separately from the "messy" community agency environment, we embrace this environment and approach it holistically. We do not aim to set up a separate shop attempting to avoid contamination by the larger clinic's way of operating. Our goal is a true integration of our services within the array of services offered in the agencies. We want to collaborate and work with the rest of the clinic. This means making collaborative decisions. It means collaboratively deciding who should stay on the case or who should take a break while I-FAST in-home services are delivered. It means collaboratively deciding how to work together when I-FAST and additional clinic services share the case. Finally, it means collaboratively deciding who should take the cases that step down after I-FAST termination, what goals should continue to be focused on, and whom to work with in the family.

GOAL TWO

To achieve goal number one while maintaining both continuity of care and not confusing families while I-FAST in home treatment is being delivered, we pursue our second goal related to fitting into these settings. We aim for influencing the way all child services are delivered within the clinic and aim to sell our principles to the larger array of clinic services. This goal is possible due to the wide applicability and flexibility of I-FAST. I-FAST can be applied to the full range of child symptoms and can be adapted to outpatient and regular case management services. Training a wide range of staff does not mean all staff in every clinic service must be trained and be faithful to I-FAST. It does mean that we seek to broaden our influence within the clinic to include staff in services likely to work on cases simultaneously to I-FAST, or receive cases after I-FAST intensive in-home services have terminated. Typically this means outpatient treatment staff and traditional case management staff.

Key Strategies

To sustain fidelity, outcomes, and the long-term use of I-FAST, we recommend the following key strategies to clinics adopting our model.

TRAINING ISSUES

- **Training a wide range of staff.** To enhance collaboration among clinic staff while sharing cases, and to enhance continuity of care once in-home I-FAST services are complete, we recommend clinics offer I-FAST training to a wider range of clinic staff than just the in-home staff. We recommend outpatient staff and case management staff also receive I-FAST training. I-FAST training packages are tailored to each clinic, but emphasize both quality and quantity. A large number of staff can be exposed to I-FAST in introductory seminars. A select, smaller group, including intensive in-home staff, outpatient staff, and traditional case management staff can receive more intensive and lengthy training. The outcome should be that the entire clinic has a familiarity with I-FAST principles and a diverse group of staff representing several services have intensive exposure. The hope is that this will "grease the wheels" for clinic supervisors who are championing I-FAST and responsible for collaboration on cases among a multitude of clinic departments. It is also a way of bringing the larger array of clinic services more in line with I-FAST treatment philosophies. This sets up the capability of sharing cases and collaborating on clinical decisions.
- **Training clinic supervisors and supervision.** Clinical supervision costs money. Spending time going over cases clinically costs money. This money can be paid to outside EB model consultants, or it can be paid to existing clinical supervisors. In I-FAST, *existing agency clinical supervisors receive the majority of I-FAST training*. This *creates an I-FAST expert within the agency*, empowering the agency to sustain I-FAST without excessive ongoing consultation costs. This model has been well supported and long advocated in the literature such as in the book *Diffusion of Innovations* (Rogers, 2003). In exchange, the agency must make a commitment to offering in-house clinical supervision. We recommend I-FAST trained supervisors offer one hour per week of I-FAST supervision to I-FAST staff. Thus, I-FAST operates on a "trainer of trainers" model. We seek to create *clinic I-FAST champions* (Rogers, 2003) by focusing the majority of our training on clinic supervisors. Training supervisors is a strategic decision done for a multitude of purposes.

  - **Reduce costs.** By creating an internal trainer, ongoing EB consultation costs can be reduced or eliminated.
  - **Empowering supervisors.** The clinic supervisor is empowered by becoming the I-FAST "expert" within the clinic. The status of existing clinic supervisors is enhanced by training, not undermined by it.
  - **Continuity of care.** Most importantly, continuity of care for families is aided when a clinic supervisor who supervises staff from multiple services such as in-home services, outpatient services, and case management services is trained in I-FAST. Training supervisors with multiple responsibilities is one way for I-FAST principles to have influence in the larger clinic environment, not just with the in-home staff.

I-FAST supervision itself is designed to fit easily into the diverse professional environment of a typical community agency. As noted in our last chapter, I-FAST supervision aims at utilizing staff's existing treatment beliefs and skills. This gives supervisors the flexibility to apply I-FAST principles with a divergent staff from multiple clinic departments.

By training supervisors and offering a supervision model that is flexible and if agencies will commit to offering this type of supervision, the "messy" environment of the mental health clinic can be positively influenced. A singular general philosophy and approach to treatment in general is championed within multiple departments and programs of the clinic by a clinic staff member who has been empowered by both the clinic and I-FAST training to exert influence on how the clinic functions overall.

This enhances the ability of staff to share a case when home-based services are involved. They all share the same supervisor. The supervisor can coordinate services so continuity of care is not compromised. Decisions on who should stay on the case and how the case will be dealt with can be truly negotiated among staff members who share the same supervisor. The principle of collaboration can be applied to the issue of who works on each case.

Working this way, when I-FAST treatment is complete, the case can easily be transitioned back to professionals who share similar treatment philosophies. The family does not have to endure a drastic change in how they are worked with.

- **Team day and group supervision.** We recommend a commitment to monthly or bimonthly team supervision and consultation. Team supervision, especially done by the existing clinical supervisor, allows for staff members from different departments to come together to focus on shared cases. This allows for development of shared treatment philosophies and collaborative decision making on shared cases. Team day establishes an organized, clinic procedure that promotes collaboration on cases, integration of I-FAST within the larger array of services and focus on clinical faithfulness to I-FAST.

  Organizing a "team day" (most often a half-day large group meeting) to offer group case consultation, live supervision interviews and demonstration interviews is also a strategic decision aimed at multiple goals:
    - **Maintain I-FAST fidelity.** In addition to providing weekly individual I-FAST supervision, providing a biweekly or monthly team supervision meeting is one more clinic procedure that is recommended as a way of maintaining fidelity to I-FAST.
    - **Hands-on learning.** When combined with live-supervision, or live demonstration interviews, team day can stress hands on learning and intensify staff skills at delivering I-FAST treatment. Hands-on learning has been identified as a preferred method of EB training that enhances long- term fidelity to the model (Beidas & Kendall, 2010).
    - **Influencing larger staff.** By including staff from outpatient and case management services in team day, larger staff gains continuous exposure to I-FAST principles.
    - **Enhance collaboration.** A multiservice team day promotes collaboration on cases among staff who share those cases. Collaboration can be facilitated by the I-FAST trained clinical supervisor, ensuring that clinical decisions among a group of staff sharing cases are consistent with I-FAST principles.
    - **Improve staff morale.** Team day, or typically a half day, should be a time staff looks forward to. The emphasis should be on learning, offering

creative services, and focusing on successfully resolving the families' difficulties. Team day should be fun and effective. When done this way, staff morale is improved. When morale is high, staff turnover is low, and productivity is high. The clinic investment in team day is paid for by staff who do not leave the agency and whose productivity does not suffer.

In our original I-FAST study, at the six-month post-termination follow-up, relapses had not occurred. Family functioning as measured on several scales remained at the levels measured at termination (Lee, Uken, & Sebold, 2007). In this original I-FAST study, we trained agency teams that consisted of intensive in-home staff, outpatient staff, and case managers. The training was delivered in a "team day" format. By training a wide range of staff in a "team day" format, we influenced a wide range of clinic services and created a team of professionals who shared and collaborated on cases. When in-home treatment terminated, the cases were passed to other members of these teams who were already familiar with and perhaps sharing the cases. The cases were passed to like-minded colleagues. Continuity of care did not suffer. We believe this is a major reason our intensive in-home outcomes were sustained on these cases.

- **Agency training curriculum.** To obtain certification, agencies must develop their own I-FAST training curriculum, supplemented by and organized around the I-FAST manual, and approved by I-FAST trainers. This curriculum becomes the property of the agency to be utilized when training new staff.
  - After receiving I-FAST certification, to further reduce costs, agencies are empowered to train new staff in I-FAST themselves. In addition to being issued an official I-FAST manual, one requirement to obtaining I-FAST agency certification is the development of an I-FAST training curriculum by the agency's I-FAST trained supervisors. Example tapes of well-orchestrated I-FAST sessions are accumulated as well as didactic materials put together by the agency supervisors. Tapes of agency supervisors and staff competently conducting I-FAST family sessions highlight those agency staffs' expertise in I-FAST. Clinical supervisors are empowered to train new staff in I-FAST using materials developed by the agency itself and approved of by I-FAST trainers. This empowerment further enhances agency investment and participation in I-FAST. By participating in the development of their training materials the agency is further committing to sustaining I-FAST long term.
  - Second, it is recommended that a minimum of two agency supervisors are certified in I-FAST. If one supervisor leaves the clinic, the clinic still has one supervisor trained in I-FAST and it becomes this supervisor's responsibility to train the new supervisor in I-FAST. These two requirements help reduce the need for additional I-FAST training from the I-FAST trainers and therefore reduce costs. These procedures also intensify the commitment of the agency supervisors to I-FAST, helping to ensure sustainability.
- **Reducing costs.** I-FAST seeks to provide training and aid agencies to sustain I-FAST long term within the parameters of existing community mental health funding streams. I-FAST seeks to reduce costs in multiple ways:

- **Generalist model.** I-FAST is a generalist model. I-FAST is designed to be effective with the full range of child and adolescent diagnoses. Clinics certified to implement I-FAST can assure stakeholders that EB is being done, but need only purchase one EB model to cover a large array of mental health difficulties. This alone eliminates the need to purchase multiple EB models for numerous diagnoses.
- **Training the trainer.** I-FAST eliminates ongoing consultation costs by using a trainer of trainer model. Existing clinic supervisors are trained and certified in the model. The clinic supervisor becomes an internal expert on I-FAST. Ongoing consultation costs with model trainers is drastically reduced or eliminated.
- **Training new staff.** Once certified and armed with their own training curriculum and the I-FAST training manual, agencies are empowered to train their own new staff. They are welcome but not required to include I-FAST trainers in the training of new staff.
- **Controlling hidden costs.** I-FAST seeks to keep hidden costs minimized by requiring as little additional paperwork of staff as possible. I-FAST paperwork requirements have minimal impact on staff productivity. In-home staff's caseloads need not be reduced to make room for additional paperwork responsibilities. Outcome data that clinics already collect are used as much as possible to track the effectiveness of the model. Requiring agency personnel to spend time tracking additional data is kept to a minimum.
- **Productivity/training balance.** I-FAST training programs seek to strike a balance between providing intensive and effective training while reducing impact on staff productivity. Although we strongly encourage a wide range of clinic staff receive I-FAST training, the core training group consists of clinic supervisors and in-home treatment staff. Outpatient staff members are encouraged to participate, but to minimize training impact on clinic productivity, outpatient staff can rotate in and out of training during the duration of the training package.

Strategically Designed I-FAST Training Packages

I-FAST training packages are designed with all of the above agency/EB training fit issues in mind. The training packages are designed as a first step at organizing the entire clinic to integrate I-FAST within its system and to sustain the model once training is complete.

- The training begins with all-staff seminars. This aims to familiarize the entire staff with I-FAST's basic premises and concepts. The ultimate goal is enhancing continuity of care as cases pass through different clinic services and personnel.
- Next, supervisors only receive training in how to do I-FAST treatment. They are taught to do what they will eventually have to supervise and train others to do. Live supervision and review of videotapes are the preferred training methods. This provides hands on, experiential learning, and begins to institutionalize live-supervision and videotape supervision as clinic procedures.

By beginning with supervisors, their credibility among their staff is enhanced, and they are given a leg up on the training.
- Next, groups of up to 10 agency practitioners receive I-FAST training. These groups consist of the clinical supervisors, in-home treatment staff, and outpatient staff. This further enhances continuity of care by creating a larger staff of likeminded practitioners. Again, live supervision and videotape review are the preferred training methods. During this phase of training, I-FAST trainers offer the live and videotape supervision. Disruption of productivity of outpatient staff can be minimized by having different staff members rotate in and out of the training. I-FAST training begins to institutionalize procedures in the agency that will continue once official I-FAST training is complete. For example, these biweekly or monthly training days (most often half-days) will eventually be replaced by a team day facilitated by the I-FAST clinic supervisor.
- The final phase of training returns to a focus on clinical supervisors. In this final phase, clinic supervisors take over the staff training, live supervision and videotape supervision, under the guidance of the I-FAST trainers. The training ends with clinic supervisors having skills at teaching, supervising, and providing I-FAST treatment with their own staff. They become the clinic experts in I-FAST eliminating the need for ongoing consultation. In addition, in-home staff members have received intensive training in I-FAST, and outpatient staff members have had intensive exposure to the model. By completing this training package, cases can move through I-FAST certified clinics with continuity of care, and larger I-FAST clinical oversight of each case. By completing this training package, clinic hierarchies and working relationships among staff are enhanced, not disrupted.

DISCUSSION

Traditionally, EB models have focused on the problem of how to implement their models in a community agency setting and be able to sustain fidelity within these "messy" treatment environments. The standard approach for sustaining fidelity has been to set up trained EB staffs and perhaps an in-house EB trained supervisor for that staff to operate separately from the rest of the clinic and be the exclusive provider while on the case. This method has successfully dealt with the problem of sustaining fidelity, but it has not dealt with the problem of sustaining outcomes and sustaining the model long term in community agency settings.

We are arguing that the concept of sustaining EB models within community agency settings must be broadened from the narrow focus of sustaining fidelity. How to sustain EB models in community agencies must also include how to sustain outcomes obtained by those models and how to sustain the model in the agency on a long-term basis. When including these additional factors, the issues of cost and how to integrate EB services within the larger array of clinic services must be considered. How the cost of these models is handled and reduced, and the impact of training specific staff on clinic functioning has been reviewed. How these settings function clinically and the implications of this functioning on the use of EB models within them have been discussed. How to design a training package and ongoing post-training clinic procedures that enhances sustainability of EB models has been shown. Failure to address these issues at this level of detail can result in treatment procedures as usual within these settings, contradicting, interfering with, overtaking, and perhaps undoing treatment outcomes obtained by EB models implemented in them. If EB models are truly to be widely disseminated and sustained within community mental health settings, the models must be fit to these organizations and these organizations must be fit to them.

We recommend a different approach for simultaneously addressing all three levels of sustainability.

- I-FAST is a training of the trainer model that allows costs to be drastically reduced.
- We are offering methods for I-FAST to operate as a truly integrated service within the larger array of services offered at the agency/clinic.
- Instead of operating separately and exclusively on cases, I-FAST in-home staff members collaborate with and share cases with clinic colleagues.
- To avoid confusing families and contaminating fidelity by operating this way, our training seeks to have wide influence on clinic services. We achieve this by offering intensive training to existing clinic supervisor who have supervisory responsibilities over numerous clinic services.
- The clinic supervisor becomes the I-FAST champion within the agency and champions I-FAST throughout the agency.
- We also offer training to a larger range of clinic staff than just the in-home staff. We are offering strategies for how to create continuity of care for families as they pass from I-FAST in-home services to other less intensive clinic services.
- We are also offering strategies for how collaboration between in-home staff and clinic colleagues can be enhanced. We suggest these strategies will result in less relapses after in-home termination and allow for the long-term sustainability of I-FAST with agencies.

RESEARCH ON I-FAST

4

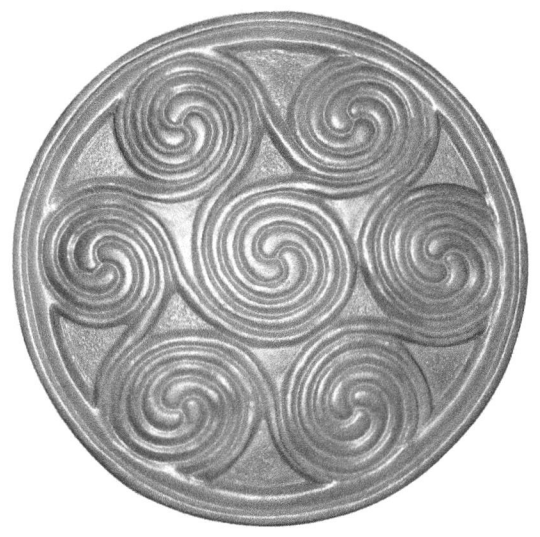

RESEARCH ON INTEGRATIVE FAMILY AND SYSTEMS TREATMENT

12

M. Y., Lee, G. J. Greene, K. S. Hsu, S. Fraser, B. Teater,
A. Solovey, D. Grove, S. Edwards, P. Scott,
P. Washburn, and C. Liu

WE NEED TO OFFER A CAUTION TO practitioners using this practitioner's guidebook regarding this final chapter on research. Most practitioners have chosen practice over research because of a passion for helping others in distress. In so doing, we have all gotten further away from the technical aspects of clinical research and experimental design. However, such research offers a strong platform to evaluate what we may feel makes sense and is useful clinically yet that may or may not prove to be effective. This chapter goes into more of the technical issues that underlie the research to date evaluating the I-FAST perspective. To do so, more technical language and data simply must be offered. With that caution in mind, we proceed with the rationale for our research program on I-FAST followed by some more detailed description of studies completed to date and others in the analysis and planning stages. We hope that this chapter will help to further inform you as a practitioner while presenting our research for others to evaluate.

RATIONALE FOR THE RESEARCH PROGRAM

The rationale for our research program is guided by existing knowledge of evidence-based intervention development (Nezu & Nezu, 2008) as applied to developing I-FAST as an effective treatment approach. Intervention development can be considered to have three stages: (1) conceptualizing an intervention based on theory and empirical research, (2) developing and standardizing the intervention, and (3) pilot testing.

In defining the I-FAST approach, we have also sought to develop what Wampold (Benish, Imel, & Wampold, 2007; Wampold et al., 1997) has described as a bona fide treatment approach. From this perspective, to determine if a treatment condition is a bona fide psychotherapy treatment, the treatment must have been delivered by a trained therapist and include an interaction in which the patient developed a relationship with the therapist and the treatment is tailored to the patient. Second, the treatment needs to satisfy two of the following four criteria: (1) the treatment is closely related to an established psychological approach or approaches, (2) a description of the therapy is provided and based on psychological principles, (3) a manual or guidelines for treatment is available and used to guide treatment, and (4) active ingredients of treatments are named and citations for these ingredients provided. We have built the I-FAST framework to satisfy these criteria as a bona fide treatment approach.

The I-FAST research program has also closely followed the stage model for psychotherapy manual development as described by Carroll and colleagues (Carroll & Nuro, 2002; Carroll & Rounsaville, 2008; Rounsaville, Carroll, & Oken, 2001). I-FAST has already moved through the Stage I manual development phase covering issues such as the overview, description, theoretical justification of I-FAST, description of the distinctiveness of I-FAST from other treatment models for similar client populations, and defining the structure and programmatic aspects of I-FAST (Carroll & Rounsaville, 2008; Rounsaville et al., 2001). Our article (Fraser, Grove, Lee, Greene, & Solovey, 2012) describing and differentiating the I-FAST approach from alternative specific factor approaches offers a summary of our Phase I work.

Our current work has focused on Stage II of manual development by refining the I-FAST treatment protocol so that it can serve as the basis of a larger randomized controlled trial in future research. Stage II has focused on developing guidelines for troubleshooting; managing common clinical problems arising in the treatment process (e.g., exacerbation of problems, low motivation, clinical transition points); clear differentiation of I-FAST from other treatment approaches with similar populations (such as Functional Family Therapy [FFT] or Multisystemic Therapy [MST], with I-FAST being more flexible in addressing a broader range of diagnoses among other differences); developing clear procedures and standards for recruiting, training, and supervising I-FAST staff; and refining and pilot-testing an observation-based fidelity measurement protocol for I-FAST, which measures treatment adherence and treatment competence (Carroll et al., 2000; Nezu & Nezu, 2008).

Our most recent work in this phase includes two articles with one article currently under review. The first article is currently under review by *The Clinical Supervisor*, and clearly describes and differentiates the I-FAST approach to training and supervision in contrast to alternative specific factor approaches to at-risk youths and families (Grove, Lee, Greene, Fraser & Solovey, unpublished manuscript). This step has addressed the refinement of the I-FAST training and supervisory format through Phase II development. The second article was published in *Research on Social Work Practice* (Lee et al., 2013). This research represents some of our work on the last transitional elements of Phase II development, wherein we have taken the first step toward head to head clinical trials of the I-FAST framework. This study examined the treatment outcomes of I-FAST, a moderated common factors approach, in reference to MST, an established specific factor approach, for treating at-risk children and adolescents and their families in an intensive community-based setting. This study used a non-randomized non-inferiority trial design to compare the outcomes of 79 families who received I-FAST, the test intervention, to 47 families who have received MST, the reference intervention. I-FAST was non-inferior or essentially comparable to MST in reducing *Problem Severity* and improving *Functioning* based on youths', parents', and workers' assessments. Although the non-randomized design of this study precludes any definitive conclusions, implications of the study were discussed with respect to the debate regarding common factors and specific factor approaches to family treatment and implementation of evidence-based treatments. Although this comparison method is now commonly used and supported in the medical literature, this approach to comparison also represents the first step to more rigorous randomized clinical trials planned for the approach.

Our most current studies, now in the analysis and manuscript preparation phase, analyze several other aspects of the I-FAST approach. The first of these addresses effectiveness with African American versus Caucasian youths and family cohorts. The second study addresses any differential effectiveness of I-FAST with internalizing versus externalizing youth problems. The final study examines the I-FAST contention that the model is sustainable with fidelity and effectiveness even after direct training and consultation have ended. The outcomes and fidelity from a large center network that had ongoing training and consultation during their use of the I-FAST approach are being compared with those of two other centers now operating independently of such supervision and consultation. Preliminary results on all three studies remain very supportive of the I-FAST framework.

We feel that the body of research thus far in our research program offers a strong grounding to support the I-FAST framework as a moderated common factor approach to at-risk youths and families. Our next steps are to begin the final Phase III studies, which will include randomized clinical trials. Publication of the current book offering treatment guidelines for practitioners further bolsters this effort. Not only does it represent a step to broader dissemination of the I-FAST approach, but it also offers a widely available treatment overview to guide these clinical trials and to be accessed by others evaluating the approach.

MORE DETAIL ON STUDIES TO DATE

A number of studies have been conducted on different aspects of I-FAST since 2003. This section of the chapter provides a detailed description of the original efficacy study on I-FAST funded by The Ohio Department of Mental Health from 2003 to 2007 (Lee et al., 2009) and the I-FAST outcome study that included additional data from two child mental health agencies that have received I-FAST training and adopted I-FAST in their intensive community-based program. It also reports a non-randomized non-inferiority trial that examined the treatment outcomes of I-FAST; a moderated common factors approach, in reference to MST; and an established specific factor approach, for treating at-risk children and adolescents and their families in an intensive community-based setting (Lee et al., 2013). Finally, it provides a brief summary of other additional studies on different aspects of I-FAST.

Study 1: The Original Efficacy Study

This is the first feasibility study[1] of I-FAST that used a one-group pre- and post-test design with a six-month follow-up to explore the efficacy of I-FAST in treating families with children at risk of out-of-home placement and receiving home-based treatment (Lee et al., 2009). This study was funded by The Ohio Department of Mental Health from 2003 to 2007. We hypothesized that effective I-FAST treatment would lead to improved functioning, reduced problem severity in the child, reduction in out-of-home placement of the child, improved family functioning, increased parental competency in addressing their child's problems, and increased family participation in the treatment process.

RESEARCH PARTICIPANTS

Research participants were from two mental health agencies in a Midwestern state; one agency serves five counties and another serves six counties. Participating families were mostly low-income families and approximately 98% of the treatment costs were paid by Medicaid and other public funds. The Court, Children's Services, hospitals, or other mental health agencies referred families to the programs. Families participating in the study received home-based services up to a six-week period with additional six-week increments negotiated based on the family's needs and progress. Families completing intake, post-treatment, and six-month follow-up received $40 in compensation.

Seventy-five families completed the program and provided data at pre-treatment and post-treatment. Among the 77 children, 64.9% were boys (50) and 35.1% girls (27). The majority of child participants were students at middle school (41.9%) and elementary schools (32.3) while 14.5% were high school students and 11.3% were in kindergartens or preschools. Child participants were predominantly Caucasian (93.2%), with 2.6% African Americans, and 5.2% biracial. The ages of the children ranged from 4 to 17 (mean: 11.8, SD 3.3) with 2.6% age 4, 19.5% between 5 and 8, 29.9% between 9 and 12, 31.2% between 13 and 14, and 16.9% between 15 and 17. Mental status examination was conducted by licensed mental health professionals. Using *DSM–IV* criteria, almost half of the child participants had a diagnosis of Hyperactive Attention Deficit Disorder (48.4%), 12.9% Adjustment Disorder, 11.3% Mood Disorder, 8.1% Depression Disorder NOS, 4.8% Oppositional Defiant Disorder, 3.2% Bipolar, 3.2% Disruptive Disorder, 1.6% Impulse-Control Disorder, 1.6% Dysthymic Disorder, 1.6% Anxiety Disorder, 1.6% Posttraumatic Stress Disorder, and 1.6% Trichotillomania. Regarding child participants' placement status, 41.3% had been in out-of-home placement before receiving I-FAST. Children who were in placement were most frequently placed in psychiatric hospitals (40%) and juvenile detention centers (32%), which was followed by foster care (16%), other youth facilities (8%), and residential treatment facilities (4%) (Table 12-1).

Method of Data Collection

TREATMENT FIDELITY

Treatment fidelity was measured by the I-FAST Checklist, which is a 31-item measure that assesses core treatment components of I-FAST: therapeutic alliance (items 1–20), second-order change strategies (items 21–25), and systems collaboration (items 26–31) (Lee et al., 2003, updated in 2011). I-FAST fidelity evaluation resemble procedures used by Knutson, Forgatch, and Rains in their study (Knutson, Forgatch, & Rains, 2003). The focus of rating with the initial family session was on the development of the therapeutic alliance. The focus of rating of the week 6 family session was on second-order change strategies and systems collaboration. The focus of rating of the consultation sessions was on all three core treatment components as suggested by I-FAST. Two independent raters, who had received the fidelity training, rated the adherence and competence of the interventions of each core treatment component on a three-point Likert scale: (0) absence, (1) some, and (2) excellent. The *I-FAST Checklist* was scored by summing individual items and ranges from 0 to 62, with higher scores indicating greater adherence to and competence of implementing I-FAST in the treatment process by clinicians or in the consultation process by clinical consultants. We had tapes from 35 initial family sessions and 17 week 6 family sessions. The study used intra-class correlation (ICC) to assess inter-rater reliability of I-FAST. Findings of ICC showed a satisfactory level of inter-rater reliability. The intra-class coefficient for therapeutic alliance was .84, for second-order change was .86, and for systems collaboration was .88. We had tapes on nine consultation sessions. Findings of ICC showed

Table 12-1

Demographics of study participants (N = 77)

Variable	Category	N (%)
Gender	Male	64.9
	Female	35.1
Age	Mean: 11.8, SD 3.3, range: 4–17	
Race/ethnicity	White	93.2
	African American	2.6
	Biracial	5.2
Education	Preschool or kindergarten	11.3
	Elementary school	32.3
	Middle school	41.9
	High school	14.5
Diagnosis	Attention–deficit/hyperactivity disorder	48.4
	Adjustment disorder	12.9
	Mood disorders	11.3
	Depression disorder NOS	8.1
	Oppositional defiance disorder	4.8
	Bipolar disorder	3.2
	Disruptive disorders	3.2
	Posttraumatic stress disorder	1.6
	Impulse-control disorder	1.6
	Dysthymic disorder	1.6
	Anxiety disorder	1.6
	Trichotillomania	1.6

a satisfactory level of inter-rater reliability. The intra-class coefficient for therapeutic alliance was .82, for second-order change .88, and for systems collaboration .80. The intra-class coefficient for the overall I-FAST was .88.

OUTCOME VARIABLES

Child's Outcomes

Child's outcomes referred to the level of emotional and behavioral functioning of the child and were operationally defined as the scores the child had on the *Problem Severity* and *Functioning* subscales of *The Ohio Scale-Short Form*. The Ohio Scales were developed to provide multisource, multicontent measures of clinical outcomes of youths ages 5 to 18 (Ogles, Lambert, & Masters, 1996). Multiple reporting sources are included in the process of data collection: the youths (if age 12 and older), parents or primary caretakers, and I- FAST case managers.

The Problem Severity Scale comprises 20 items covering common problems associated with children who receive mental health services. Raters are asked to rate the degree to which the child has experienced the problem in the past 30 days on a six-point scale (from 0, "Not at all" to 5, "All the time"). The scores range from 0 to 100, with a higher score indicating a more severe problem.

The Functioning Scale comprises 20 items designed to rate the child's level of functioning in a variety of areas of daily activity. Raters are asked to rate the current level of functioning of the youths using a five-point scale (from 0, "Extreme troubles" to 4, "Doing very well"). The scores range from 0 to 80, with a higher score indicating a higher level of functioning in the youth. Ogles, Melendez, Davis, and Lunnen (2001) report satisfactory reliability coefficients of *The Ohio Scales* across multiple reporting sources that range from .65 to .97 (Cronbach's alpha) with the test–retest reliabilities ranging from .43 to .88. In addition, *The Ohio Scale* ratings have been found to significantly correlate with several other well-established related measures. *The Ohio Scales* ratings statistically significantly correlated with *Child and Adolescent Functional Assessment Scales* (Hodges & Wong, 1996) and *Child Behavior Checklist CBCL* (Ogles et al., 2001).

Child's Placement Status

Child's placement status was operationally defined by the location and frequency of out-of-home placement pre-treatment, at post-treatment, and six-month follow-up.

Family Functioning

FACESII, which measures the level of cohesion and adaptability of a family, was used in this study to evaluate family functioning. FACESII is 30-item scale with 16 items measuring cohesion and 14 items measuring adaptability (Olson, Portner, & Bell, 1982). Respondents are requested to rate how frequently the described behavior occurs in his/her family on a five-point Likert scale that ranges from 1 (almost never) to 5 (almost always). Scoring procedures are described in the *Family Inventories Manual* (Olson, 1992). Olson (1992) reported satisfactory Cronbach's alpha of .90 for the total scale, .87 for Cohesion, and .78 for Adaptability. Test–retest reliability was .83 for Cohesion and .80 for Adaptability. Good concurrent validity was also established for FACESII (Hampson, Hulgus, & Beavers, 1991).

Parental Competence with Children

Parental competence with children was operationally defined by the scores on the *Parental Efficacy Scale*, which is a 10-item scale adapted and modified from the *Parental Locus of Control Scale* (Campis, Lyman, & Prentice-Dunn, 1986). Parents are asked to rate their responses on a five-point Likert-type scale from "Strongly disagree" (1), "Disagree" (2), "Neither agree or disagree" (3), "Agree" (4), to "Strongly agree" (5). *The Parental Efficacy Scale* is scored by summing individual items with the scores ranging from 5 to 50, with a higher score indicating greater parental competence in relation to children. Norms for the original *Parental Efficacy Scale* are not reported although means for parents who did not report difficulties in the parenting role (17.62) are distinguished from means of parents who had requested counseling services for parental problems (19.27) (Campis et al., 1986). Good internal consistency has been found for the *Parental Efficacy Scale* (Campis et al., 1986).

Family Participation

Family participation was operationally defined as the scores on the *Family Participation Measure* as completed by the parents (Friesen, 2001; Friesen & Pullman, 2002). The

Family Participation Scale consists of seven items and is designed to measure a caregiver's impression of his or her level of participation in planning for a child's service and treatment. Respondents are asked to answer the questions on a four-point Likert-type scale from "Not at all" (1), "A little" (2), "Some" (3), to "A lot" (4). Psychometric properties have not been reported by the authors because this is a relatively new scale. On the other hand, the scale was developed in a large-scale national study that investigates experiences of families whose children received services for severe emotional and behavioral disorders.

DATA ANALYSES

Data collected from various instruments were checked and coded for data processing and statistical analyses. The *Statistical Package for Social Sciences* was used for this purpose. Regarding treatment fidelity, the study used intra-class correlation (ICC) to assess inter-rater reliability of I-FAST. The study used paired-sample t-tests to examine the within-subject changes from pre-treatment to post-treatment and repeated measures analysis of variance to assess the within-subject changes during the three assessments of pre-treatment, post-treatment, and six-month follow-up. In addition, the study used the Wilcoxon signed rank tests to assess the within-subject changes during the three assessments of pre-treatment, post-treatment, and six-month follow-up for the categorical variable of child's placement status.

To address the problem of attrition, we had used multiple imputation method to simulate value for the missing assessments to reduce the adverse effect of missing observations in the data analyses. When there were a valid pre-treatment assessment and at least one valid assessment at post-treatment or six-month follow-up, we imputed the missing assessment with available valid results along with the age and gender of the client. Details for the imputation are provided in the footnotes of Tables 12-2 and 12-3. We used PROC MI from SAS to create five imputed datasets and combined these results to simulate value with PROC MIANALYZE for the missing observations (Graham, Cumsille, & Elek-Fisk, 2003; Schafer & Olsen, 1998).

FINDINGS

Child's Outcomes: The Ohio Scales

Based on parents' assessment, the mean score of *Problem Severity* at pre-treatment was 40.4 (SD = 20.6), meaning that the child, on average, on several occasions exhibited each of the listed problem behaviors in the past 30 days (Table 12-2). The mean score of the *Functioning Scale* was 35.0 (SD = 17.3) at pre-treatment, indicating a relatively low level of functioning in the children. Based on findings from paired-sample t-tests of the parents' evaluations, there was a significant decrease in the severity of problem behaviors in the child [$t = 8.557$, df = 75, $p < .001$], significant improvement in child's level of functioning [$t = -6.839$, df = 72, $p < .001$] from pre-treatment to post-treatment (Table 12-3).

The youths in the program reported a different pattern in evaluating their problem severity and level of functioning at pre-treatment. On average the youths assessed themselves at a lower level of problem severity (30.7 vs. 40.4) and a higher level of functioning (47.6 vs. 35.0) as compared to their parents. The differences between the youths and their parents on evaluating problem severity and level of functioning, however, were reduced at post-treatment. The mean scores for differences in problem severity as rated by youths and parents were 12.9 and 18.1 respectively. Youths,

Table 12-2

Paired-sample *t*-Tests of The Ohio Scales (parents', youths' and case managers' assessments), Parental Competence, and Family Participation at Pre-Treatment and Post-Treatment

	Pre-treatment	Post-treatment	t	df	p
Ohio Scales					
Parents' assessment					
Problem Severity (N = 76)	40.4 (SD = 20.6)	22.3 (SD = 16.2)	8.557	75	.000
Functioning (N = 73)	35.0 (SD = 17.3)	48.5 (SD = 15.5)	−6.839	72	.000
Youths' assessment					
Problem Severity (N = 39)	30.7 (SD = 19.4)	17.8 (SD = 12.1)	4.178	38	.000
Functioning (N = 38)	47.6 (SD = 19.4)	57.6 (SD = 10.7)	−3.275	37	.002
Case managers' assessment					
Problem Severity (N = 72)	37.9 (SD = 15.1)	16.7 (SD = 10.0)	12.409	71	.000
Functioning (N = 68)	34.1 (SD = 12.7)	49.7 (SD = 12.0)	−9.056	67	.000
Parental Competence with Children (N = 64)	34.2 (SD = 6.4)	36.2 (SD = 5.3)	−2.509	63	.015
Family participation (N = 70)	25.9 (SD = 3.0)	25.4 (SD = 3.7)	1.089	69	.280

Note:
Data were imputed for missing assessments:
Problem Severity (parent rating): 57 completed all three assessments, 2 missing in post-treatment only and 17 missing in six-months follow-up only.
Problem Severity (worker rating): 53 completed all three assessments, 4 missing in post-treatment only and 15 missing in six-month follow-up only.
Problem Severity (youth rating): 29 completed all three assessments, 1 missing in post-treatment only and 9 missing in six-month follow-up only.
Functioning (parent rating): 54 completed all three assessments, 2 missing in post-treatment only and 17 missing in six-month follow-up only.
Functioning (worker rating): 51 completed all three assessments, 3 missing in post-treatment only and 14 missing in six-month follow-up only.
Functioning (youth rating): 28 completed all three assessments and 10 missing in six-month follow-up only.
Parent competence with children: 44 completed all three assessments, 7 missing in post-treatment only and 13 missing in six-month follow-up only.
Family Participation: 51 completed all three assessments, 3 missing in post-treatment only and 16 missing in six-month follow-up only.

however, still rated themselves at a higher level of functioning at post-treatment than their parents (57.6 vs. 48.5). Paired-sample *t*-tests found that there was a significant decrease in the severity of problem behaviors in the youths [$t = 4.178$, df $= 38$, $p < .001$], significant improvement in their level of functioning [$t = -3.275$, df $= 37$, $p < .01$] from pre-treatment to post-treatment based on the youths' evaluations (Table 12-2).

The case managers' rating of *The Ohio Scale* indicated a significant improvement in the areas of assessment of Problem Severity and Functioning from pre-treatment to post-treatment. Based on findings from paired-sample t-tests on the case managers' evaluations, there was a significant decrease in the severity of problem behaviors in the child [$t = 12.409$, df = 71, $p < .001$] and significant improvement in child's level of functioning [$t = -9.056$, df = 67, $p < .001$] from pre-treatment to post-treatment (Table 12-2).

Figure 12-1 shows the mean scores of problem severity and level of functioning at pre-treatment, post-treatment, and six-month follow-up based on parents', youths', and case managers' reports. Across multiple reporting sources, findings based on pairwise comparisons indicated there were significant changes from pre-treatment to post-treatment, significant changes from pre-treatment to six-month follow-up, and nonsignificant changes from post-treatment to six-month follow-up for problem severity and level of functioning in children (Table 12-3). In other words, significant positive changes in the children's behavioral outcomes from pre-treatment to post-treatment were maintained six months after the families terminated from the program.

Placement Status

Data were obtained on the placement status of 75 children prior to their receiving treatment and at post-treatment. Among the 75 children, 41.3% (31) had been in out-of-home placement before receiving home-based services in such settings as psychiatric hospitals (40%), juvenile detention centers (32%), foster care (16%), other youth facilities (8%), and residential treatment facilities (4%). At post-treatment, only 5.3% (4) of child participants were in out-of-home placement. Three of them were placed in psychiatric hospitals and one was in a residential treatment facility. Findings based on Wilcoxon signed-rank tests indicated significant differences in the pattern of distribution of placement status of children from pre-treatment to post-treatment, with significantly higher percentage of children in out-of-home placement pre-treatment than at post-treatment ($p < .001$).

Of these 75 children, complete data were obtained on 59 of them regarding their placement status at pre-treatment, post-treatment, and six-month follow-up. Among these 59 children, 40.7% were assigned to out-of-home placement before treatment. Only 5.1% (3) and 15.3% (9) were in out-of-home placement at post-treatment and six-month follow-up respectively (Figure 12-2). Specifically, three children were placed in psychiatric hospitals at post-treatment. At six-month follow-up, five children were placed in psychiatric hospitals, one in a residential treatment facility, and three in juvenile detention centers. Findings based on using the Wilcoxon signed-rank tests indicated significant differences in the pattern of distribution of placement status of children from pre-treatment to post-treatment, post-treatment to six-month follow-up, and pre-treatment to six-month follow-up. A significantly higher proportion of the children were in out-of-home placement at pre-treatment than at post-treatment. In addition, there were also a higher percentage of children in placement at six-month follow-up than at post-treatment. There was still a significantly lower percentage of children in placement at six-month follow-up than at pre-treatment (Figure 12-2).

Family Functioning

FAMILY COHESION

Data were obtained from 60 families regarding family cohesion at pre-treatment, post-treatment, and six-month follow-up. Figure 12-4 shows the distribution

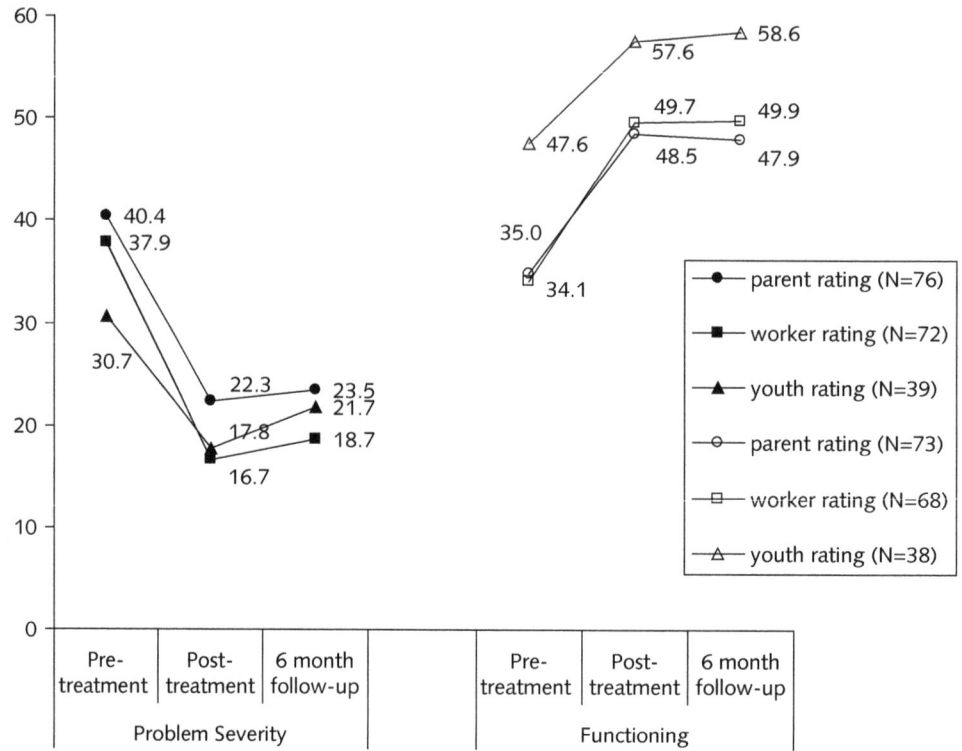

FIGURE 12-1
The Ohio Scales: Pre-treatment, post-treatment, and six-month follow-up.
Note: Data were imputed for missing assessments; see note in Table 12-1.

of families for each family type at pre-treatment, post-treatment, and six-month follow-up. At pre-treatment as well as at post-treatment approximately one-third of these families were found to be "Disengaged" (35.0% and 33.3% respectively). At post-treatment fewer families were found to be "Separated" (23.3%) than at pre-treatment (31.7%), and more families (31.7%) were found to be "Connected Separated" at post-treatment than at pre-treatment (26.7%). In addition, the percentage of families considered to be "Very Connected" nearly doubled from pre-treatment to post-treatment (6.7% vs. 11.7%). Regarding changes between post-treatment and six-month follow-up, there were more families in the categories of "Connected Separated" and "Separated" and fewer families in the categories of "Very Connected" and "Disengaged" at six-month follow-up than at post-treatment. Patterns of distribution also showed the families in the category of "Very Connected" stayed the same (6.7% vs. 6.7%) but more were classified as "Connected Separated" (26.7% vs. 36.7%) from pre-treatment to six-month. There were also slightly fewer families in the categories of "Separated" and "Disengaged" at six-month follow-up than at pre-treatment (Figure 12-3).

Findings based on pairwise comparisons indicated there were significant changes from pretreatment to post-treatment, nonsignificant changes from post-treatment to 6-month follow-up, and marginal significant changes from pre-treatment to six-month follow-up in terms of family cohesion (Table 12-3). Overall, families tended to become connected and less separated and/or disengaged from pre-treatment to post-treatment and 6 month follow-up.

Table 12-3

Pairwise Comparisons of the Ohio Scales (parents', youths', and case managers' assessments), FACEII, Parental Competence, and Family Participation: Pre-Treatment (T1), Post-Treatment (T2), and Six-month Follow-up (T3)

	T1-T2				T2-T3				T1-T3			
	Mean Difference	Std. Error	Sig.	95% Confidence Interval for Difference	Mean Difference	Std. Error	Sig.	95% Confidence Interval for Difference	Mean Difference	Std. Error	Sig.	95% Confidence Interval for Difference
Ohio Scales—Parents' assessment												
Problem Severity (N = 76)	−18.1	2.1	.000	−22.3 −13.9	1.2	1.9	.536	−2.5 4.8	−17.0	2.1	.000	−21.1 −12.8
Functioning (N = 73)	13.6	2.0	.000	9.6 17.5	−0.6	1.7	.730	−4.0 2.8	13.0	2.1	.000	8.9 17.1
Ohio Scales—Youths' assessment												
Problem Severity (N = 39)	−12.9	3.1	.000	−19.1 −6.7	3.9	3.0	.199	−2.2 10.0	−9.0	3.1	.006	−15.2 −2.7
Functioning (N = 68)	9.9	3.0	.002	3.8 16.1	1.0	1.9	.595	−2.9 5.0	11.0	3.6	.004	3.7 18.2
Ohio Scales—Case managers' assessment												
Problem Severity (N = 72)	−21.3	1.7	.000	−24.7 −17.8	2.1	1.3	.127	−0.6 4.7	−19.2	1.7	.000	−22.5 −15.9
Functioning (N = 68)	15.6	1.7	.000	12.2 19.1	0.2	1.2	.163	−2.1 2.5	15.8	2.0	.000	11.9 19.7
FACEII												
Family Cohesion (N = 60)	3.4	1.6	.039	0.2 6.7	0.1	1.0	.956	−2.0 2.1	3.5	1.8	.057	−0.1 7.1
Family Adaptability (N = 54)	3.2	1.3	.016	0.6 5.8	−0.9	0.8	.264	−2.6 0.7	2.3	1.3	.075	−.02 4.8
Parental Competence with Children (N = 64)	2.0	0.8	.015	0.4 3.5	0.2	0.7	.805	−1.3 1.6	2.2	0.8	.006	0.6 3.7
Family Participation (N = 70)	−0.6	0.5	.280	−1.6 0.5	1.0	0.4	.018	0.2 1.8	0.9	0.5	.073	1.8 −.08

Note:
Data were imputed for missing assessments; see note in Table 12-1.
Family Cohesion: 43 completed all three assessments, 5 missing in post-treatment only and 12 missing in six-month follow-up only. Family Adaptability: 37 completed all three assessments, 7 missing in post-treatment only and 10 missing in six-month follow-up only.

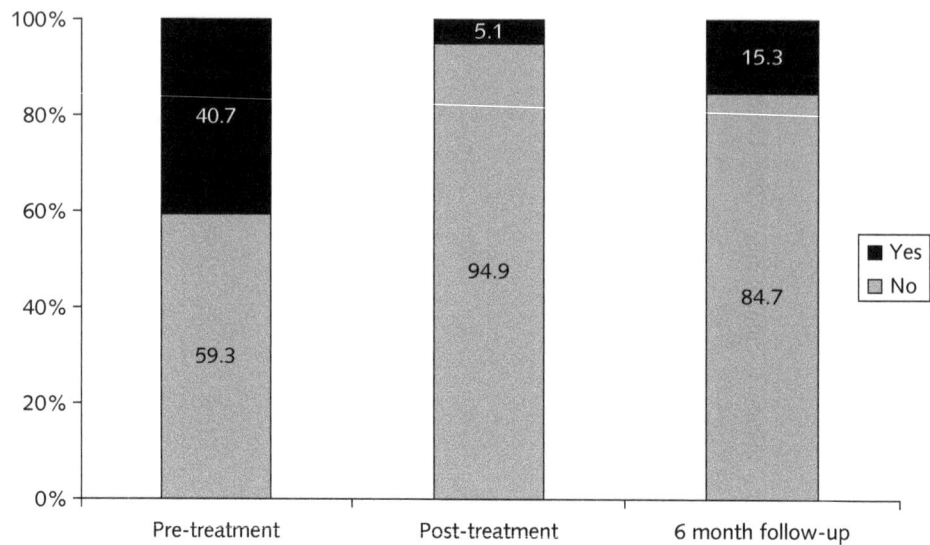

FIGURE 12-2
Placement status of children: Pre-treatment, post-treatment, and six-month follow-up (N = 59).
Note: Pre-treatment and post-treatment: Asymp. sig. (two-tailed) from Wilcoxon signed-rank test = .000 post-treatment and six-month follow-up: Asymp. sig. (two-tailed) from Wilcoxon signed-rank test = .026 pre-treatment and six-month follow-up: Asymp. sig. (two-tailed) from Wilcoxon signed-rank test = .224.

FAMILY ADAPTABILITY

Data were obtained from 54 families at pre-treatment, post-treatment, and six-month follow-up. Figure 12-4 shows the distribution of families for each family type at pre-treatment, post-treatment, and six-month follow-up. At pre-treatment and at post-treatment slightly more than a quarter of these families were found to be the "Structure" type (27.8% and 29.6%). There were fewer families in the categories of "Rigid" at post-treatment than at pre-treatment (16.7% vs. 29.6%) and more families in the categories of "Very Flexible" at post-treatment than at pre-treatment (16.7% vs. 3.7%). Regarding changes between post-treatment and six-month follow-up,

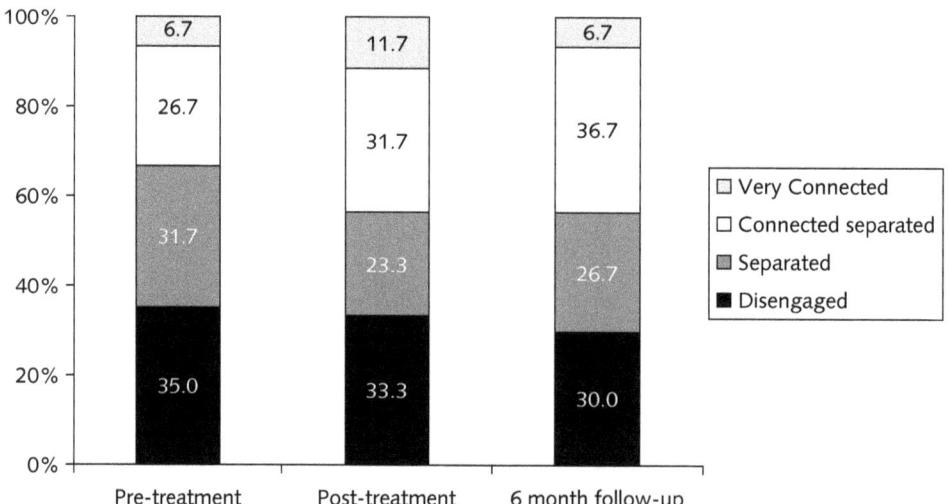

FIGURE 12-3
FACESII: Family Cohesion at pre-treatment, post-treatment, and six-month follow-up (N = 60).
Note: Data were imputed for missing assessments; see note in Table 12-2.

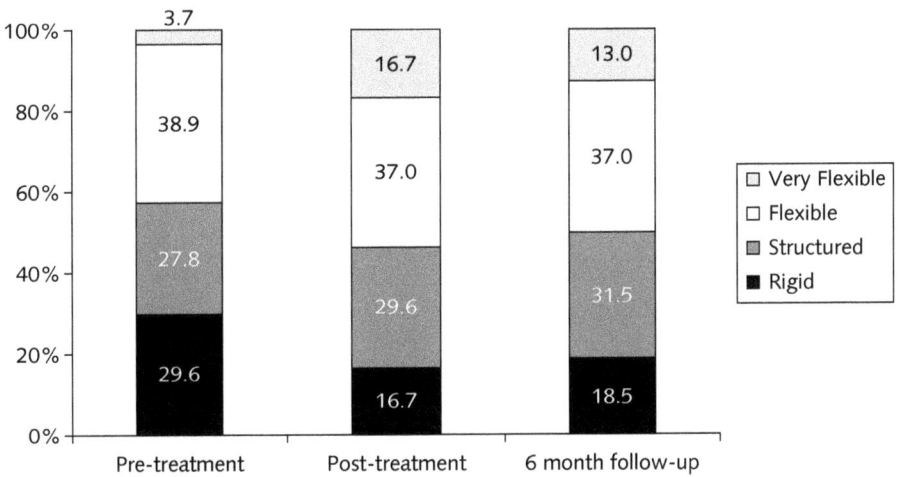

FIGURE 12-4
FACEII: Family Adaptability at pre-treatment, post-treatment, and six-month follow-up (N = 54).
Note: Data were imputed for missing assessments; see note in Table 12-2.

while the percentage of families in the category of "Flexible" remained unchanged, there was a slight decrease for families in the categories of "Very Flexible" at six-month follow-up than at post-treatment. In addition, there were slightly more families in the category of "Structure" (31.5% vs. 29.6%) and "Rigid" (18.5% vs. 16.7%) at six-month follow-up than at post-treatment. Findings based on pairwise comparisons indicated there were significant changes from pre-treatment to post-treatment in family adaptability and nonsignificant changes from post-treatment to six-month follow-up in terms of family adaptability (Table 12-3). Overall, families showed a trend of becoming more flexible and less rigid with treatment, with these changes being maintained at six-month follow-up.

Parental Competence with Children
Data were obtained from 64 families on the *Parental Competence with Children* measure. The mean score of 36.2 (SD = 5.3) at post-treatment compared favorably with the mean score of 34.2 (SD = 6.4) at pre-treatment. Based on findings from the paired-sample *t*-test of the parents' evaluations, parents increasingly perceived themselves as being competent in parenting their children from pre-treatment to post-treatment and these improvements were statistically significant [$t = -2.509$, df = 63, $p < .01$) (Table 12-2).

Figure 12-5 shows the mean scores of *Parental Competence with Children* at pre-treatment, post-treatment, and six-month follow-up. There was a continuous increase in the mean scores from pre-treatment to post-treatment to six-month follow-up (34.2 vs. 36.2 vs. 36.4). Findings based on pairwise comparisons indicated there were significant changes from pre-treatment to post-treatment, as well as from pre-treatment to six-month follow-up, with nonsignificant changes from post-treatment to six-month follow-up on the *Parental Competence with Children* measure (Table 12-3). In sum, parents perceived themselves as becoming significantly more competent in addressing problems with their children with treatment and they were able to maintain these positive changes at six-month follow-up.

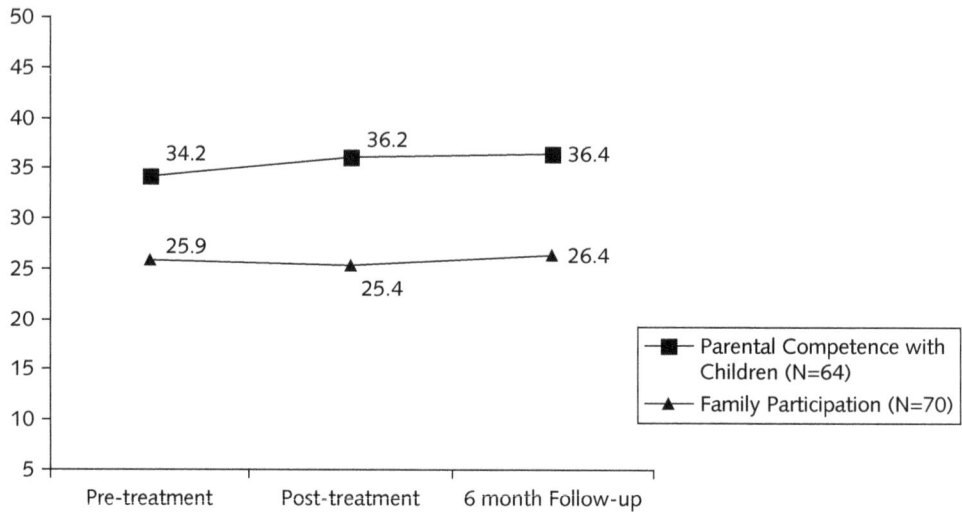

FIGURE 12-5

Parents' evaluation of Parental Competence and Family Participation: Pre-treatment, post-treatment, and six-month follow-up.
Note: Data were imputed for missing assessments; see note in Table 12-1.

Family Participation

Seventy families provided data on the *Family Participation* measure at pre-treatment and post-treatment as reported by the parents. At the pre-treatment these families already reported very high level of participation in the treatment process (25.9, SD = 3.0). At post-treatment these parents continued to report a high level of family participation (25.4, SD = 3.7) despite a slight but nonsignificant decrease in the mean scores from pre-treatment to post-treatment (25.9 vs. 25.4). Findings from the paired-sample t-test did not indicate significant differences in parental competence with service providers from pre-treatment to post-treatment based on the evaluation of parents [t = 1.089, df = 69, p = .280) (Table 12-2).

Figure 12-6 shows the mean scores on the *Family Participation* measure at pre-treatment, post-treatment, and six-month follow-up. There was a slight decrease in mean scores from pre-treatment to post-treatment and an increase in the mean scores from post-treatment to six-month follow-up (25.9 vs. 25.4 vs. 26.4). Findings based on pairwise comparisons indicated there were significant changes from pre-treatment to six-month follow- up in family participation while nonsignificant changes from pre-treatment to post-treatment and from post-treatment to six-month follow-up in (Table 12-3). In sum, families reported a significantly higher level of participation in the treatment process from pre-treatment to six-month follow-up.

DISCUSSION AND SUMMARY

The study measured fidelity by having two independent raters who used the I-FAST Checklist to rate videotaped or audiotaped sessions of family sessions and consultation sessions. We used intra-class correlation to assess inter-rater reliability of I-FAST. The findings of ICC showed a satisfactory level of inter-rater reliability.

Findings of this feasibility trial provided initial empirical evidence that supported the effectiveness of I-FAST for reducing a child's problem, improving a child's functioning, reducing out-of-home placements, improving family functioning, and parental competence with their children. In terms of child's behavioral outcomes, findings indicated that there was a significant decrease in problem severity and a significant increase in the level of functioning in children from pre-treatment to post-treatment as reported by parents, the youth, and I-FAST case managers. Children were able to maintain their positive changes at six-month follow-up. In addition, there was a significant decrease in the number of children in out-of-home placement at post-treatment than at pre-treatment. Despite significantly more children were placed in out-of-home placement at six-month follow-up than at post-treatment, the number was still significantly less than the number of children in out-of-home placement before they participated in the program. In terms of family functioning, findings from FACESII showed significant increases in the level of cohesion and adaptability in these families. Specifically, there was a trend of families becoming more connected and less separated and/or disengaged, more flexible and less rigid, more balanced and less extreme with treatment. All observed changes were significant from pre-treatment to post-treatment and/or from pre-treatment to six-month follow-up. In addition, families were able to maintain these positive changes at six-month follow-up. Regarding parental competence with children, parents became significantly more competent in addressing problems with their children from pre-treatment to post-treatment, and they were able to maintain these positive changes at six-month follow-up. Findings regarding family participation in the treatment process indicated a high level of participation throughout the evaluation period. In addition, there was significantly greater family participation in treatment from pre-treatment to six-month follow-up.

Study 2: Efficacy of I-FAST from 2004 to 2012

Since the initial efficacy study of I-FAST, a total of 15 agencies had received training on I-FAST. Two child mental health agencies in a Midwestern state that had adopted I-FAST in their home-based programs systematically collected data for program evaluation purposes. Data were collected when the agencies had completed I-FAST training and were completely on their own to sustain I-FAST. One community-based program received training on I-FAST from July, 2007 to December, 2008. Following the completion of the training, data on treatment outcomes were collected from January, 2009 to September, 2010 to evaluate the efficacy of I-FAST in improving outcomes for children and families. The other agency received training from January 2010 to June 2011. Data were collected from September 2011 to October 2012 for program evaluation purpose. The initial I-FAST efficacy study was approved by a university Institutional Review Board. For the two program evaluation studies, the Board reviewed and exempted these studies from IRB because the data were provided as secondary de-linked data with no direct or indirect identifiers of the clients. This study examines the accumulative efficacy of I-FAST including data from the two agencies that have adopted I-FAST in their home-based programs.

RESEARCH PARTICIPANTS

Two hundred and ten families who received I-FAST services and provided data at pre-treatment and/or post-treatment were included in the study. Among the 210 children, 68.7% were boys (144) and 31.4% girls (66). The majority of child participants were students at middle school (38.0%) and high school (34.0%) while 23.0% were elementary school students and 5.0% were in kindergartens or preschools. Two-thirds of child participants were Caucasian (62.4%), with 27.6% African Americans, 2.4% Hispanic/Latino Americans, 0.5% Asian Pacific Islanders, and 6.2% biracial. The ages of the children ranged from 5 to 18 (mean: 13.1, SD 3.1). Mental status examination was conducted by licensed mental health professionals. Using *DSM–IV* criteria, almost one-third of the child participants had a diagnosis of Hyperactive Attention Deficit Disorder (31.0%), 22.4% Mood Disorder, 18.6% Conduct and Disruptive Disorders, 13.3% Oppositional Defiant Disorder, 7.6% Adjustment Disorder, 4.8% Bipolar, and 2.4% Posttraumatic Stress Disorder (Table 12-4).

TREATMENT ADHERENCE

Treatment fidelity of the agencies who received I-FAST training was ensured by requiring the participating service professionals to adhere to a standard treatment as defined by each treatment approach. I-FAST requires agency to develop some of their own procedures for monitoring model fidelity that include agency I-FAST supervisors providing ongoing consultation with I-FAST case managers and using the *I-FAST Fidelity Scale* to monitor model fidelity (Lee, Fraser, Greene, Solovey, & Grove, 2003, updated in 2011). Although there is minimal involvement from I-FAST model developers in the day-to-day monitoring of the model fidelity, the agency is required to seek recertification biennially. Part of the recertification process requires the agency to submit videotapes of treatment sessions as well as videotapes of supervision sessions to the model developers for fidelity check purpose.

Table 12-4

Demographics of study participants

Variable	N	Category	Count	%
Gender	210	Male	144	68.6
		Female	66	31.4
Age	210	Mean: 13.1, SD, 3.1, range: 5–18		
Race/ethnicity	210	White	131	62.4
		African American	58	27.6
		Hispanic/Latino	5	2.4
		Asian/Pacific Islander	1	0.5
		Biracial	13	6.2
		Others	2	1.0
Education	200	Preschool or kindergarten	10	5.0
		Elementary school	46	23.0
		Middle school	76	38.0
		High school	68	34.0
Diagnosis	210	Conduct and disruptive disorders	39	18.6
		Attention–deficit/hyperactivity disorder	65	31.0
		Bipolar disorder	10	4.8
		Oppositional defiance disorder	28	13.3
		Mood disorders	47	22.4
		Adjustment disorder	16	7.6
		Posttraumatic stress disorder	5	2.4

METHOD OF DATA COLLECTION

Assessment of children's level of functioning and level of problem severity were obtained at pre- and termination from parents, youths 12 years or older, and case managers using The Ohio Scales.

Child's Outcomes

Child's outcomes were operationally defined as the scores the child had on the *Problem Severity* and *Functioning* subscales of The Ohio Scale-Short Form. The Ohio Scales were developed to provide multisource, multicontent measures of clinical outcomes of youths ages 5 to 18 (Ogles et al., 1996). Multiple reporting sources are included in the process of data collection: the youths (if age 12 and older), parents or primary caretakers, and I-FAST case managers. Psychometric properties of the scales have been described in Study 1.

DATA ANALYSES

Data collected from various instruments were checked and coded for data processing and statistical analyses. The Statistical Package for Social Sciences was used for this purpose. The study used paired sample *t*-test analysis to assess within-subject change from pre-treatment and post-treatment of each group. In addition, Reliable Change Indexes (RCIs) were calculated for the primary outcome measures on child behavioral outcomes. To address the problem of attrition, we had used multiple imputation method to simulate value for the missing assessments to reduce the adverse effect of missing observations in the data analyses. When there was a valid pre-treatment assessment or post-treatment assessment, we imputed the missing assessment with available valid results along with profile information (Gender, Race, Age, Grade, Diagnosis) and measurement information (both pre-treatment and post-treatment scores form parents', youths', and workers' ratings on *Problem Severity* and *Functioning Scale*) for best use of information (Allison, 2000). This study used Multiple Imputation to create five imputed datasets. Independent sample *t*-test was used in each imputed dataset separately and these results of analysis are recombined to averaged values for inference (Graham et al., 2003; Schafer & Olsen, 1998). Details for the imputation are provided in the footnote of Tables 12-2 and 12-3.

FINDINGS

Baseline Characteristics

Table 12-5 shows the mean scores of *Problem Severity* of clients at pre-treatment based on parents', youths', and case managers' reports. Despite differences across multiple reporting sources, the mean scores of *Problem Severity* at pre-treatment were above the clinical cutoff score of 20, meaning the level of problem severity on average, as assessed by parents, youths, and case managers, reached clinical significance as a problem (35.75, 27.96, 33.85). The mean scores of *Functioning* of clients at pre-treatment were below the clinical cutoff score of 50 for parents and workers and 60 for youth. In other words, the level of functioning on average, as assessed by parents, youths, and case managers, reached clinical significance as a problem (39.14, 55.16, 38.57).

Treatment Efficacy

Clients showed reduction in *Problem Severity* and improvement in *Functioning* for pre-treatment to post-treatment. The mean scores of *Problem Severity* at

Table 12-5

Paired Sample *t*-Test

		N	Pre-test	Post-test	t	df	p	Cohen's d
Problem Severity	Parent	208	35.75 ± 19.63	20.61 ± 16.51	11.44	207	.000	0.79
	Youth	151	25.96 ± 17.19	17.52 ± 13.45	5.80	150	.000	0.47
	Worker	209	33.85 ± 15.99	17.70 ± 12.33	13.71	208	.000	0.95
Function	Parent	207	39.14 ± 16.43	49.10 ± 16.09	−8.32	206	.000	−0.58
	Youth	151	55.16 ± 14.33	61.88 ± 12.19	−5.83	150	.000	−0.47
	Worker	209	38.57 ± 13.57	51.11 ± 14.56	−11.54	208	.000	−0.80

Notes:

Plus-and-minus values are means ± SD.

Data were imputed for missing assessments:

Problem Severity (parent rating): 176 completed both two assessments, 2 missing in both pre-treatment and post-treatment, 11 missing in pre-treatment only, 20 missing in post-treatment only.

Problem Severity (youth rating): 110 completed both two assessments, 59 missing in both pre-treatment and post-treatment, 9 missing in pre-treatment only, 30 missing in post-treatment only.

Problem Severity (worker rating): 185 completed both two assessments, 1 missing in both pre-treatment and post-treatment, 7 missing in pre-treatment only, 17 missing in post-treatment only.

Functioning (parent rating): 171 completed both two assessments, 3 missing in both pre-treatment and post-treatment, 12 missing in pre-treatment only, 23 missing in post-treatment only.

Functioning (youth rating): 112 completed both two assessments, 59 missing in both pre-treatment and post-treatment, 10 missing in pre-treatment only, 28 missing in post-treatment only.

Functioning (worker rating): 175 completed both two assessments, 1 missing in both pre-treatment and post-treatment, 16 missing in pre-treatment only, 18 missing in post-treatment only.

post-treatment were below or very close to the clinical cutoff score of 20, meaning the level of problem severity on average, as assessed by parents, youths, and case managers, did not reach clinical significance as a problem (20.61, 17.52, 17.70). Similarly, the mean scores of *Functioning* at post-treatment were above or very close to the clinical cutoff scores of 50 for parents and case managers and 60 for youths, meaning the level of *Functioning* on average did not reach clinical significance as a problem based on multiple reporting sources (49.10, 61.88, 51.11).

The study used paired-sample *t*-tests to examine within-group changes in scores from pre-treatment to post-treatment. Regarding *Problem Severity*, clients showed significant reduction in *Problem Severity* based on parents' [$t = 11.44$, df = 207, $p = .000$], youths' [$t = 5.80$, df = 150, $p = .000$], and case managers' assessments [$t = 13.71$, df = 208, $p = .000$]. Cohen's *d* were .79 and .95 based on parents' and case managers' assessment indicating large effect sizes. Cohen's *d* was .44 based on youths' assessment indicating a small effect size. Regarding *Functioning*, clients showed significant improvement based on parents' [$t = -8.32$, df = 206, $p = .000$], youths' [$t = -5.83$, df = 150, $p = .000$], and case managers' assessments [$t = -11.54$, df = 208, $p = .000$]. Cohen's *d* ranged from −.58 to −.80 based on parents' and case managers' assessment indicating large effect sizes. Cohen's *d* was −.47 based on youths' assessment indicating a small effect size.

The study also calculated the RCI for all measurements. Using the method suggested by Jacobson and Truax (1991), the established RCI for *Problem Severity* is 10 and 8 for *Functioning* (Ohio Department of Mental Health, 2006). Regarding *Problem Severity*, approximately 57.2% and 63.2% of clients achieved reliable change based on parents' and case managers' assessments. Youths reported a lower percentage of clients achieving reliable change (45.7%). On *Functioning*, about two-thirds of clients achieved reliable change based on case managers' assessments (64.1%). Parents' and youths' reports indicated slightly lower percentages of clients achieving reliable improvement in *Functioning* (52.7% and 43.7%) (Table 12-6). To note, findings also showed a small percentages of clients experience deterioration in their symptoms. Based on parents', youths', and case managers' assessments, 7.7%, 15.2%, and 6.2% of clients experienced deterioration in *Problem Severity* from pre-treatment to post-treatment. In addition, 14.0%, 11.3%, and 9.6% of clients experienced deterioration in *Functioning* from pre-treatment to post-treatment.

DISCUSSION AND SUMMARY

This study used a one-group pre-test–post-test design to examine treatment efficacy of I-FAST. Findings were based on data collected from the original I-FAST efficacy study and two child mental health agencies that had received training and adopted I-FAST in their intensive community-based services. A total of 210 children and adolescents received I- FAST services. At pre-treatment, the clients on average showed clinical significant problems in both *Problem Severity* and *Functioning*. At post-treatment, clients as a group did not show clinical significant problems in both *Problem Severity* and *Functioning*. Based on parents', youths', and case managers' reports, there were significant decreases in *Problem Severity* and significant increases in *Functioning* in child and adolescent clients from pre-treatment and post-treatment. In addition, approximately 60% of clients achieved reliable changes in *Problem Severity* and *Functioning* from pre-treatment to post-treatment based on parents' and case managers' assessments. Overall, findings based on youths' assessments indicated a more conservative evaluation. Approximately 45% of clients achieved reliable changes in *Problem Severity* and *Functioning* from pre-treatment to post-treatment based on youths' assessment. To note, a small group of clients (between 6% and 15%) experienced deterioration in *Problem Severity* or *Functioning* based on multiple reporting sources (see Table 12-6).

Study 3: Comparison of Efficacy of I-FAST and MST for Treating At-risk Youth

This is a non-inferiority study[2] that compared treatment outcomes of I-FAST, a moderated common factors approach, to Multisystemic Therapy (MST), which is a well-established specific factors approach, for treating at-risk children and adolescents and their families.[3] This study hypothesized that I-FAST was non-inferior to MST in the youth outcomes of *Problem Severity* and *Functioning*. MST was selected as the active control because it is one of the most established evidence-based family treatments (EBFTs) with at-risk youths with behavioral and emotional problems (Henggeler et al., 1999; Huey et al., 2004; Klietz, Borduin, & Schaeffer, 2010;

Table 12-6

Reliable Change

	RCI	N	n	%
Problem Severity—Parents	10	208		
Reliable change			119	57.2
No change			73	35.1
Deterioration			16	7.7
Problem Severity—Youth	10	151		
Reliable change			69	45.7
No change			59	39.1
Deterioration			23	15.2
Problem Severity—Workers	10	209		
Reliable change			132	63.2
No change			64	30.6
Deterioration			13	6.2
Function—Parents	8	207		
Reliable change			109	52.7
No change			69	33.3
Deterioration			29	14.0
Function—Youth	8	151		
Reliable change			66	43.7
No change			68	45.0
Deterioration			17	11.3
Function—Workers	8	209		
Reliable change			134	64.1
No change			55	26.3
Deterioration			20	9.6

Note:
Data were imputed for missing assessments; see note in Table 12-5.

Schaeffer & Borduin, 2005). A meta-analysis of MST outcome studies reported the average standardized measure of effect size of MST as .55 and concluded that youths and families treated with MST were functioning better than 70% of youths and families in the comparison groups (Curtis, Ronan, & Borduin, 2004).

RESEARCH PARTICIPANTS

The study was based on data collected by a large child mental health agency in a Midwestern state for program evaluation purposes. Community-based programs at the agency received training in I-FAST from July 2007 to December 2008. Following the completion of the training, data on treatment outcomes were collected from January, 2009 to September, 2010 to evaluate the efficacy of I-FAST in improving outcomes for children and families when the agency was completely on its own to provide I-FAST services with minimal support from the original I-FAST developers. During the same period, the agency also collected data on its MST program for at-risk youths since 2007. A university Institutional Review Board (IRB) reviewed and exempted the study from IRB because the data were provided as secondary de-linked data with no direct or indirect identifiers of the clients.

From January 2009 to September 2010, the agency provided I-FAST to 79 clients and their families and MST to 47 clients and their families. Clients in both I-FAST and MST groups ranged from 12 to 18 years old, with a mean age of 15.9 for the I-FAST group and 15.5 for the MST group. Two-thirds of clients in both the I-FAST and MST groups were males and one-third were females (Table 12-7). Clients were predominantly African American (53.9% in I-FAST and 55.3% in MST) and Caucasian Americans (46.1% in I-FAST and 40.4% in MST). The majority of clients in the I-FAST group and the MST group were students in high school (59.25% and 68.1%) and middle school (39.4% and 29.8%). Only 1.4% of clients in the I-FAST group and 2.1% in the MST group were in elementary school (Table 12-7). Clients in both treatment conditions had *DSM–IV* diagnoses. The most predominant types of diagnoses related to attention–deficit/hyperactivity disorder and disruptive behavior disorders including oppositional defiant disorder and conduct disorder (87.3% in I-FAST and 87.2% in MST) (Table 12-7). On average, the length of treatment for the I-FAST group was 162.4 days, and for the MST group it was 151.2 days. There were no statistically significant differences between the two treatment conditions on age, gender, race, education, *DSM–IV* diagnoses, and length of treatment.

Intervention and Treatment Adherence

The two interventions were I-FAST and MST. Both approaches were used to provide intensive home-based treatments for at-risk families. Depending on the needs and progress of the families I-FAST practitioners initially go into the home two to three times a week for a total of up to four to six hours a week; as families make progress the number of hours and visits may be reduced until termination or transfer of the case. For MST practitioners they go into the home two to three times a week for four to six hours throughout the duration of treatment. Treatment fidelity was insured by requiring the participating service professionals to adhere to a standard treatment as defined by each treatment approach. As a well-established evidence-based treatment model MST has clear procedures for monitoring model fidelity that requires agency supervisors to maintain ongoing consultation with MST consultants certified by the model developers and MST clinicians to complete progress reports and fidelity paperwork. I-FAST requires agencies to develop their own procedures for monitoring model fidelity that include agency I-FAST supervisors providing ongoing consultation with I-FAST workers and using the *I-FAST Fidelity Scale* to monitor model fidelity (Lee et al., 2003, updated in 2011). Although there is minimal involvement from I-FAST model developers in the day-to-day monitoring of the model fidelity, the agency is required to seek recertification biennially. Part of the recertification process requires the agency to submit videotapes of treatment sessions as well as videotapes of supervision sessions to the model developers for fidelity check purposes. In brief, based on the recertification requirements of both approaches, model developers and the agency carefully monitored model fidelity of both I-FAST and MST.

Table 12-7

Baseline Characteristics of Youth Clients in I-FAST and MST Groups

	I-FAST (N = 79)		MST (N = 47)			df	p
Gender—N (%)							
Male		52 (65.8)		31 (66.0)	$\chi^2 = .00$	1	.988[1]
Female		27 (34.2)		16 (34.0)			
Race—N (%)							
White		35 (46.1)		19 (40.4)	$\chi^2 = .35$	2	.178
Black		41 (53.9)		26 (55.3)			
Others				2 (4.3)			
Education—N (%)							
High school		42 (59.2)		32 (68.1)	$\chi^2 = 1.19$	2	.553
Middle school		28 (39.4)		14 (29.8)			
Elementary		1 (1.4)		1 (2.1)			
Primary DSM:IV Diagnosis—N (%)							
ADHD & Disruptive Behavior Disorders		65 (87.3)		41 (87.2)	$\chi^2 = 2.01$	3	.571
Adjustment Disorders		2 (2.5)		2 (4.3)			
Mood Disorders		11 (13.9)		3 (6.4)			
All Other Diagnoses		1 (1.3)		1 (2.1)			
Age at Pre-treatment Assessment	n = 79	15.2 ± 1.5	n = 47	15.5 ± 1.3	t = −.96	124	.339
Length of treatment (days)	n = 79	162.4 ± 82.1	n = 47	151.2 ± 66.5	t = .796	124	.431
OS Problem Severity Pre-treatment							
Youth	n = 66	23.2 ± 14.9	n = 20	15.0 ± 14.0	t = 2.19	84	**.032**
Parent	n = 68	28.1 ± 19.9	n = 40	23.6 ± 13.7	t = 1.27	106	.208
Worker	n = 74	27.4 ± 15.2	n = 34	26.7 ± 11.5	t = .25	106	.801
OS Functioning Pre-treatment							
Youth	n = 65	56.3 ± 13.3	n = 20	61.9 ± 12.0	t = −1.66	83	.101
Parent	n = 69	42.4 ± 16.7	n = 40	45.1 ± 17.1	t = −.79	107	.429
Worker	n = 73	44.1 ± 14.0	n = 34	42.1 ± 14.3	t = −.67	105	.505

Note:
Plus-and-minus values are means ± SD.
[1] Fisher's Exact Test p = 1.000.

METHOD OF DATA COLLECTION

As part of the program evaluation, the agency used *The Ohio Scales* to assess the youths' level of problem severity and level of functioning at pre-treatment and termination. As mentioned earlier, *The Ohio Scales* ratings statistically significantly correlated with *Child and Adolescent Functional Assessment Scales* (Hodges & Wong, 1996) and *Child Behavior Checklist CBCL* (Olges et al., 2001), which were two outcome measurements used by MST in its randomized clinical trials (e.g., Timmons-Mitchell, Bender, Kishna, & Mitchell, 2006; Henggeler et al., 1999).

Pre-treatment data were collected at the time of intake and post-treatment data were collected at six months or at the time of termination, whichever came earlier. There was no difference between I-FAST and MST group in the data collection process.

DATA ANALYSES

The study used *Statistical Package for Social Sciences* 19.0 for data analyses purposes. Chi-squared tests and independent *t*-tests were used to compare demographic and baseline characteristics between I-FAST and MST groups at baseline. The study adopted the non-inferiority test for two proportions using a difference to compare treatment outcomes of I-FAST to MST on *Problem Severity* and *Functioning* from pre-treatment to termination. Specifically, the study used the RCI (Jacobson & Traux, 1991) of *The Ohio Scales* as a criterion of successful treatment. We then calculated the proportion of clients who achieved an improvement between the two assessments at or above the RCI of *The Ohio Scales* from both the I-FAST group and the MST group. Non-inferiority of a proposed treatment (I-FAST) with reference to a proven treatment (MST) is established by showing a treatment difference is likely smaller than a prespecified non-inferiority margin. For I-FAST to be considered as a non-inferior treatment to MST, the study accepted a margin of equivalence (δ) of 15% from the proportion of success achieved by the reference group MST. In other words, the study would consider I-FAST as a non-inferior treatment to MST if the difference in proportion of success in I-FAST to MST were not less than –15% to the proportion achieved by the MST. Taking an alpha of .025, I-FAST would be judged non-inferior to MST if the lower limit of the two-sided 95% confidence interval (CI) for the difference in successful proportion between I-FAST and MST was above –15% of that from MST. The statistical hypothesis to be tested is: $H_0: p_{I\text{-FAST}} - p_{MST} \leq -\delta$ versus $H_1: p_{I\text{-FAST}} - p_{MST} > -\delta$ where δ is the acceptable margin of equivalence.

A 15% non-inferiority margin was used in this analysis. Based on clinical judgment and historical data, non-inferiority margins were usually set between 5% and 15% for most studies (European Medicines Agency, 2005; U.S. Department of Health and Human Services Food and Drug Administration, 2010). As this is an exploratory study and in consultation with three experienced home-based treatment providers, a 15% non-inferiority margin is viewed as acceptable in this study because of the perceived benefits of the test treatment (European Medicines Agency, 2005) in enhancing adaptability and sustainability of the model. In addition, historical data based on the systematic review conducted by Curtis and his associates (2004) concluded that youths and families treated with MST were functioning better than 70% of youths and families in the comparison groups. Because a non-inferiority margin is chosen as the smallest value that would be a clinically important effect (Wiens, 2002), a 15% non-inferiority margin for this study was consistent with and supported by the historical data (Curtis et al., 2004). A post hoc power analysis with PASS v12 was conducted to examine the power of the present analysis to detect differences with the current sample.

RESULTS

Baseline Characteristics

Table 12-1 displays the baseline measurements for I-FAST and MST at pre-treatment. With the exception of the mean scores on *Problem Severity* based on youths' assessment [$t = 2.19$, df = 84, $p = .032$], there were no statistical significant differences on all baseline measurements between the I-FAST group and the MST group based on youths', parents', and workers' ratings on *Problem Severity* and *Functioning*. In addition, the baseline mean scores of *Problem Severity* were above the clinical cutoff score of 20 across multiple reporting sources, meaning that these clients had clinically significant problems at pre-treatment (Table 12-7). Likewise, the baseline mean scores of *Functioning* were below the clinical cutoff score of 60 for youths and 50 for parents and workers, meaning that these clients had clinically significant lower level of functioning at pre-treatment. The only exception was based on youths' ratings of the MST group; the baseline mean score of 15 on *Problem Severity* was below the clinical cutoff score of 20 and the baseline mean score of 61.9 on *Functioning* was above the clinical cutoff score of 60. In other words, youths in the MST group did not rate themselves as having a clinically significant problem or clinically significant lower level of functioning at pre-treatment (Table 12-7).

Non-Inferiority Tests for Two Proportions Using a Difference: I-FAST and MST

This study used non-inferiority tests for two proportions using a difference to compare the treatment outcomes of I-FAST and MST on *Problem Severity* and *Functioning*. This study used reliable change as indicated by RCIs of *Problem Severity* and *Functioning* to establish treatment effectiveness. Table 12-8 shows the proportion of youths who had achieved reliable change using RCIs in both the MST and I-FAST groups. Overall, the I-FAST group showed a higher proportion in achieving RCI in all measures than the MST group. In the I-FAST group, 47.1%, 43.9%, and 50% accomplished reliable reduction in *Problem Severity* from pre-treatment to post-treatment based on parents', youths', and workers' assessments. In addition, 53.7%, 49.2%, and 58.9% accomplished reliable improvement in *Functioning* from pre-treatment to post-treatment based on parents', youths', and workers' assessments. In the MST group, 37.5%, 20%, and 41.2% accomplished reliable reduction in *Problem Severity* based on parents', youths', and workers' assessments. In addition, 42.5%, 20%, and 35.3% accomplished reliable improvement in *Functioning* based on parents', youths', and workers' assessments.

A margin of equivalence of 15% with reference to the MST proportion of success was identified from each measure. Because the success proportion based on workers', parents', and youths' assessments varied, the non-inferiority margin was identified for each measure, which were .062, .056, and .030 on *Problem Severity* and .053, .064, and .030 on *Functioning* (see Table 12-8).

The differences in the proportion of youths who had achieved reliable change on *Problem Severity* and *Functioning* as based on workers', parents', and youths' assessments between the I-FAST and MST groups are presented in Figures 12-6 and 12-7. Results from all six assessments showed I-FAST was non-inferior to MST. Figure 12-1 presented findings of the non-inferiority tests for two proportions using a difference on *Problem Severity*. Non-inferiority of I-FAST to MST was established because the lower bound of the two-sided 95% CI for the difference of proportion of youths achieving reliable change between I-FAST and MST groups were greater than the non-inferiority margin for each measure. In addition, based on youths' assessment, the lower bound of the two-sided 95% CI interval for the difference of proportion of youths achieving reliable change between I-FAST and MST groups was greater than zero, thus indicating superiority of I-FAST to MST.

Table 12-8

Reliable Change Index Results of Youth Clients in I-FAST and MST Groups

		N	Proportion Achieving RCI	Margin of Equivalence[α]	95% CI
Problem Severity					
Ohio Scale Worker (OSW)	MST	34	.412	.062	
	IFAST	74	.500		.381–.619
Ohio Scale Parent (OSP)	MST	40	.375	.056	
	IFAST	68	.471		.348–.596
Ohio Scale Youth (OSY)	MST	20	.200	.030	
	IFAST	66	.439		.317–.567
Functioning					
Ohio Scale Worker (OSW)	MST	34	.353	.053	
	IFAST	73	.589		.468–.703
Ohio Scale Parent (OSP)	MST	40	.425	.064	
	IFAST	67	.537		.411–.660
Ohio Scale Youth (OSY)	MST	20	.200	.030	
	IFAST	65	.492		.366–.619

[α] The Non-Inferiority Margin is the acceptable difference in success rate between the new treatment group, i.e., in this case I-FAST, and the reference group, i.e., MST. In this analysis a –15% of the proportion of the reference group is adopted as the margin of equivalence for each measure.

Figure 12-7 presents findings of the non-inferiority test for two proportions on *Functioning* based on workers', parents', and youths' assessments. Non-inferiority of I-FAST to MST was established because the lower bound of the two-sided 95% CI interval for the difference of proportion of youths achieving reliable change between I-FAST and MST groups were greater than the non-inferiority margin. Based on

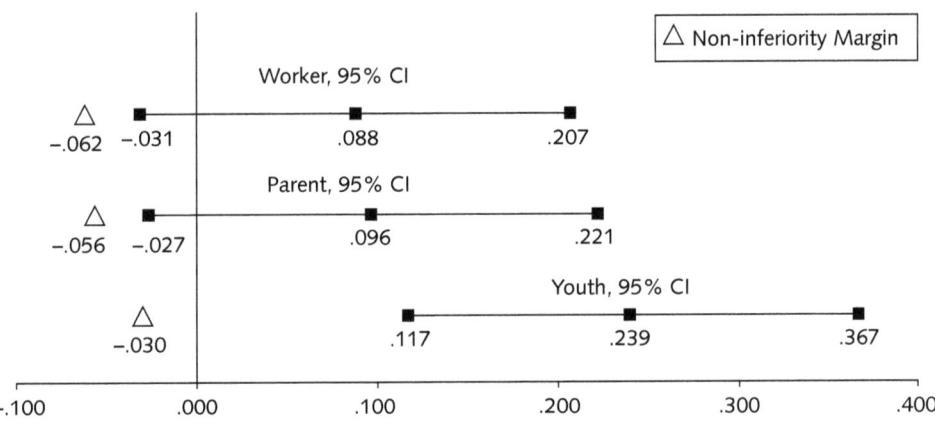

Difference in rate of achieving RCI in reducing Problem Severity between I-FAST and MST

FIGURE 12-6 **Non-inferiority tests on for two proportions using a Difference Problem Severity.**

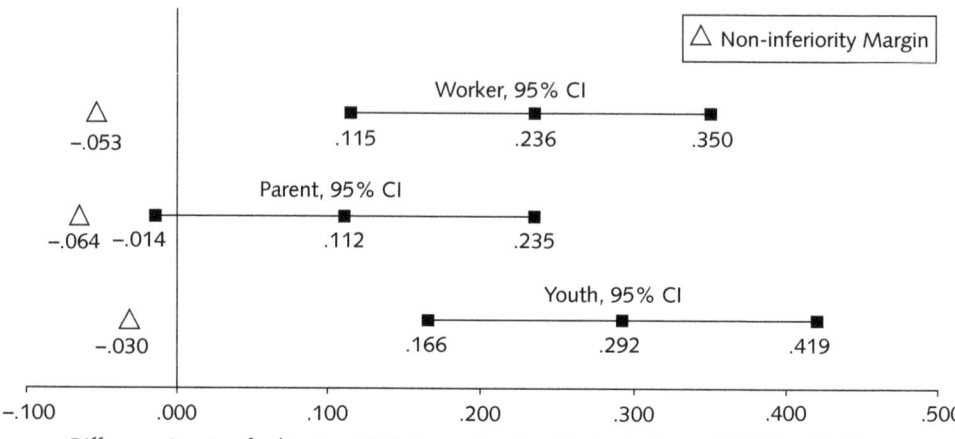

FIGURE 12-7 **Non-inferiority tests for two proportions using a Difference on Functioning.**

workers' and youths' assessments, the lower bound of the two-sided 95% CI intervals for the difference of proportion of youths achieving reliable change between I-FAST and MST groups were greater than zero, and thus indicating superiority of I-FAST to MST.

A post hoc power analysis with PASS v12 showed the power of the present analysis as .65, .71, and .92 for the *Problem Severity* subscale with workers, parents, and youths. For the *Functioning* subscale, the power results were .96, .75, and .97 for workers, parents, and youths.

DISCUSSION AND SUMMARY

Limitations of this study need to be acknowledged. This study used secondary data collected for program evaluation purposes. As such, random assignment procedures were not utilized in the study. Consequently, there were selection biases between clients in the I-FAST group and MST group. For instance, many clients in the MST group were court-referred while clients in the I-FAST group were referred by diverse referral sources including the courts, schools, child welfare, criminal justice systems, and other social service agencies. However, there were no statistical significant differences between the clients participating in I-FAST and MST on demographic characteristics including age, gender, race, and educational attainment; primary *DSM–IV* diagnoses; pre-treatment level of *Problem Severity* and *Functioning* as measured by *The Ohio Scales* and assessed by parents and workers; as well as treatment duration (Table 12-1). In addition, all data were collected during the same time period, that is, from January 2009 to September 2010 at the same mental health agency. The only statistically significant difference was found in *Problem Severity* based on youths' assessments where youths in the MST group self-reported a significantly lower level of *Problem Severity* than youths in the I-FAST group. Second, while model fidelity of MST was closely monitored by the model developers, and I-FAST fidelity was closely monitored by the agency as well as the I-FAST recertification requirements, this study has no direct access to the results of the fidelity evaluation. In view of the cited limitations, we treated the present study providing preliminary evidences for further exploration of the effectiveness of I-FAST in family therapy with at-risk youths within a community mental health service agency setting.

This was a non-randomized non-inferiority study to compare the effectiveness of I-FAST, a moderated common factors approach, in reference to MST, a specific factors approach, in treating at-risk children and adolescents and their families. As a group, findings of the study indicated that approximately 35% to 60% of youths in I-FAST and MST achieved reliable change in *Problem Severity* and *Functioning* based on workers' and parents' assessments. Findings of this study provided initial support to the study hypothesis that I-FAST was non-inferior to MST. I-FAST was non-inferior to MST in reducing *Problem Severity* and improving *Functioning* in clients based on parents' assessments. I-FAST was non-inferior to MST in reducing *Problem Severity* in clients based on workers' assessments. In addition, findings indicated the superiority of I-FAST to MST in reducing *Problem Severity* and *Functioning* in youths based on youths' assessments, and superiority of I-FAST to MST in improving *Functioning* based on workers' assessments (Figures 12-1 and 12-2). However, findings of superiority of I-FAST compared to MST based on youths' assessments will need to be interpreted with caution. One plausible explanation for such findings is that MST youths had self-rated *Problem Severity* below the clinical cutoff score and *Functioning* above the clinical cutoff score at pre-treatment (Table 12-1). A lack of recognition of their problems among MST youths might influence their assessment of treatment outcomes.

Additional Studies on I-FAST

- **Lee, M. Y., Teater, B., Greene, G. J., Hsu, K. S., Fraser, J. S., Solovey, A., & Washburn, P. (2012). Key processes, ingredients and components of successful systems collaboration: Working with severely emotionally or behaviorally disturbed children and their families.** *Administration and Policy in Mental Health and Mental Health Services Research, 39*(5), 394–405.

Through qualitative data, this study explored the process of and the skill components involved in interagency collaboration when providing Integrative Family and Systems Treatment (I-FAST) for families with severely emotionally or behaviorally disturbed children who were at risk of out-of-home placement. Data were collected through a series of eight focus groups with 26 agency collaborators across 11 counties in Ohio. Data analysis revealed two emergent phenomena: the process of developing collaboration, which consisted of making initial contact, a trial period, and developing trust; and the key ingredients of collaboration, which focused on interpersonal and professional qualities. Practice implications of each theme are discussed.

- **Lee, M. Y., Teater, B., Hsu, K. S., Greene, G. J., Fraser, J. S., Solovey, A., Grove, D. (2013). Systems collaboration with schools and treatment of SED children or adolescents.** *Children & Schools, 35*(3), 155–168.

This study explored the relationship between the level of systems collaboration with schools and outcomes for severely emotionally or behaviorally disturbed children and families involved in the I-FAST, a home-based treatment program. Using data collected from 38 clients and their families, this study utilized a structural equation model to explore how systems collaboration with schools influenced children's behavioral outcomes, parental competence, and family functioning. The Squared Multiple Correlations from endogenous variables of the final model accounted for

31% of the variance in *Problem Severity in Children*, 38% of the variance in *Level of Functioning in Children*, 30% of the variance in *Parental Competence with Children*, and 41% of the variance in *Family Functioning*. The final model indicated the following: *Systems Collaboration with Schools* positively influenced *Parental Competence with Children*, which positively predicted *Level of Functioning in Children* and negatively predicted *Problem Severity in Children*. While the limited sample size of the study precludes any definitive conclusions, implications of the study on the potential role of systems collaboration with schools in treating families with at-risk children or adolescents are explored and discussed.

CONCLUSION

This section of the chapter has provided a detailed description of findings of three studies and a brief summary of two additional I-FAST studies that focused on the role of systems collaboration, which is a major treatment component of I-FAST. The two outcome studies provide initial empirical evidence that I-FAST treatment tends to lead to improved functioning and reduced problem severity in the child, reduction in out-of-home placement of the child, improved family functioning, increased parental competency in addressing their child's problems, and increased family participation in the treatment process. Approximately 60% of children and adolescents showed reliable changes in their level of problem severity and functioning from pre-treatment to post-treatment as assessed by parents and case managers. In addition, I-FAST was non-inferior to MST in reducing *Problem Severity* and improving *Functioning* in clients. Findings also indicated the superiority of I-FAST to MST in reducing *Problem Severity* and *Functioning* in youths based on youths' assessments, and superiority of I-FAST to MST in improving *Functioning* based on workers' assessments.

The effectiveness of I-FAST will still need to be tested further in a large-scale study with an experimental design that will provide more conclusive evidence of I-FAST as an alternative, feasible, and effective home-based treatment model. Specific recommendations for the future large scale effectiveness study include: (1) include control or comparison groups using randomized assignment procedures in effectiveness and non-inferiority studies; (2) increase the rigor of the fidelity procedures by using observation-based approaches with a refined, specific, and rigorous fidelity measurement protocol of I-FAST; (3) use established instruments to measure outcomes at the family and agency level in addition to child behavioral outcomes to explore further the impact of I-FAST on diverse stakeholders; (4) include multiple research sites that serve ethnically/racially diverse populations; and (5) use multiple research methods, both quantitative and qualitative, to identify the mechanisms of change associated with I-FAST.

NOTE

[1] This study and the tables are from an article originally published as: Lee, M. Y., Greene, G. J., Hsu, K. S., Solovey, A., Grove, D., Fraser, S., Washburn, P., Teater, B. (2009). *Utilizing family strengths and resilience: Integrative family and systems treatment (I-FAST) with children and adolescents with severe emotional and behavioral problems*. Family Process, 48(3), 395–416.

[2] This study was originally published in Lee, M. Y., Greene, G. J., Fraser, S., Grove, D, Solovey, A., Edwards, S., & Scott, P. (2013). *Common and specific factors approaches to home-based treatment: I-FAST and MST*. Research on Social Work Practice, 23(4), 407–418.

[3] This study was sponsored by The Buckeye Ranch.

REFERENCES

Adams, J. F. (1997). *Questions as interventions in therapeutic conversation.* Journal of Family Psychotherapy, *8*, 17–35.
Alexander, J. F., & Sexton, T. L. (2002). Functional family therapy: A model for treating high-risk, acting-out youth. In F. W. Kaslow (Ed.), *Comprehensive handbook of psychotherapy: Integrative/eclectic* (Vol. 4, pp. 111–132). Hoboken, NJ: John Wiley & Sons.
Allison, P. D. (2000). *Multiple imputation for missing data: A cautionary tale.* Sociological Methods and Research, *28*, 301–309.
Anderson, H., Goolishian, H. A., & Winderman, L. (1986). *Problem-determined systems: Towards transformation in family therapy.* Journal of Strategic & Systemic Therapies, *5*, 1–13.
Aspinwall, L. G., & Staudinger, U. M. (2002). A psychology of human strengths: Some central issues of an emerging field. In L. G. Aspinwall & U. M. Staudinger (Eds.), *A psychology of human strengths: Fundamental questions and future directions for a positive psychology* (pp. 9–22). Washington, DC: American Psychological Association.
Atteneave, N. (1969). *Treating the troubled family.* New York, NY: Basic Books.
Bandura, A. (1986). *Social foundations of thought and action: A social-cognitive theory.* Englewood Cliffs, NJ: Prentice Hall.
Barkley, R. A. (1997). *ADHD and the nature of self-control.* New York, NY: Guilford Press.
Barlow, D. H. (1981). *On the relation of clinical research to clinical practice: Current issues, new directions.* Journal of Consulting and Clinical Psychology, *49*, 147–155.
Bateson, G. (1955). *A theory of play and fantasy.* A.P.A. Psychiatric Research Reports II, 39–51.
Bateson, G. (1972). *Steps to an ecology of mind.* New York, NY: Ballantine Books.
Bateson, G. (1979). *Mind and nature: A necessary unity.* New York, NY: E. P. Dutton.
Bavelas, J. B., McGee, D., Phillips, B., & Routledge, R. (2000). *Microanalysis of communication in psychotherapy.* Human Systems, *11*, 47–66.
Beck, A. T. (1976). *Cognitive therapy and the emotional disorders.* Oxford, UK: International Universities Press.
Beidas, R. S., & Kendal, P. C. (2010). *Training practitioners in evidence-based practice: A critical review of studies from a systems-contextual perspective.* Clinical Psychology, *17*, 1–30.
Benish, S. F., Imel, Z. E., & Wampold, B. E. (2007). *The relative efficacy of bona fide psychotherapies for treating post-traumatic stress disorder: A meta-analysis of direct comparisons.* Clinical Psychology Review, *28*, 746–758. Doi:10.1016/j,cpr.2008.06.001
Berg, I. K. (1994). *Family-based services: A solution-focused approach.* New York, NY: W. W. Norton.
Berg, I. K., & De Jong, P. (1996). *Solution-building conversations: Co-constructing a sense of competence with clients.* Families in Society, *77*, 376–391.
Berg, I. K., & Dolan, Y. (2001). *Tales of solutions: A collection of hope-inspiring stories.* New York, NY: W. W. Norton.
Berg, I. K., & Gallagher, D. (1991). Solution-focused brief treatment with adolescent substance abusers. In T. C. Todd & M. D. Selekman (Eds.), *Family therapy approaches with adolescent substance abusers* (pp. 93–111). Boston, MA: Allyn and Bacon.
Berg, I. K., & Kelly, S. (2000). *Building solutions in child protective services.* New York, NY: W. W. Norton.
Berg, I. K., & Miller, S. D. (1992). *Working with Asian American clients: One person at a time.* Families in Society, *73*, 356–363.
Berger, P. L., & Luckman, T. (1966). *The social construction of reality: A treatise in the sociology of knowledge.* New York, NY: Anchor Books.
Beutler, L. E. (1973). *The therapy dyad: Yet another look at diagnostic assessment.* Journal of Personality Assessment, *37*, 303–308.
Beutler, L. E., Engle, D., Oro-Beutler, M. E., Daldrup, R., & Meredith, K. (1986). *Inability to express intense affect: A common link between depression and pain?* Journal of Consulting and Clinical Psychology, *54*, 752–759.
Beutler, L. E., Johnson, D. T., Neville, C. W., & Workman, S. N. (1972). *"Accurate empathy" and A-B dichotomy.* Journal of Consulting and Clinical Psychology, *38*, 372–375.
Biswas-Diener, R., & Dean, B. (2007). *Positive psychology coaching: Putting the science of happiness to work for your clients.* Hoboken, NJ: John Wiley & Sons.
Bohart, A. C. (2002). *How does the relationship facilitate productive client thinking?* Journal of Contemporary Psychotherapy, *32*, 61–69.
Bohart, A. C., & Tallman, K. (2010). Clients: The neglected common factor in psychotherapy. In B. L. Duncan, S. D. Miller, B. E. Wampold, & M. A. Hubble (Eds.), *The heart & soul of change: Delivering what works in therapy* (2nd ed., pp. 83–111). Washington, DC: American Psychological Association.
Borah, P. (2011). *Conceptual issues in framing theory: A systematic examination of a decade's literature.* Journal of Communication, *61*, 246–263.
Bordin, E. S. (1979). *The generalizability of the psychoanalytic concept of the working alliance.* Psychotherapy: Theory, Research and Practice, *16*, 252–260.
Bowen, M. (1974). *Alcoholism as viewed through family systems theory and family therapy.* Annals of the New York Academy of Sciences, *233*, 115–122.
Bowen, M. (1978). *Family therapy in clinical practice.* New York, NY: Jason Aronson.

Breulin, D. C. (1989). Clinical implications of oscillation theory: Family development and the process of change. In C. N. Ramsey, Jr. (Ed.), *Family systems in medicine* (pp. 135–149). New York, NY: Guilford Press.

Bronfenbrenner, U. (1979). *The ecology of human development: Experiments by design and nature.* Cambridge, MA: Harvard University Press.

Brown, K. W., & Ryan, R. M. (2004). Fostering health self-regulation from within and without: A self-determination theory perspective. In P. A. Linley & S. Joseph (Eds.), *Positive psychology in practice* (pp. 1005–1124). New York, NY: John Wiley & Sons.

Budman, S. H., & Burman, A. S. (1988). *Theory and practice of brief therapy.* New York: Guilford Press.

Busseri, M. A., & Tyler, J. D. (2004). *Client-practitioner agreement on target problems, working alliance, and counseling outcome.* Psychotherapy Research, *14*, 77–88.

Campbell, J. M. (2000). *Becoming an effective supervisor: A workbook for counselors and psychotherapists.* Philadelphia, PA: Accelerated Development.

Campis, L. K., Lyman, R. D., & Prentice-Dunn, S. (1986). *The Parental Locus of Control Scale: Development and validation.* Journal of Clinical Child Psychiatry, *15*, 260–267.

Capra, F. (1996). *The web of life: A new scientific understanding of living systems.* New York, NY: Anchor Books.

Carroll, K., Nich, C., Sifrey, R., Frankforter, T., Nuro, K., & Rounsaville, B. J. (2000). *A general system for evaluating therapist adherence and therapist competence in psychotherapy research in the addictions.* Drug and Alcohol Dependence, *57*, 225–238.

Carroll, K. M., & Nuro, K. F. (2002). *One size cannot fit all: A Stage model for psychotherapy manual development.* Clinical Psychology: Science and Practice, *9*, 396–406.

Carroll, K. M., & Rounsaville, B. J. (2008). *A vision of the next generation of behavioral therapies research in addictions.* Addiction, *102*, 850–862.

Castonguay, L. G., Goldfried, M. R., Wiser, S., Raue, P. J., & Hayes, A. M. (1996). *Predicting the effect of cognitive treatment for depression: A study of unique and common factors.* Journal of Consulting Psychology, *64*, 497–504.

Cheavens, J. S., Feldman, D. B., Gum, A., Michael, S. T., & Snyder, C. R. (2006). *Hope therapy in a community sample: A pilot investigation.* Social Indicators Research, *77*, 61–78.

Claiborn, C. D., & Dowd, E. T. (1985). *Attributional interpretations in counseling: Content versus discrepancy.* Journal of Counseling Psychology, *32*, 188–196.

Coppock, T. E., Owen, J. J., Zagarskas, E., & Schmidt, M. (2010). *The relationship between therapist and client hope with therapy outcomes.* Psychotherapy Research, *20*, 619–626.

Curtis, N. M., Ronan, K. R., & Borduin, C. M. (2004). *Multisystemic treatment: A meta-analysis of outcome studies.* Journal of Family Psychology, *18*, 411–419.

Deci, E. L., & Ryan, R. M. (2002). Self-determination research: Reflections and future directions. In E. L. Deci & R. M. Ryan (Eds.), *Handbook of self-determination research* (pp. 431–441). Rochester, NY: University of Rochester Press.

De Jong, P., & Berg, I. K. (2008). *Interviewing for solutions* (3rd ed.). Belmont, CA: Thompson Brooks/Cole.

de Shazer, S. (1985). *Keys to solution in brief therapy.* New York, NY: W. W. Norton.

de Shazer, S. (1994). *Words were originally magic.* New York, NY: W. W. Norton.

de Shazer, S., Berg, I. K., Lipchik, E., Nunnally, E., Molnar, A., Gingerich, W. J., & Weiner-Davis, M. (1986). *Brief therapy: Focused solution development.* Family Process, *25*, 207–222.

Diamond, G. S., & Diamond, G. M. (2002). Studying a matrix of change mechanisms: An agenda for family-based process research. In H. A. Liddle, D. A. Santisteban, R. F. Levant, & J. H. Bray (Eds.), *Family psychology: Science-based interventions* (pp. 41–66). Washington, DC: American Psychological Association.

Echterling, L. G., Presbury, J. H., & McKee, J. E. (2005). *Crisis intervention: Promoting resilience and resolution in troubled times.* Upper Saddle River, NJ: Pearson Education.

Eiser, J. R. (2000). *The influence of question framing on symptom report and perceived health status.* Psychology and Health, *15*, 13–20.

Elliot, A. J., & Church, M. (2002). *Client-articulated avoidance goals in the therapy context.* Journal of Counseling Psychology, *72*, 218–232.

Elliot, A. J., & Harackiewicz, J. M. (1996). *Approach and avoidance achievement goals and intrinsic motivation: A meditational analysis.* Journal of Personality and Social Psychology, *73*, 171–185.

Ellis, A. (1962). *Reason and emotion in psychotherapy.* Oxford, UK: Lyle Stuart.

Escudero, V., Heatherington, L., & Friedlander, M. L. (2010). Therapeutic alliances and alliance building in family therapy. In J. C. Muran & J. P. Barber (Eds.), *The therapeutic alliance: An evidence-based guide for practice* (pp. 240–262). New York, NY: Guilford Press.

European Medicines Agency (27 July 2005). *Guideline on the choice of the non-inferiority margin.* London, UK: Committee for Medicinal Products for Human Use, EMEA.

Fairhurst, G. T. (2011). *The power of framing: Creating the language of leadership.* San Francisco, CA: Jossey-Bass.

Fairhurst, G. T., & Sarr, R. A. (1996). *The art of framing: Managing the language of leadership.* San Francisco, CA: Jossey-Bass.

Falender, C. A., & Safranske, E. P. (2004). *Clinical supervision: A competency-based approach.* Washington, DC: American Psychological Association.

Fast, B., & Chapin, R. (2000). *Strengths-based care management for older adults*. Baltimore, MD: Health Professions Press.

Feist, S. C. (1999). *Practice and theory of professional supervision for mental health counselors*. Directions in Mental Health Counseling, 9(9), 105–120.

Feldman, P. (1994). *The use of therapeutic questions to restructure dysfunctional triangles in marital therapy: A psychodynamic family therapy approach*. Journal of Family Psychotherapy, 5, 55–67.

Fine, M., & Turner, J. (2002). Collaborative supervision: Minding the power. In T. Todd & C. Storm (Eds.), *The complete systemic supervisor*. New York, NY: Authors Choice Press.

Fisch, R., Weakland, J. H., & Segal, L. (1982). *The tactics of change: Doing therapy briefly*. San Francisco, CA: Jossey-Bass.

Fitzsimmons, G. J., & Williams, P. (2000). *Asking questions can change choice behavior: Does it do so automatically or effortfully?* Journal of Experimental Psychology: Applied, 6, 195–206.

Frank, J. D. (1961). *Persuasion and healing: A comparative study of psychotherapy*. Baltimore, MD: Johns Hopkins University Press.

Frank, J. D., & Frank, J. B. (1991). *Persuasion and healing: A comparative study of psychotherapy* (3rd ed.). Baltimore, MD: Johns Hopkins University Press.

Fraser, J. S. (1995). *Process, problems, and solutions in brief therapy*. Journal of Marital and Family Therapy, 21(3), 265–279.

Fraser, J. S., & Solovey, A. (2007). *Second-order change in psychotherapy: The golden thread that unifies effective treatments*. Washington, DC: American Psychological Association.

Fraser, S., Solovey, A., Grove, D., Lee, M. Y., & Greene, G. J. (2012). *Integrative Families and Systems Treatment: A Middle Path Towards Integrating Common and Specific Factors in Evidence Based Family Therapy*. Journal of Marital and Family Therapy, 38(3), 518–528.

Friedlander, M. L., Escudero, V., & Heatherington, L. (2006). *Therapeutic alliances in couple and family therapy: An empirically-informed guide to practice*. Washington, DC: American Psychological Association.

Friedlander, M. L., Escudero, V., Heatherington, L., & Diamond, G. M. (2011). *Alliance in couple and family therapy*. Psychotherapy, 48, 25–33.

Friedlander, M. L., Escudero, V., Heatherington, L., & Diamond, G. M. (2011). Alliance in couple and family therapy. In J. C. Norcross (Ed.), *Psychotherapy relationships that work: Evidence-based responsiveness* (2nd ed., pp. 92–109). New York, NY: Oxford University Press.

Friesen, B. J. (2001). *Family participation measure*. Portland, OR: Regional Research Institute for Human Services, Research and Training Center on Family Support and Children's Mental Health.

Friesen, B. J., & Pullman, M. (2002). Family participation in planning services: A brief measure. In C. Newman, C. Liberton, K. Kutash, & R. Friedman (Eds.), 14th Annual Research Conference Proceedings: *A system of care for children's mental health: Expanding the research base* (pp. 353–358). Tampa, FL: Louis de la Parte Florida Mental Health Institute, Research and Training Center on Children's Mental Health.

Galassi, J. P., & Akos, P. (2007). *Strengths-based school counseling: Promoting student development and achievement*. Mahwah, NJ: Lawrence Erlbaum.

Garfinkle, H., & Sacks, H. (1970). On formal structures of practical actions. In J. C. McKinney & E. A. Tiryakin (Eds.), *Theoretical sociology* (pp. 337–366). New York, NY: Appleton-Century-Crofts.

Gassman, D., & Grawe, K. (2006). *General change mechanisms: The relation between problem activation and resource activation in successful and unsuccessful therapeutic interactions*. Clinical Psychology and Psychotherapy, 13, 1–11.

Gergen, K. J. (1999). *An invitation to social construction*. Thousand Oaks, CA: SAGE.

Gergen, K. J. (2009). *Relational being: Beyond self and community*. New York, NY: Oxford University Press.

Glisson, C., Schoenwald, S. K., Kelleher, K., Landsverk, J., Hoagwood, K. E., Mayberg, S., & Greene, P. (2008). *Therapist turnover and new program sustainability in mental health clinics as a function of organizational culture, climate, and service structure*. Administration and Policy in Mental Health, 35, 124–133.

Godin, G., Sheeran, P., Conner, M., & Germain, M. (2008). *Asking questions changes behavior: Mere measurement effects on frequency of blood donation*. Health Psychology, 27, 179–184.

Goffman, E. (1974). *Frame analysis*. New York, NY: Free Press.

Goin, M., Yamamoto, J., & Silverman, J. (1965). *Therapy congruent with class-linked expectations*. Archives of General Psychiatry, 13, 133–137.

Goldberg, M. C. (1998). *The art of the question: A guide to short-term question-centered therapy*. New York, NY: John Wiley & Sons.

Goldenberg, H., & Goldenberg, I. (2008). *Family therapy: An overview* (7th ed.). Belmont, CA: Thomson Brooks/Cole.

Goldman, H. H., Ganju, V., Drake, R. E., Gorman, P., Hogan, M., Hyde, P. S., & Morgan, O. (2001). *Policy implications for implementing evidence-based practices*. Psychiatric Services, 52, 1591–1597.

Goodyear, R. K., & Nelson, M. L. (1997). The major formats of psychotherapy supervision. In C. E. Watkins Jr. (Ed.), *Handbook of psychotherapy supervision* (pp. 328–344). New York, NY: John Wiley & Sons.

Gore, J. S., & Cross, S. E. (2011). *Task frame and perceived fit: The role of personality, task label, and partner involvement*. Motivation and Emotion, 35, 368–382.

Graham, J. W., Cumsille, P. E., & Elek-Fisk, E. (2003). Methods for handling missing data. In J. A. Schinka, W. F. Velicer, & R. B. Weiner (Eds.), *Handbook of Psychology* (Vol. 2, pp. 87–114). New York, NY: John Wiley & Sons.

Greene, R. (2001). *The explosive child*. New York: Harper Collins.

Greene, G. J., & Lee, M. Y. (2011). *Solution-oriented social work practice: An integrative approach to working with client strengths*. New York, NY: Oxford University Press.

Greene, R. W., & Ablon, J. S. (2001). *What does the MTA study tell us about effective psychosocial treatment for ADHD?* Journal of Clinical Child Psychology, 30, 114–121.

Greene, R. W., & Ablon, J. S. (2006). *Treating explosive kids: The collaborative problem-solving approach*. New York, NY: Guilford Press.

Greene, R., Ablon, S. J., Goring, G. C. et al. (2004b). *Effectiveness of collaborative problem solving in affectively dysregulated children with oppositional-defiant disorder: Initial findings*. Journal of Consulting & Clinical Psychology, 72(6), 1157–1164.

Grove, D. (2009). Introduction to why a mental health clinic should avoid family therapy. In M. Richeport-Haley & J. Carlson (Eds.), *Jay Haley revisited*. New York, NY: Routledge.

Grove, D., & Haley, J. (1993). *Conversations on therapy*. New York, NY: W. W. Norton.

Haffner, J. (1983). *Agoraphobic women married to abnormally jealous men*. British Journal of Medical Psychology, 52, 99–104.

Hafner, R. J., & Ross, M. W. (1983). *Predicting the outcome of behavior therapy for agoraphobia*. Behaviour Research and Therapy, 21, 375–382.

Haley, J. (1963). *Strategies of psychotherapy*. New York, NY: Grune & Stratton.

Haley, J. (1973). *Uncommon therapy: The psychiatric techniques of Milton H. Erickson, M.D.* New York, NY: W. W. Norton.

Haley, J. (1976). *Problem solving therapy*. San Francisco, CA: Jossey Bass.

Haley, J. (1980). *Leaving home: The therapy of disturbed young people*. New York: McGraw-Hill.

Haley, J. (1985). *Ordeal therapy*. San Francisco, CA: Jossey-Bass.

Haley, J. (1987). *Problem-solving therapy* (2nd ed.). San Francisco, CA: Jossey-Bass.

Haley, J. (1996). *Learning and teaching therapy*. New York, NY: Guilford Press.

Haley, J. (1997). *Leaving home: The therapy of disturbed young people* (2nd ed.). New York, NY: Brunner/Mazel.

Ham, M. A. (1987). Client behavior and counselor empathic performance. In G. A. Gladstein & Associates, *Empathy and counseling: Explanations in theory and research* (pp. 31–50). New York: Springer-Verlag.

Hampson, R. B., Hulgus, Y. F., & Beavers, W. R. (1991). *Comparisons of self-report measures of the Beavers Systems Model and Olson's Circumplex Model*. Journal of Family Psychology, 4, 326–340.

Hansen, N. B., Lambert, M. J., & Forman, E. V. (2002). *The psychotherapy dose-response effect and its implications for treatment delivery services*. Clinical Psychology: Science and practice, 9, 329–343.

Haynes, R., Corey, G., & Moulton, P. (2003). *Clinical supervision in the helping professions: A practical guide*. Pacific Grove, CA: Thompson Brooks/Cole.

Henderson, C. E., Cawyer, C. S., & Watkins. C. E. (1999). *A comparison of student and supervisor perceptions of effective practicum supervision*. The Clinical Supervisor, 18, 47–74.

Henggeler, S. W., Rowland, M. D., Randall, J., Ward, D. M., Pickrel, S. G., Cunningham, P. B., Miller, S. l., Edwards, J., Zealberg, J. J., Hand, L. D., & Santos, A. B. (1999). *Home-based Multisystemic therapy as an alternative to the hospitalization of youths in psychiatric crisis: Clinical outcomes*. Journal of American Academy of Child and Adolescent Psychiatry, 38, 1331–1339.

Henggeler, S. W., Schoenwald, S. K., Rowland, M. D., & Cunningham, P. B. (2002). *Serious emotional disturbance in children and adolescents: Multisystemic therapy*. New York, NY: Guilford Press.

Henry, P. W., Sprenkle, D. H., & Sheehan, R. (1986). *Family therapy training: Student and faculty perceptions*. Journal of Marital and Family Therapy, 12, 249–258.

Heritage, J., & Watson, R. (1979). Formulations as conversational objects. In G. Pasathas (Ed.), *Everyday language: Studies in ethnomethodology* (pp. 123–162). New York, NY: Irvington.

Hoagwood, K., Hibbs, E., Brent, D., & Jensen, P. (1995). *Introduction to the special section: Efficacy and effectiveness in studies of child and adolescent psychotherapy*. Journal of Consulting and Clinical Psychology, 63, 683–687.

Hodges, K., & Wong, M. M. (1996). *Psychometric characteristics of a multidimensional measure to assess impairment: The child and adolescent functional assessment scale*. Journal of Child and Family Studies, 5, 445–467.

Hogue, A., Liddle, H. A., & Becker, D. (2002). Multidimensional family prevention for at-risk adolescents. In F. W. Kaslow (Series Ed.) & T. Patterson (Vol. Ed.), *Comprehensive handbook of psychotherapy*, Vol. 2: *Cognitive-behavioral approaches* (pp. 141–166). New York. NY: John Wiley & Sons.

Hogue, A., Liddle, H. A., Becker, D., & Johnson-Leckrone, J. (2002). *Family-based prevention counseling for high-risk young adolescents: Immediate outcomes*. Journal of Community Psychology, 30, 1–22.

Horigan, V. E., Suarez-Morales, L., Robbins, M. S., Zarate, M., Mayorga, C. C., Mitrani, V. B., & Szapocznik, J. (2005). Brief strategic family therapy for adolescents with behavior problems. In J. L. Lebow (Ed.), *Handbook of clinical family therapy* (pp. 73–102). Hoboken, NJ: John Wiley & Sons.

Horvath, A. O., & Bedi, R. P. (2002). The alliance. In J. C. Norcross (Ed.), *Psychotherapy relationships that work: Therapist contributions and responsiveness to patients* (pp. 37–69). New York, NY: Oxford University Press.

Horvath, A. O., & Greenberg, L. S. (1986). The development of the working alliance inventory. In L. S. Reenberg & W. M. Pinsof (Eds.), *The therapeutic process: A research handbook* (pp. 529–556). New York, NY: Guilford Press.

Howard, K. I., Kopta, S. M., Krause, M. S., & Orlinsky, D. E. (1986). *The dose-effect relationship in psychotherapy.* American Psychologist, *41*, 159–164.

Howard, K. L., Moras, K. Brill, P. L., Martinovich, Z., & Lutz W. (1996). *Evaluation of psychotherapy: Efficacy, effectiveness, and patient progress.* American Psychologist, *51*(10), 1059–1064.

Huey, S. J., Jr., Henggeler, S. W., Rowland, M. D., Halliday-Boykins, C. A., Cunningham, P. B., & Pickrel, S. G., & Edwards, J. (2004). *Multisystemic therapy effects on attempted suicide by youths presenting psychiatric emergencies.* Journal of American Academy of Child and Adolescent Psychiatry, *43*, 183–190.

Irving, L. M., Snyder, C. R., Cheavens, J., Gravel, L., Hanke, J., Hilberg, P., & Nelson, N. (2004). *Therelationship between hope and outcomes at the pretreatment, beginning, and later phases of psychotherapy.* Journal of Psychotherapy Integration, *14*, 419–443.

Jackson, D. D. (1957). *The question of family homeostasis.* The Psychiatric Quarterly Supplement, *31*, 79–90.

Jacobson, N. S., & Truax, P. (1991). *Clinical significance: A statistical approach to defining meaningful change in psychotherapy research.* Journal of Consulting and Clinical Psychology, *59*, 12–19.

Jones, C. W. (1986). *Frame cultivation: Helping new meanings take root in families.* The American Journal of Family Therapy, *14*, 57–68.

Kazdin, A. E. (2008). *The Kazdin method for parenting the defiant child: With no pills, no therapy, no contest of wills.* Boston, MA: Houghton Mifflin.

Keeney, B. P. (1983). *Aesthetics of change.* New York, NY: Guilford Press.

Kelly, A. (2000). *Helping clients construct desirable identities: A self-presentational view of psychotherapy.* Psychological Bulletin, *126*, 475–494.

Kinney, J. H., Booth, D. A., & Booth, C. (1991). *Keeping families together: The homebuilders model.* Hawthorne, NY: Aldine de Gruyter.

Kirsch, I. (1990). *Changing expectations: A key to effective psychotherapy.* Pacific Grove, CA: Brooks/Cole.

Klietz, S. J., Borduin, C. M., & Schaeffer, C. M. (2010). *Cost–benefit analysis of multisystemic therapy with serious and violent juvenile offenders.* Journal of Family Psychology, *24*, 657–666.

Knutson, N. M., Forgatch, M. S., & Rains, L. A. (2003). *Fidelity of Implementation Rating System (FIMP): The training manual for PMTO.* Eugene, OR: Oregon Social Learning Center.

Koss, M. P., & Shiang, J. (1994). In Bergin, A. E. & Garfield, S. L. (Eds). *Handbook of psychotherapy and behavior change (4th Ed).* Oxford, England: John Wiley & Sons (pp. 644–700).

Kral, R., & Kowalski, K. (1989). *After the miracle: The second stage in solution-focused brief therapy.* Journal of Strategic and Systemic Therapies, *8*, 73–76.

Ladenay, N., Elliks, M. V., & Friedlander, M. L. (1999). *The supervisory working alliance, t trainee self-efficacy, and satisfaction.* Journal of Counseling and Development, *77*, 447–455.

Ladenay, N., & Friedlander, M., L. (1995). *The relationship between the supervisory working alliance and trainees' experience of role conflict and role ambiguity.* Counselor Education and Supervision, *34*, 220–231.

Lakoff, G. (2006). *Thinking points: Communicating our American values and vision.* New York, NY: Farrar, Straus & Giroux.

Lakoff, G. (2008). *The political mind: Why you can't understand 21st-century American politics with an 18th-century brain.* New York, NY: Viking.

Lambert, M. (2007). *Presidential address: What we have learned from a decade of research aimed at improving psychotherapy outcome in routine care.* Psychotherapy Research, *17*(1), 1–14.

Larsen, D. J., & Stege, R. (2010a). *Hope-focused practices during early psychotherapy sessions: Part I: Implicit approaches.* Journal of Psychotherapy Integration, *20*, 271–292.

Larsen, D. J., & Stege, R. (2010a). *Hope-focused practices during early psychotherapy sessions: Part II: Explicit approaches.* Journal of Psychotherapy Integration, *20*, 293–311.

Larson, L. M., Clark, M. P., Wesley, L. H., Koraleski, S. F., Daniels, J. A., & Smith, P. L. (1999). *Videos versus role plays to increase counseling self-efficacy in perpractica trainees.* Counselor Education and Supervision, *38*(4), 237–248.

Latham, G. P., Winters, D., & Locke, E. A. (1994). *Cognitive and motivational effects of participation: A mediator study.* Journal of Organizational Behavior, *15*, 49–63.

Lazare, A., Eisenthal, S., & Wasserman, L. (1975a). *The customer approach to patienthood: Attending to patient requests in a walk-in clinic.* Archives of General Psychiatry, *32*, 553–558.

Lazare, A., Eisenthal, S., & Wasserman, L. (1975b). *Patient requests in a walk-in clinic.* Comprehensive Psychiatry, *16*, 467–477.

Lee, M. Y. (2013). An exploratory study comparing common to specific factors approaches to home-based treatment of at-risk children and adolescents: Integrative Family and Systems Treatment (I-FAST) and Multi-Systemic Therapy (MST). Presentation at 2013 Annual Conference of the Society for Social Work and Research, San Diego, CA, January 16–20, 2013.

Lee, R. E., & Everett, C. A. (2004). *The integrative family therapy supervisor*. New York, NY: Routledge.

Lee, M. Y., Fraser, S., Greene, G. J., Solovey, A., & Grove, D. (2003, updated in 2011). I-FAST Fidelity Scale. Unpublished Manuscript.

Lee, M. Y., & Greene, G. J. (2003). A teaching framework for transformative multicultural social work education. Journal of Ethnic & Cultural Diversity in Social Work, *12*(3), 1–28.

Lee, M. Y., & Greene, G. J. (November 16, 2010). Integrative Family and Systems Treatment (I-FAST). Evaluation Report. Submitted to The Buckeye Ranch, Columbus, OH.

Lee, M. Y., Greene, G. J., Fraser, J. S., Grove, D, Solovey, A., Edwards, S., & Scott, P. (2014). *Common and specific factors approaches to home-based treatment: I-FAST and MST*. Research on Social Work Practice, *23*(4), 407–418.

Lee, M. Y., Greene, G. J., Hsu, K. S., Solovey, A., Grove, D., Fraser, S., Washburn, P., Teater, B. (2009). *Utilizing Family Strengths and Resilience: Integrative Family and Systems Treatment (I-FAST) with Children and Adolescents with Severe Emotional and Behavioral Problems*. Family Process, *48*(3), 395–416.

Lee, M. Y., Sebold, J., & Uken, A. (2003). *Solution-focused treatment of domestic violence offenders: Accountability for change*. New York, NY: Oxford University Press.

Lee, M. Y., Teater, B., Greene, G. J., Hsu, K. S., Fraser, S., Solovey, A., . . . , & Washburn, P. (2012). *Key processes, ingredients and components of successful systems collaboration: Working with severely emotionally or behaviorally disturbed children and their families*. Administration and Policy in Mental Health and Mental Health Services Research, *39*(5), 394–405.

Lee, M. Y., Teater, B., Hsu, K. S., Greene, G. J., Fraser, J. S., Solovey, A., & Grove, D. (2013). *Systems collaboration with schools and treatment of SED children or adolescents*. Children & Schools, *35*(3), 155–168.

Lee, M. Y., Uken, A., & Sebold, J. (2007). *Role of self-determined goals in predicting recidivism in domestic violence offenders*. Research on Social Work Practice, *17*, 30–41.

Lehman, P., & Simmons, C. A. (2009). *Strength-based batterer intervention: A new paradigm in ending family violence*. New York, NY: Springer.

Levav, J., & Fitzsimmons, G. J. (2006). *When questions change behavior: The role of ease of representation*. Psychological Science, *17*, 207–213.

Lewis, S., Passmore, J., & Cantore, S. (2011). *Appreciative inquiry for change management: Using AI to facilitate organizational development*. London, UK: Kogan Page.

Liddle, H. A. (1991). Training and supervision in family therapy: A comprehensive and critical analysis. In A. S. Gurman & D. P. Kniskern (Eds.), *Handbook of family therapy* (Vol. 2, pp. 638–697). Philadelphia, PA: Brunner/Mazel.

Liddle, H. A., Rodriguez, R. A., Dakof, G. A., Kanzki, E., & Marvel, F. A. (2005). Multidimensional family therapy: A science-based treatment for adolescent drug abuse. In Jay L. Lebow (Ed.), *Handbook of clinical family therapy* (pp. 128–163). Hoboken, NJ: John Wiley & Sons.

Liddle, H. A., & Saba, G. (1984). The isomorphic nature of training and therapy: Epistemologic foundations for a structural-strategic family therapy. In J. Schwartzman (Ed.), *Families and other systems*. New York, NY: Guilford Press.

Liddle, H. A., & Schwartz, R. C. (1983). *Live supervision/consultation: Conceptual and pragmatic guidelines*. Family Process, *22*, 477–490.

Lindblad-Goldberg, M., Dore, M. M., & Stern, L. (1998). *Creating competence from chaos: A comprehensive guide to home-based services*. New York, NY: W. W. Norton.

Linehan, M. M. (1993). *Cognitive-behavioral treatment of borderline personality disorder*. New York, NY: Guilford Press.

Linley, P. A., Harrington, S., & Garcea, N. (2010). *Oxford handbook of positive psychology and work*. New York, NY: Oxford University Press.

Little, J. H. (1997). *Effects of the duration, intensity and breadth of Family Preservation services: A new analysis of data from the Illinois family first experiment*. Children and Youth Services Review, *19*, 17–39.

Little, J. H., & Schuerman, J. (1995). *A synthesis of research on family preservation and family reunification programs*. Washington, DC: Evaluation of Family Preservation Services, U.S. Department of Health and Human Services.

Locke, E. A. (1996). *Motivation through conscious goal setting*. Applied and Preventive Psychology, *5*, 117–124.

Locke, E. A., & Bryan, J. F. (1969a). *The directing function of goals in task performance*. Organizational Behavior & Human Performance, *4*, 35–42.

Locke, E. A., & Bryan, J. F. (1969b). *Knowledge of score and goal level as determinants of work rate*. Journal of Applied Psychology, *53*, 59–65.

Locke, E. A., & Latham, G. P. (1990). *A theory of goal setting and task performance*. Englewood Cliffs, NJ: Prentice Hall.

Locke, E. A., & Latham, G. P. (2002). *Building a practically useful theory of goal setting and task motivation: A 35-year odyssey*. American Psychologist, *57*, 705–717.

Long, J. R. (2001). *Goal agreement and early therapeutic change*. Psychotherapy, *38*, 219–232.

Madanes, C. (1990). *Sex, love, and violence: Strategies for transformation*. New York, NY: W. W. Norton.
Madanes, C. (1995). *The violence of men*. San Francisco, CA: Jossey-Bass.
Marshall, W. L., Marshall, L. E., Serran, G. A., & O'Brien, M. D. (2011). *Rehabilitating sexual offenders: A strength-based approach*. Washington, DC: American Psychological Association.
Massatti, R. R., Sweeney, H. A., Panzano, P. C., & Roth, D. (2008). *The de-adoption of innovative mental health practice (IMHP): Why organizations choose not to sustain an IMPH*. Administration and Policy in Mental Health, 35, 50–65.
Maton, K. I., Schellenbach, C. J., Leadbeater, B. J., & Solarz, A. L., Eds. (2004). *Investing in children, youth, families, and communities: Strengths-based research and policy*. Washington, DC: American Psychological Association.
Mazzucchelli, T. G., & Sanders, M. R. (2010). *Facilitating practitioner flexibility within an empirically supported intervention: Lessons from a system of parenting support*. Clinical Psychology, 17, 238–252.
McCambridge, J., & Kypri, K. (2011). *Can simply answering research questions change behavior? Systematic review and metaanylysis of brief alcohol intervention trials*. PLoS ONE, 6, 1–9.
McCollum, E. E., & Wetchler, J. L. (1995). *In defense of case consultation: Maybe "dead" supervision isn't dead after all*. Journal of Marital and Family Therapy, 21, 155–166.
McGee, D., Del Vento, A., & Bavelas, J. B. (2005). *An interactional model of questions as therapeutic interventions*. Journal of Marital and Family Therapy, 31, 371–384.
McGruder, J. H. (1999). *Madness in Zanzibar: "Schizophrenia" in three families in the "developing" world. (Tanzania, Third World)*. Dissertation Abstracts International Section A: Humanities and Social Sciences, Vol. 60 (4-A), pp. 1208 [dissertation].
McQuaide, S., & Ehrenreich, J. H. (1997). *Assessing client strengths*. Families in Society, 78, 201–212.
Michalak, J., & Holtforth, M. G. (2006). *Where do we go from here? The goal perspective in psychotherapy*. Clinical Psychology, 13, 346–365.
Miller, G. (1997). *Becoming miracle workers: Language and meaning in brief therapy*. New York, NY: Aldine De Gruyter.
Minuchin, S. (1974). *Families and family therapy*. Cambridge, MA: Harvard University Press.
Minuchin, S. (1984). *Family kaleidoscope*. Cambridge, MA: Harvard University Press.
Minuchin, S., & Fishman, H. C. (1981). *Family therapy techniques*. Cambridge, MA: Harvard University Press.
Mohr, J. J., & Woodhouse, S. S. (2000, June). *Clients' visions of helpful and harmful psychotherapy: An approach to measuring individual differences in therapy priorities*. Paper presented at the 31st Annual meeting of the Society for Psychotherapy Research, Chicago, IL.
Molnar, A., & de Shazer, S. (1987). *Solution-focused therapy: Toward the identification of therapeutic tasks*. Journal of Marital and Family Therapy, 13, 349–358.
Montalvo, B. (1973). *Aspects of live supervision*. Family Process, 12, 343–359.
Montalvo, B., & Storm, C. (2002). Live supervision revolutionizes the supervision process. In T. C. Todd & C. L. Storm (Eds.), *The complete systemic supervisor* (pp. 283–297). New York, NY: Authors Choice Press.
Mosher, L. R. (1999). *Soteria and other alternatives to acute psychiatric hospitalization: A personal and professional review*. Journal of Nervous and Mental Diseases, 187, 142–149.
Najavits, L. M., & Strupp, H. H. (1994). *Differences in the effectiveness of psychodynamic therapists: A process-outcome study*. Psychotherapy, 31, 114–123.
Napier, A. Y. (1978). *The rejection-intrusion pattern: A central family dynamic*. Journal of Marriage and Family Counseling, 4, 5–12.
Nardone, G., & Watzlawick, P. (1993). *The art of change: Strategic therapy and hypnotherapy without trance*. San Francisco, CA: Jossey-Bass.
Nezu, A. M., & Nezu, C. M. (2008). *Evidence-based outcome research: A practical guide to conducting randomized controlled trails for psychosocial interventions*. New York: Oxford University Press.
Nichols, W. C. (1988). An integrative psychodynamics and systems approach. In H. A. Liddle, D. C. Breunlin & R. C. Schwartz, (Eds.), *Handbook of family therapy training and supervision* (pp. 110–127). New York, NY: Guilford Press.
Nichols, W. C., & Lee, R. E. (1999). Mirrors, cameras and blackboards: Modalities of supervision. In R. E. Lee & S. Emerson (Eds.), *The eclectic trainer* (pp. 45–61). Galena, Il: Geist & Russel.
Nickerson, R. S. (1998). *Confirmation bias: A ubiquitous phenomenon in many guises*. Review of General Psychology, 2, 175–220.
Norcross, J. C. (2002). Empirically supported therapy relationships. In J. C. Norcross (Ed.), *Psychotherapy relationships that work: Therapist contributions and responsiveness to patients* (pp. 3–16). New York: Oxford University Press.
Norcross, J. C. (2010). The therapeutic relationship. In B. L. Duncan, S. D. Miller, B. E. Wampold & M. A. Hubble (Eds.), *The heart & soul of change: Delivering what works in therapy* (2nd ed., pp. 113–141). Washington, DC: American Psychological Association.
Ogles, B. M., Lambert, M. J., & Masters, K. S. (1996). Assessing outcome in clinical practice. Boston, MA: Allyn & Bacon.
Ogles, B. M., Melendez, G., Davis, D., & Lunnen, K. M. (2001). *The Ohio Scales: Practical Outcome Assessment*. Journal of Child and Family Studies, 10, 199–212.

O'Hanlon, B. (1984). *Framing interventions in therapy: Deframing and reframing*. Journal of Strategic & Systemic Therapies, *3*, 1–4.

O'Hara, M. M. (1984). Person-centered gestalt: Towards a holistic synthesis. In R. F. Levant & J. M. Shlien (Eds.), *Client-centered therapy and the person-centered approach: New directions in theory, research, and practice* (pp. 203–221). New York, NY: Praeger.

O'Hearn, T. C., & Gatz, M. (2002). *Going for the goal: Improving youth's problem-solving skills through a school-based intervention*. Journal of Community Psychology, *30*, 281–303.

Ohio Department of Mental Health. (2006). *The Statewide Report, Vol. 12*. Columbus, OH: Author.

Olson, D. H. (1992). *Family inventories manual*. Minneapolis, MN: Life Innovations.

Olson, D. H., Portner, J., & Bell, R. Q. (1982). *FACESII: Family adaptability and cohesion evaluation scales*. St. Paul, MN: Family Social Sciences, University of Minnesota.

Orlinsky, D. E., Grawe, K., & Parks, B. K. (1994). Process and outcome in psychotherapy: Noch einmal. In A. E. Bergin & S. L. Garfield (Eds.), *Handbook of psychotherapy and behavior change* (4th ed., pp. 270–376). Oxford, UK: John Wiley & Sons.

Patton, M. J., & Kivilghan, D. M. J. (1997). *Relevance of the supervisory alliance to the counseling alliance and to treatment adherence in counselor training*. Journal of Counseling Psychology, *44*, 109–111.

Pomeroy, E., & Garcia, R. (2008). *The grief assessment and intervention workbook: A strengths perspective*. Belmont, CA: Brooks/Cole.

Price, J. (1999). *Power and compassion: Working with difficult adolescents and abused parents*. New York, NY: Guilford Press.

Protinsky, H. (1997). Dismounting the tiger: Using tape in supervision. In C. L. Storm & T. C. Todd (Eds.), *The reasonably complete systemic supervisor resource guide* (pp. 298–308). Needham Heights, MA: Allyn & Bacon.

Quinn, W. H., Kuehl, B. P., Thomas, F. N., & Joanning, H. (1988). *Families of adolescent drug abusers: Systemic interventions to attain drug-free behavior*. The American Journal of Drug and Alcohol Abuse, *14*, 65–87.

Quinn, W. H., Kuehl, B. P., Thomas, F. N., & Joanning, H. (1989). *Family treatment of adolescent drug abuse: Transitions and maintenance of drug-free behavior*. American Journal of Family Therapy, *17*, 229–243.

Rand, K. L., & Cheavens, J. S. (2009). Hope theory. In S. J. Lopez & C. R. Snyder (Eds.), *Oxford handbook of positive psychology* (2nd ed., pp. 323–333). New York: Oxford University Press.

Rapp, C. A., & Goscha, R. J. (2011). *The strengths model: A recovery-oriented approach to mental health services* (3rd ed.). New York, NY: Oxford University Press.

Rath, T., & Conchie, B. (2006). *Strengths-based leadership*. Washington, DC: Gallup Press.

Reiter, M. D. (2010). *Hope and expectancy in solution-focused brief therapy*. Journal of Family Psychotherapy, *21*, 132–148.

Rogers, C. R. (1980). *A way of being*. Boston, MA: Houghton Mifflin.

Rogers, E. M. (2003). *Diffusion of innovations* (5th ed.). New York, NY: Free Press.

Ronch, J. L., & Goldfield, J., Eds. (2003). *Mental wellness in aging: Strengths-based approaches*. Baltimore, MD: Health Professions Press.

Rooney, C., Higgins, E. T., & Shah, J. (1995). *Goals and framing: How outcome focus influences motivation and emotion*. Personality and Social Psychology Bulletin, *21*, 1151–1160.

Rounsaville, B. J., Carroll, K. M., & Onken, L. S. (2001). *A stage model of behavioral therapies research: Getting started and moving on from stage I*. Clinical Psychology: Science and Practice, *8*, 133–142.

Rowe, C. L., & Liddle, H. A. (2003). *Substance abuse*. Journal of Marital and Family Therapy, *29*, 97–120.

Ryan, R. M., & Deci, E. L. (2000a). *Self-determination theory and the facilitation of intrinsic motivation, social development, and well-being*. American Psychologist, *55*, 68–78.

Ryan, R. M., & Deci, E. L. (2000b). *Intrinsic and extrinsic motivations: Classic definitions and new directions*. Contemporary Educational Psychology, *25*, 54–67.

Ryan, R. M., & Deci, E. L. (2008). *A self-determination theory approach to psychotherapy: The motivational basis for effective change*. Canadian Psychology, *49*, 186–193.

Ryan, T. A. (1970). *Intentional behavior*. New York, NY: Ronald Press.

Saleebey, D. (2002). *The strengths perspective in social work practice* (3rd ed.). Boston, MA: Allyn and Bacon.

Saltzburg, S., Greene, G. J., & Drew, H. (2010). *Using live supervision in field education: Preparing social work students for clinical practice*. Families in Society, *91*, 293–299.

Schaeffer, C. M., & Borduin, C. M. (2005). *Long-term follow-up to a randomized clinical trial of multisystemic therapy with serious and violent juvenile offenders*. Journal of Consulting and Clinical Psychology, *73*, 445–453.

Schafer, J. L., & Olsen, M. K. (1998). *Multiple imputation: A primer*. Statistical Methods in Medical Research, *8*, 3–15.

Schoenwald, S. K., & Henggeler, S. W. (2005). Multisystemic therapy for adolescents with serious externalizing problems. In J. L. Lebow (Ed.), *Handbook of clinical family therapy* (pp. 103–127). Hoboken, NJ: John Wiley & Sons.

Seikkula, J. (2006). *Five-year experience of first-episode nonaffective psychosis in open-dialogue approach: Treatment principles, follow-up outcomes, and two case studies*. Psychotherapy Research, *16*, 214–228.

Selvini Palazzoli, M., Boscolo, L., Cecchin, G. F., & Prata, G. (1978). *Paradox and counterparadox: A new model in the therapy of the family in schizophrenic transaction*. New York, NY: Jason Aronson.

Selvini-Palazzoli, M., Boscolo, L., Cecchin, G., & Prata, G. (1980). Hypothesizing-circularity and neutrality: Three guidelines for the conductor of the session. Family Process, *19* (1), 3–12.

Semin, G. R., & De Poot, C. J. (1997). The question-answer paradigm: You might regret not noticing how a question is worded. Journal of Personality and Social Psychology, *73*, 472–480.

Sexton, T. S. (2011). *Functional family therapy in clinical practice*. New York: Routledge/ Taylor & Francis Group.

Sexton, T. L., & Alexander, J. F. (2002). Functional family therapy for at-risk adolescents and their families. In F. W. Kaslow & T. Patterson (Eds.), *Comprehensive handbook of psychotherapy: Cognitive-behavioral approaches* (Vol. 2, pp. 117–140). Hoboken, NJ: John Wiley & Sons.

Sexton, T. L., & Alexander, J. F. (2004). *Functional family therapy clinical training manual*. Seattle, WA: Annie E. Casey Foundation.

Sexton, T. L., & Alexander, J. F. (2005). Functional family therapy for externalizing disorders in adolescents. In J. L. Lebow (Ed.), *Handbook of clinical family therapy* (pp. 164–191). Hoboken, NJ: John Wiley & Sons.

Shapiro, D. A., Barkham, M. Stiles, W. B., Hardy, G. E., Reese, A., Reynolds, S., & Startup, M. (2003). Psychology and Psychotherapy: Theory, Research and Practice, *76*, 211–235.

Snyder, C. R., Feldman, D. B., Taylor, J. D., Schroeder, L. L., & Adams, V. III. (2000). *The roles of hopeful thinking in preventing problems and enhancing strengths*. Applied and Preventative Psychology, *15*, 262–295.

Snyder, C. R., Ilardi, S., Michael, S. T., & Cheavens, J. (2000). Hope theory: Updating a common process for psychological change. In C. R. Snyder & R. E. Ingram (Eds.), *Handbook of psychological change: Psychotherapy processes & practices for the 21st century* (pp. 128–153). New York: John Wiley & Sons.

Snyder, C. R., Michael, S. T., & Cheavens, J. S. (1999). Hope as a psychotherapeutic foundation of common factors, placebos, and expectancies. In M. A. Hubble, B. L. Duncan, & S. D. Miller (Eds.), *The heart & soul of change: What works in therapy* (pp. 179–200). Washington, DC: American Psychological Association.

Snyder, C. R., & Taylor, J. D. (2000). Hope as a common factor across psychotherapy approaches: A lesson from the Dodo's verdict. In C. R. Snyder (Ed.), *Handbook of hope: Theory, measures & applications* (pp. 89–108). San Diego, CA: Academic Press.

Snyder, M. (1984). When belief creates reality. In L. Berkowitz (Ed.), *Advances in experimental social psychology* (Vol. 18, pp. 248–305). New York: Academic Press.

Snyder, M., & Stukas, A. A., Jr. (2000). Self-fulfilling prophecy. In A. E. Kazdin (Ed.), *Encyclopedia of psychology* (Vol. 3, pp. 216–218). New York, NY: Oxford University Press.

Snyder, M., & Thomsen, C. J. (1988). Interactions between therapists and clients: Hypothesis testing and behavioural confirmation. In D. C. Turk & P. Salovey (Eds.), *Reasoning, inference, and judgement in clinical psychology* (pp. 124–152). New York, NY: Free Press.

Sparks, J. A., & Duncan, B. L. (2010). Common factors in couple and family therapy: Must all have prizes? In B. L. Duncan, S. D. Miller, B. E. Wampold & M. A. Hubble (Eds.), *The heart & soul of change: Delivering what works in therapy* (2nd ed., pp. 357–391). Washington, DC: American Psychological Association.

Sprenkle, D. H., Blow, A. J., & Dickey, M. H. (1999). Common factors and other nontechnique variables in marriage and family therapy. In M. A. Hubble, B. L. Duncan, & S. D. Miller (Eds.), *The heart and soul of change: What works in therapy* (pp. 329–360). Washington, DC: American Psychological Association.

Sprenkle, D. H., Davis, S. D., & Lebow, J. L. (2009). *Common factors in couple and family therapy: The overlooked foundation for effective practice*. New York, NY: Guilford Press.

Stanton, M. D. (1980). *A critique of the Wells and Dezen review of the results of nonbehavioral family therapy*. Family Process, *19*, 169–176.

Stanton, M. D., & Todd, T. C., & Associates. (1982). *The family therapy of drug abuse and addiction*. New York, NY: Guilford Press.

Szapocznik, J., Robbins, M. S., Mitrani, V. B., Santisteban, D. A., Hervis, O., & Williams, R. A. (2002). Brief strategic family therapy. In J. Lebow (Ed.), *Comprehensive handbook of psychotherapy*, Vol. 4: *Integrative/eclectic* (pp. 83–109). New York, NY: John Wiley & Sons.

Tice, C. J., & Perkins, K. (2001). *Faces of social policy: A strengths perspective*. Belmont, CA: Brooks/Cole.

Timmons-Mitchell, J., Bender, M. B., Kishna, M. A., & Mitchell, C. C. (2006). *An independent effectiveness trial of multisystemic therapy with juvenile justice youth*. Journal of Clinical Child and Adolescent Psychology, *35*, 227–236.

Todd, T. C., & Storm, C. L. (2002). *The complete systemic supervisor*. New York, NY: Authors Choice Press.

Tomm, K. (1987). *Interventive interviewing: Part II. Reflexive questioning as a means to enable self healing*. Family Process, *26*, 167–183.

Tryon, G. S., & Winograd, G. (2002). Goal consensus and collaboration. In J. C. Norcross (Ed.), *Psychotherapy relationships that work: Therapist contributions and responsiveness to patients* (pp. 109–125). New York: Oxford University Press.

Tryon, G. S., & Winograd, G. (2011). *Goal consensus and collaboration*. Psychotherapy, *48*, 50–57.

Unru, Y. A. (1997). *Predicting use of child welfare services after intensive family preservation services*. Research on Social Work Practice, *7*, 202–215.

U.S. Department of Health and Human Services Food and Drug Administration. (March 2010). *Guidance for industry: Non-inferiority clinical trials (draft guidance)*. Washington, DC: Author.

U.S. Public Health Service, Office of the Surgeon General. (2001). *Youth violence: A report of the Surgeon General*. Available at http://www.surgeongeneral.gov/library/youth violence

Valle, M. F., Huebner, E. S., & Suldo, S. M. (2006). *An analysis of hope as a psychological strength*. Journal of School Psychology, *44*, 393–406.

Van Gorp, B. (2007). *The constructionist approach to faming: Bringing culture back in*. Journal of Communication, *57*, 60–78.

van Wormer, K., & Davis, D. R. (2007). *Addiction treatment: A strengths perspective* (2nd ed.). Belmont, CA: Brooks/Cole.

Walsh, F. (2006). *Strengthening family resilience* (2nd ed.). New York, NY: Guilford Press.

Walter, J. L., & Peller, J. E. (1982). *Becoming solution-focused in brief therapy*. New York, NY: Brunner/Mazel.

Wampold, B. E. (2001). *The great psychotherapy debate: Models, methods, and findings*. Mahwah, NJ: Lawrence Erlbaum.

Wampold, B. E. (2010a). *The basics of psychotherapy: An introduction to theory and practice*. Washington, DC: American Psychological Association.

Wampold, B. E. (2010b). The research evidence for the common factors models: A historically situated perspective. In B. L. Duncan, S. D. Miller, B. E. Wampold, & M. A. Hubble (Eds.), *The heart and soul of change: Delivering what works in therapy* (2nd ed., pp. 49–81). Washington, DC: American Psychological Association.

Wampold, B. E., Mondin, G. W., Moody, M., Stich, F., Benson, K., & Ahn, H. (1997). *A meta-analysis of outcome studies comparing bona fide psychotherapies: Empirically, "all must have prizes."* Psychological Bulletin, *122*, 203–215. Doi:10.1037/0033-2909.122.3.203

Ward, D. B., & Wampler, K. S. (2010). *Moving up the continuum of hope: Developing a theory of hope and understanding its influence in couples therapy*. Journal of Marital & Family Therapy, *36*, 212–228.

Warner, R., Ed. (1995). *Alternatives to the hospital for acute psychiatric treatment*. Washington, DC: American Psychiatric Association.

Watson, J. C. (2002). Revisioning empathy. In D. Cain & Seeman (Eds.), *Humanistic psychotherapies: Handbook of research and practice* (pp. 445–472). Washington, DC: American Psychological Association.

Watzlawick, P., Beavin, J. H., & Jackson, D. D. (1967). *Pragmatics of human communication: A study of interactional patterns, pathologies, and paradoxes*. New York, NY: W. W. Norton.

Watzlawick, P., Weakland, J. H., & Fisch, R. (1974). *Change: Principles of problem formation and problem resolution*. New York, NY: W. W. Norton.

Weakland, J. (1981). *Radical change in gerontology: Semblance & substance*. Generations, *6*, 24–25.

Weakland, J. H., Fisch, R., Watzlawick, P., & Bodin, A. (1974). *Brief therapy: Focused problem resolution*. Family Process, *13*, 141–168, 269–277.

Weinberger, J., & Eig, A. (1999). In I. Kirsch (Ed.), *How expectancies shape experience. Expectancies: The ignored common factor in psychotherapy* (pp. 357–382). Washington, DC: American Psychological Association.

Weissberg, R. P., Barton, H. A., & Shriver, T. P. (1997). The social-competence promotion program for young adolescents. In T. Gullotta & G. Albee (Eds.), *Primary prevention works* (pp. 269–289). Newbury Park, CA: SAGE.

Wells, K., & Whittington, D. (1993). *Child and family functioning after intensive family preservation services*. Social Work Review, *67*(1), 55–83.

Whiffin, R. (1982). The use of videotape in supervision. In R. Whiffen & J. Byng-Hall (Eds.), *Family therapy supervision: Recent developments in practice* (pp. 39–46). New York, NY: Grune & Stratton.

Whitaker, C., & Napier, A. (1978). *The family crucible*. London, UK: Harper and Row.

White, M., & Epston, D. (1990). *Narrative means to therapeutic ends*. New York, NY: W. W. Norton.

Wiens, B. L. (2002). *Choosing an equivalence limit for non-inferiority or equivalence studies*. Control Clinical Trials, *23*, 2–14.

Wilder, C., & Weakland, J. H. (1982). *Rigor & imagination: Essays from the legacy of Gregory Bateson*. New York, NY: Praeger.

Wittgenstein, L. (1958). *Philosophical investigations* (3rd ed.). (G. E. M. Anscombe, Trans.). New York, NY: Macmillan.

Wollburg, E., & Braukhaus, C. (2010). *Goal setting in psychotherapy: The relevance of approach and avoidance goals for treatment outcomes*. Psychotherapy Research, *20*, 488–494.

Wood, R., & Locke, E. A. (1990). Goal setting and strategy effects on complex tasks. In B. Shaw & L. Cummings (Eds.), *Research in organizational behavior* (Vol. 2, pp. 73–109). Greenwich, CT: JAI.

Zuroff, D. C., Koestner, R., Moskowitz, D. S., McBride, C., Marshall, M., & Bagby, M. (2007). *Autonomous motivation for therapy: A new common factor in brief treatments for depression*. Psychotherapy Research, *17*, 137–148.

INDEX

Note: Figures and tables are indicated by page numbers in italics.

abused children, 143–144
acceptance
   being nonjudgmental, 150
   by client of frames, 97
   by client of rationale or myth, 14
   normalizing related, 118
accommodating, 111
action phase of change, 46
active listening, 32
adaptability of model, 33
adherence, 148–149
   agency settings, 162
   supervision and, 159, 161
African American cohorts, 207
agencies, social service
   abused children, 144
   advantages of model, 33
   agency/model fit, 188
   assessing services offered, 193–194
   at-risk families and their problems, 187
   avoiding relapse after in-home treatment ends, 140
   case consultation, 164–165
   challenges of "messy" settings, 187, 188–190, 196, 198
   costs, 191–192, 195, 197, 199–200
   EB training and implementation impacting, 191–193
   improvement acknowledged by other professionals?, 141–142
   intervention by related to interactional patterns, 18
   negotiating impasses between professionals, 93–94
   settings, 162, 187, 188–190
   sustainability of effective treatments, 189–190
   training curriculum, 199
agency/model fit, 188
   enhancing, 195
   goals, 196
   I-FAST training packages, 200–201
   key principles, 195–196
   key strategies, 196–200
   strategizing, 190–191
agency thinking, 84
allegiance, 148–149, 161
   agency settings, 162
alliances. *See also* working alliances
   assumptions about, 22
all involved parties
   change process, 112
   no blame placed, 112
   use of term, 111
allowing a practitioner to vent, 165
amplifying change, practitioner's role, 134
anxiety
   indirect questions, 121
   as response to change, 135
   school phobia, 137
   at termination, 143
approach goals, 91
Aspinwall, L. G., 44
assimilating, 111

at-risk families. *See also* family
   challenges to agencies, 187
   I-FAST research, 207
   outside agencies and family patterns, 18
at-risk youth
   cost of services for, 3
   I-FAST research, 207
   multiple problems, 65
   need for family-centered treatment, 3
   new parenting behavior, 128
   participants' blaming patterns, 112–113
   research comparing I-FAST and MST, 223–231
   treatment goals, 3
   validating position of, 49
   whom to engage, 42
avoidance goals, 91

Barkley, R. A., 148, 153, 154
Barlow, D. H., 148
Bateson, G., 6
beginning treatment errors, 178–179
behavioral confirmation, 95–96
behavior as communication, 109
behind the mirror etiquette, 183–184
between-session tasks, 128–129
blaming, 64
   defensive reaction to, 150
   deleting the focus on, 123
   problem-saturated stories, 113–114
   process of change, 112
Bohart, A. C., 50
bona fide treatment approach, 205–206
bond, establishing a therapeutic, 59
Bordin, E. S., 15
Brief Strategic Family Therapy (BSFT), 187
brief therapy components, 28
Budman, S. H., 28
building resilience
   skills for, 137–139
   tips for, 144–147
Burman, A. S., 28

Carroll, K., 206
case consultation, 164–165
   goals, 165–166
Cawyer, C. S., 160
celebrating success, 165–166
Celtic spiral designs, 1
change. *See also* initiating change; stages of change model
   adjusting to rapid change, 138–139, 177–178
   ahead of families, 166–167
   amplifying, 134, 137
   amplifying incremental changes, 144
   anxiety as response, 135
   assimilation and accommodation, 9, 10–11, 111
   basic assumptions about, 174
   behind families, 167–168
   brief interventions, utility of, 28
   as constant, 10–11, 63, 111
   contextual model, 15
   control over, 86

change (*Cont.*)
   credit for change, 25, 137, 177, 180
   desired and undesired, 10
   dose-response effect, 28
   first-order, 17
   fluctuations in problems, 13
   four common factors accounting for, 14
   general process of
   goal attainment and, 86–87
   initiating, 26, 109
   not noticed, 135, 173
   parents as agents of change, 43
   path of least resistance, 110
   persistence and, 64–65
   processes summarized, 18–19
   readiness to, 115
   responses to (by type), 134–136
   restraints from, 132, 137, 168
   safety interventions and, 69
   second-order, 17
   shift in perceived problem, 109
   stage of (model), 46
   from systems perspective, 42
   three-step process for family system, 10
   tracking, 137
   tracking interactions that point to, 74
   treatment process of change, 23, *24, 27*
   who is most motivated, 46–47
change agents, parents as, 43
chapter organization (CSI), 35–36
children, engaging, 44
choice questions, 122
circular processes, feedback loops, 6, 66
client
   acceptance of frame, 20
   encouraging trust of, 41
   practitioner positive bond, 15
   relationship with, 14
client determined, 114
client feedback, 122
client frames, 103
client language
   tracking and utilizing, 103
   utilizing, 51–52, 174
clients
   diagnoses stigmatizing, 43
   frames (positions), tracking and utilizing, 105–106
   how practitioners use framing with, 99–100
   negative views of, 43
   positive view of practitioner, 45
   relationship with practitioner, 113–114
   respecting client perspectives, 22, 43–44
   response to interventions, observing and utilizing, 31–32
   strengths and ability to change, 44–45
client values, 51–52
clinical supervisors, 201
co-constructing
   frames with clients, 43
   understanding of reality, 12
   vicious cycles, 8, *8*
co-creating
   frames and reframes, 102
   multiple versions of reality, 13

cognitive behavioral approaches, questions to change frames, 120, 121
collaborating
   with all parties, 59
   with parents, 43–44
collaboration
   assumptions about, 22
   empowering relationship with one parent/caregiver, 45
   engaging with parents, 43–44
   goal consensus and, 84–85
collaboration with colleagues
   in-home treatment, 164
   negotiating impasses, 94–95
   struggles with colleagues, 168
   theory-driven disagreements, 168
   validating techniques for, 50
collaboration with family members, overall goals, 5
collaborative contract, 25
collaborative involvement, 85
collaborative supervision, 160
collaborative teamwork with community agencies, 5
common factors
   engaging and, 43–45
   goal setting, 82–84
   in I-FAST, 4
   psychotherapy, 4
   sources of, 4–5
   treatment frames summarized, 97–98
   treatment outcomes, 23
common sense of purpose, 83
communication
   as constructive, 119, 174
   as directive, 174
   directive questions leading to change, 119–120
   theories reviewed, 109
   using questions and responses, 174
community agencies. *See* agencies, social service
Comparison of efficacy of I-FAST and MST for Treating At-Risk Youth Study, 223–224
   data analyses, 227
   data collection methods, 226–227
   discussion and summary, 230–231
   intervention and treatment adherence, 225
   research participants, 224–225
   results, 227–230
comparison questions, 122
competence, developing a sense of, 82–83
complainant, 115
compliments, 101
conceptual flexibility, 150–151
conceptualizing, 35
   framing and goal setting, 80–82
conceptual level. *See* I-FAST, Level I
conceptual umbrella, 154
connection questions, 122
constructivism, 11–12. *See also* social constructivism
   expanding the constructivist context, 111
   frames and, 95–96
   framing and engaging, 43
   initiating change, 110–112

consultation, 164–165
  goals of, 165–166
  helping practitioner past an impasse, 166
contemplative phase of change, 46
context
  interactional, 164
  understanding the big picture, 47
contextual approach to client change, 15
  two-step process, 96
continuity of care, 194–195
  goals, 196
  training supervisors for, 197
coping questions, 76–77
co-practitioners, family members as, 53
creative flexibility, 154
  evolving with practice, 155
cultural context
  co-constructing reality, 12
  identifying and utilizing client language and values, 51–52
Cunningham, P. B., 187
curiosity
  outcome of tasks, 175
  questioning and, 119
Curtis, N. M., 227
customer, family as, 115

dance steps metaphor, 155–156
Davis, D., 210
Davis, S. D., 16
deals, method of striking, 89
defiance, teenage, 73, 87, 123
defiant child, 129, 154
deframing, 70. *See also* framing; reframing
  definition, 104
  practitioner understandings, 151
delete, 123, 174
demonstration interviews, 185
demoralization, 97
depression, 91
devising and offering tasks
diagnosis, definition, 81–82
diagnostic assessment, agency, 194
diagnostic labels, 66
  avoiding use of, 80–81
  specific problems versus diagnoses, 81–82
Diagnostic and Statistical Manual of Mental Disorders (DSM), 187
Dialectical Behavior Therapy "chain analysis," 71
Diamond, G. M., 16
Diamond, G. S., 16
difference questions, 122
direct observation, assessing interactional patterns, 71–72
discrepancy model, 103
disruptive behavior disorders
  literature on, 148
  motivations, 152
divorce
  as reaction to change, 136, 138–139
  as a transition, 118
domino effect, 9
  overcoming one problem creating, 110, 171
dose-response effect, 28

drug addiction cases, 53
  Narcotics Anonymous, 54

EB. *See* evidence-based (EB) approaches to treatment
Ecosystemic Structural Family Therapy (ESFT), 188
Efficacy of I-FAST from 2004 to 2012 study, 219
  data analyses, 221
  data collection methods, 221
  discussion and summary, 223
  findings, 221–223
  research participants, 219–220
  treatment adherence, 220
Ehrenreich, J. H., 13
empathy/empathizing
  definitions, 50
  engaging active client involvement with, 50
  goal consensus and, 85
  supervising and practitioner's judgment, 160–161
  varying client needs for, 51
empowerment model
  agency advantages, 33
  clear goals, 90
  identifying habitual interactions, 64
  need for, vii
  parent empowerment model, 81
  parents left out, 43–44
  practitioners empowered, 159–160
  professional aligning with parent, 118
enactment, 72
end-of-session, task frames, 101
end stage treatment errors, 178, 180
engagement
  definition, 85
  goals in early stage of, 87
  habitual interactions during stage of, 72, 73
  individual and family, 41–42
  as key and ongoing, 48
  tracking powerful family members, 57
  use of term, 41
engaging, 41
  beginning elements, 59–60
  child's input, 44
  client language and values, 51–52
  collaborating with all parties, 59–60
  common factors and, 43–45
  conceptualizing, 42–45
  core practitioner skills, 49
  framing and positive reframing, 53–56
  identifying strengths, 52–53
  implementing, 48–50
  key phases in, 23–24, 24
  practice procedures, 20
  recruiting family members to treatment, 59
  strategizing, 45–48
  tracking power, 57–58
  types of, 41–42
  validation and empathy, 50–51
  whom to engage, 42, 176–177
episodes of care
  avoiding "illness" label, 80–81
  I-FAST model as, 81
  in-home treatment, 139
  use in terminating phase, 26, 143

Erickson, M., 32, 106
Everett, C. A., 185
evidence-based (EB) approaches to treatment, vii
   "golden thread," 17
   in "messy" agency settings, 187
   models available, 3–4
   practical dilemmas posed, 4
   required by funding sources, 3
   research on, 205–207
   sustainability in agency settings, 187
evidence-based (EB) common factors, 14–15.
      See also I-FAST, Level II
   sources of, 4–5
exception questions, 62, 75, 122
exceptions. *See also* interactional exceptions
   basic skills list for identifying, 78
   as clues for solutions, 63
   dynamics of change, 11
   family strengths and resources, 11, 63
   focus as primary intervention, 74–75
   focus on strengths, 64
   following up on tasks, 126
   identifying, 52–53
   identifying, common errors, 172
   identifying current successes, 76
   identifying past successes, 75–76
   identifying strengths and resources, 11, 64
   past exceptions, 76
   in process of initiating change, 112
   questions for probing, 63–64
   tracking, core questions for, 74
   tracking, skills for, 73–74
   treatment dialogues focusing on strengths, 74
   within vicious cycles, 11
expectancy, 95
   of practitioner, 120
expert status, empowerment and, 47
exploring questions, 122
extended family members
   abused children, 143–144
   aid with between-session tasks, 129
   at termination phase, 143
externalizing the problem, 121
   research on, 207
extinction burst, 146

Fairhurst, G.T., 96, 102
Falender, C. A., 160
family
   acceptance of frames, 173–174
   additional members as additional helpers, 59
   ahead of, 166–167
   assessing if practitioner is in synch, 166–167
   assimilation and accommodation, 9
   at-risk. *See* at-risk families; at-risk youth
   behind, 167–168
   change occurs but is unrecognized by someone, 135, 173
   change occurs and worse problems occur, 136
   as circle of concentric and interconnected spirals, 1
   collaboration to attain treatment goals, 5
   conflicting goals, 86
   constant change in, 111

engagement skills needed for process, 41–42
extended family members
   feedback processes, 16
   frames (positions), tracking and utilizing, 105–106
   not taking credit for change, 177, 180
   patronizing practitioner, 169–170
   person most upset by problem, 110
   recruiting additional members to treatment, 59
   response to intervention as feedback, 32
   response to tasks by, 72–73
   shifts for adolescent stages, 9
   as systems, 16
   trust in practitioner, 159
   understanding the big picture, 47, 67
   use of term, 21
   utilize their theories about the problem, 106–107
family functioning, measures of, 210
family members as co-practitioners, 53
Family Participation Measure, 210–211, 218
family system, change in three steps, 10
family treatment, recruiting additional family members to, 59, 67
fathers, noncustodial, 56
feasibility questions, 122
feedback. *See also* negative feedback; positive feedback
   in change process, 122
   client's self-feedback process, 122
   definition, 62
   family response to intervention as, 32
   in family systems, 16
   goals and, 80
   live supervision team, 184
   practicing goal behaviors, 86
   problem circular feedback loops, 66
Feist, S. C., 161
Fine, M., 160
first-order change, 17. *See also* second-order change
   frames, 103
   identifying attempted solutions, 104
   lack of resolution, 111
   positive framing and, 55
   in small units, 68
   summarized, 18–19
Fisch, R., 70
fit, 187. *See also* agency/model fit
fits by child, 129
flexibility
   agency advantages, 33
   in approach/frame/rationale, 97–98
   choosing whom to work with, 164, 176–177
   creativity and, 154
   I-FAST as flexible meta-model, 34
   practitioner conceptual, 150–151
   practitioner views and biases, 11
   (re)framing, 102–103
   rigor and imagination of practitioner, 37
   in supervision, 159–160
   teaching to groups of practitioners, 163–164
   treatment choices, 28–29, 36
   treatment frames, 97–98
   whom to involve in treatment, 48, 176–177

Forgatch, M. S., 208
formula first session task, 130
formulations, 123
foster care, children in, 55–56
frame analyses, 19
frames
    assumptions about, 22
    client acceptance of, 20
    constructing, 101–102, 173–174
    definition, 12
    de-framing and reframing, 13
    facilitating change (steps), 114–115
    facilitating the framing process, 12
    flexibility in approach/frame/rationale, 97–98
    framing process described, 12
    guidelines for developing, 101–107
    how to frame clients and families, 43
    key phases in framing and reframing, 25
    making them acceptable, 12
    master, 96
    nature of change and focus of intervention, 111–112
    offering tasks without, 175–176
    overarching, 173
    practice procedures, 19
    practitioner and supervisor construction, 164
    skills for practitioners, 163
    supervising, 173–174
    terms interchangeable with, 95
    that set up tasks, 173
    types and purposes of, 98–99
    using clients' language, 92
    using practitioners' existing skill sets, 30
    using questions to change frames, 120
frames of reference, 95
framing, 53–54, 95. *See also* deframing; reframing
    essential elements, 107–108
    flexible, 102–103
    goals, 99
    how practitioners use it with clients, 99–100
    improvement, 101
    key phases, 25
    parents' motives, 56
    positive reframing, 54–56
    practice procedures, 20
    practitioner adjusts to client responses, 102
    practitioner understandings, 151
    priming for spontaneity, 102
    strengths related, 97
    tasks, 100–101, 125, 175–176
Frank, J. D., 4, 14, 96
Functional Family Therapy, (FFT), 188
Functioning Scale, 209, 210, 211, 221

general process of change, 17
genuineness, 153, 154
    validation of "incorrect" premises, 117
goal consensus, 79
    adapting model to attain, 33
    commitment to, 15
    essential components, 94
    key phases, 25
    skills to focus goal, 170–171
    strategizing, 84–85
    supervising role and, 170–171
    who owns goal, 170–171
goal development and consensus, key phases, 25
goals
    actions associated with, 79
    aligned with stages of change, 86–87
    aligning client, family, and larger system goals, 88
    alignment, three methods, 88–90
    approach or avoidance, 91
    behavior practiced on a regular basis, 86
    complexity of the task, 80
    conflicting, among family members, 86
    consensus about and commitment to, 15
    deals, method of striking, 89
    defining concretely, specifically, and behaviorally, 90–91
    definition, 79
    family's language used in defining, 92
    feedback on progress, 80
    frameworks compared, 154
    interpersonal in nature, 86
    mutual, 152
    parents motivated to accomplish, 85–86
    powerful agents aligned with, 57, 152
    practice procedures, 20
    prioritizing, 87–88
    reinforcing, 121
    scaling questions as small steps, 121
    stated in the present, 92–93
    stating positively, 91
    stating in process or active form, 92–93
    of systems, 6, 16
    tasks unrelated to client's, 175
    termination as goal achievement, 140–141
    treatment goals for at-risk youth, 3
    useful, characteristics of, 90
    within client's control, 86
goal setting
    agreeing on a priority goal, 87–88
    basic concepts, 79–80
    essential components, 94
    focus on common sense of purpose, 83
    goal commitment, 79
    guidelines for, 85–87
    pre-suppositional language in, 92
    process form, 92–93
    self-efficacy, 79
godparents for abused children, 143–144
Goldman, H. H., 187
grandparents, 127–128
Grawe, K., 50
Greene, R., 148, 152, 154
    three-basket approach, 154

habitual interactional patterns (HIPs), 61
    identifying, 64
    in-home observation, 71–72
    interruption or redirection of, 112
    lack of resolution of problem, 111–112
    reasons families get stuck, 100
    task frames, 100–101
    tasks, 124–133
    tracking, 70
    tracking skills, 73

Haley, J., 57, 81, 138, 152, 154
hands-on learning, 198
hard restraints from change, 132
helpfulness questions, 122
Henderson, C. E., 160
Henggeler, S. W., 187
hierarchical interviews, 57
Homebuilders model, 190
hope, promoting
    coping questions, 76–77
    deconstructing experience of reality, 73–74
    goal setting and treatment outcome, 83–84
    "hope treatment," 84
    initiating change and, 26
    three interrelated components of hope, 84
Howard, K. I., 28
hyperactivity, 127–128
hypnotherapy, 32

identifying exceptions, list of basic skills, 78
identifying interactional exceptions, list of basic skills, 78
identifying strengths, 64
I-FAST Checklist, 208, 218
I-FAST Fidelity Scale, 220, 225
I-FAST (Integrative Family and Systems Treatment)
    agency advantages, 33
    collaboration with fellow professionals, 50, 93–94
    described, 1
    development of model, vii
    efficacy, original study, 207–219
    efficacy, second (2002-12) study, 219–223
    efficacy, study comparing I-FAST and MST, 223–231
    elements of effective treatment, 96
    as episode of care model, 81
    episode versus illness issue, 82
    essence of intervention, 19
    evaluating practitioner's skills, 162–163
    five steps for sustaining model in agency setting, 191
    as flexible meta-model, 34
    focus of change in, 112
    foundation concepts summarized, 18–19
    as generalist model, 200
    guidelines for practice, 27–28
    Level I (meta-frame), 5–13, 5, 34
    Level II (meta-frame), 5, 14–19, 34–35
    Level III (meta-frame), 5, 19–20, 35
    major assumptions, 22–23
    as meta-model, 4, 5
    methods for identifying interactional patterns, 70
    minimum practitioner requirements, 164–165
    observing and utilizing how clients respond to interventions, 31–32
    parameters and presupposition, 124–125
    practice procedures, 19–20
    premises of, 13
    protocol phases and procedures, 3–27
    rationale for research program, 205–207
    recommendations for further study, 232
    research on effectiveness of, 37, 207–231
    research on, additional, 231–232
    research program overview, 205–207
    skills chapter organization (CSI), 35–36
    skills listed, 150–153
    structure of meta-model, 34–35
    supervision as collaboration, 186
    supervisory role with assumptions of change, 174
    sustainability in agency settings, 187
    tasks available, 133
    termination as successful, 140
    as time-limited approach, 27–28
    training information, vii
    treatment decisions and choices, 28–30
    treatment focus, 84
    treatment process, 23
    use of acronym "FAST," 27, 28
    utilizing practitioners' skill sets, 30–31
    weekly consultation suggestions, 165–168
    whom to include in treatment, 45–46
implementation level. See I-FAST, Level III
implementing, 36
    collaborating with all parties, 59
    frames and reframes, 101–107
    framing and positive reframing, 53–56
    goal setting, 90–94
    identifying strengths and engagement, 52–53
    identifying and utilizing client language and values, 51–52
    interventions (change), 116–133
    through matching, 154–156
    recruiting family members to treatment, 59
    specific skills overview, 48
    tracking power, 57–58
    understanding and validating client perspectives and dilemmas, 49–50
indicator questions, 122
in-home
    agency staff retention, 192
    assessing interactional patterns, 72
    collaboration with colleagues, 164
    difficulty letting practitioner disengage, 178
    evidence-based treatment models, 187–188
    flexibility in approach, 48
    in-office versus, 116
    in-session tasks, 127
    other systems involved, 139
    practitioner as teammate, 144
    prioritizing goals, 87–88
    professionals acknowledging improvement, 141–142
    relapses after treatment, 139–140
    safety and interactions, 69–70
    terminating treatment, 139
    treatment model common elements, 139
initiating change, 29, 109
    essential elements, 133
    facilitating change, 114–115
    joining change versus, 114
    master frames, 110
    strategizing, 113–116
    systems theory, 109–110
in-office
    flexibility in approach, 48
    in-home versus, 116

in-session tasks, 72–73
   between-session tasks, 128–129
   how families typically respond, 128
   range of, 127
   tracking responses to, 125–126
integration/integrating, 21
integrative
   nature of I-FAST, 148
   use of term, 21
interaction, spirals of. *See* spirals of interaction
interactional assessment
   persistence and, 65
   summary of basic skills, 77
interactional context, 164
interactional exceptions. *See also* exceptions
   amplifying, 130, 172
   developing skills, 61–62
   frame or rationale for change, 15
   identifying, 61
   identifying, common errors, 172
   tasks for amplifying, 130
   tracking, as focused skill, 73–77
   virtuous cycles, 9, *9*
interactional focus, 123
interactional patterns, 61
   changing, 17
   direct observation skills, 71–72
   frame or rationale for change, 15
   interconnectedness, 62–63
   interviews to assess, 70–71
   methods for identifying, 70
   "mine field," 70
   observing responses to tasks, 72–73
   parenting practices and, 16
   pattern shift procedures, 20
   practitioner errors with, 171–172
   removal of child, 18
   as rules of system, 62
   systems theory, 16
   tracking, 70
   tracking, practice procedures, 20
   vicious cycles, 7–8
interactional understanding, 64
   of the problem, 171
interactions, 61–62
   adult-to-adult about the child, 66
   adult-to-child, 66
   habitual or exceptional, 61, 64
   identifying, 171–172
   identifying strengths, 64
   safety and, 69–70
   as series of messages, 62
   two types, 66
interconnectedness and wholeness, 9–10
interpersonal influence of communication, 109
intervener support, 23
interventions
   assumptions about main task of, 22
   basic I-FAST tenets, 113
   brief, utility of, 28
   client response, observing and utilizing, 31–32, 116
   early and intensive, 28
   essence of, in I-FAST model, 19
   following up on, 176
   framing in, 99
   goal of, 9, *9*, 140–141
   guidelines for choosing how to intervene, 115–116
   learning what types to avoid, 70
   least restrictive, 116–117
   linear, 10
   observation of ongoing change, 10
   practitioner's skill set and knowledge, 115–116
   steps prior to, 114–115
   supervising, 164
   systems theory implications, 9–10
   therapeutic relationship and, 113–114
   three stages, 205
   use of questions as a procedure, 119
   validation as crossover intervention, 117
interviews
   assessing interactional patterns, 70–71, 72
   demonstration, 185
   for exceptions, skills, 74
   first break, 185
   hierarchical, 57
   live supervision, 182–185
   organizing, 152
   planning, 182–183, 185
   processing, 184, 185
   session break, 184
   specific skills for, 71
intrinsic motivation and self-determination, 82–83
involuntary behavior, 131

joining
   joining change versus initiating change, 114
   lack of, 169
   understanding and validating processes, 49

Kinney, 190
Knutson, N. M., 208
Koss, M. P., 28
Kowalski, K., 74
Kral, R., 74

Lakoff, G., 12
language. *See also* client language
   of deframing, 104–105
   of family in describing and defining goals, 92
   family's, listening to, 151–152, 174
   for frames and reframes, 101
   of practitioner, for framing, 105
   role of, 63–64
Lebow, J. L., 16
Lee, R. E., 184
life as one damned thing after another, 140, 146
life as a roller coaster, 140, 145
linear intervention, 10
listening
   before framing or reframing, 102
   skills of practitioner, 151–152
   by supervisors, 160
live supervision, 182–185
   steps, 182–185
Lunnen, K. M., 210

Madanes, C., 144
maintenance phase of change, 46
manual development, 206
master frames, 96
   initiating change, 110
maximum flexibility, 154
Mazzucchelli, T. G., 148, 149
McQuaide, S., 13
Medicaid, 194
medical neglect of child, 72
medications, 142
Melendez, G., 210
mental health clinics. *See* agencies, social service
mental health problems, labeling, 80–81
Mental Research Institute (MRI)
   think in opposites, 131
   use of questions, 120
mere measurement effect, 119
meta-frames
   individual viewpoints as, 13
   on practice techniques, 5
meta-frames for practice, Level III, 35
meta-framework, 155
meta-ideas, 37
meta-level treatment approach, vii
   I-FAST as, 4
   process of change theory, 148
meta-model
   I-FAST as, 34
   rigor and imagination, 34–35
   three levels, 34–35
middle treatment errors, 178, 179–180
Minuchin, S., 57, 118
Mohr, J. J., 51
Montalvo, B., 182
Mosher, L. R., 80
motivation for change
   goals parents are motivated by, 85–86
   intrinsic, and self-determination, 82–83
Multidimensional Family Therapy (MDFT), 187
multiple systems
   assumptions about, 22
   embedded, 17–18
multisystemic
   assumptions about, 23
   practice procedures, 20
multisystemic practice procedures, time devoted to, 28
Multisystemic Therapy (MST), 187, 206
   research comparing with I-FAST, 223–231
mutual goals, 152

narrative practitioner questions to change frame, 121
natural environment, 20, 143
natural resources/supports, 143
negative feedback, attempts at stability, 6
negative feedback loops, as deviation reducing, 6
nonjudgmental, being, 150, 154
normalizing, 118–119

objectivity, 12
observation, assessing interactional patterns, 71–73
Ogles, B. M., 210
O'Hanlon, B., 70

O'Hara, M. M., 51
Ohio Scales, 209–210, 211, *212*, *214*, *215*, 221, 226–227, *229*, 230
Olson, D. H., 210
Open Dialogue Treatment, 81
Original Efficacy Study, 207
   data analyses, 211
   data collection methods, 208–209
   discussion and summary, 218–219
   findings, 211–218
   outcome variables, 209–211
   research participants, 207–208
Orlinsky, D. E., 50
out-of-control teenagers
   credit for improvement, 137, 141
   girls, 188–189
   safety measures, 69
out-of-session responses to tasks, 126
ownership questions, 122

paradoxical tasks, 131
parallel processes, 159
Parental Competence with Children measure, 217, *218*
Parental Efficacy Scale, 210
parental primacy, assumptions about, 23
parent empowerment model, 81. *See also* empowerment model
parent friendly
   practitioners as, 164
   support system, 143
parenting, social constructivism and, 11
parenting practices, as mechanism of change, 16
parents. *See also* divorce; family
   as agents of change, 43
   agreement on focus, 164
   blamed for children's problems, 56
   child improves but parental interaction does not change, 136
   engaging and collaborating with, 43–44
   giving them credit, 137
   goals and safety issues, 89
   goals they are motivated by, 85–86
   linear interventions with teens, 10
   seeing their children in foster care, 55–56
   who yell a great deal, 151
Parks, B. K., 50
partnership, client-practitioner, 16
pathways thinking, 84
patronizing behavior, by client, 169–170
patterns, exceptions to problem patterns, 11
pattern shift, 20
phone calls, 183
physical abuse, 88
physical discipline, 93
planning questions, 122
positive feedback
   described, 62
   use of term, 6–7
positive feedback loops
   as deviation amplifying, 6
   in family system, 16
   simple example, 62, *62*

as vicious cycles, 7
as virtuous cycles, 7
positive reframing, 54–56
    definition, 54–55
    examples of, 55–56
    how practitioners use, 99–100
posttraumatic stress disorder (PTSD)
    case, 29–30
    exposure therapy, 82
power
    family member with (definition), 57
    figuring out who has, 48, 57–58
    process of establishing goals and, 152
    of questions, 119–123
power struggles, 106, 154
practitioners
    assessing if in synch with family, 166–167
    beginning, 161, 171–172, 176
    buy-in to a model, 162
    client response to intervention interactional sequence, 31–32
    clinical choices available to, 29–30
    consultations with supervisor, 165–168
    "devil's advocate" position, 87
    disengaging from family after terminating, 142–143
    effective, form followed by, 149
    effective treatment rationales, 151
    empowered by I-FAST model, 159–160
    expanding skills of, 162–163
    family trusting, 159
    framing language, 105
    frustrations possible with model, 34
    genuineness, 153
    helping practitioners get unstuck, 178–179
    how to frame clients and families, 43
    imaginative response of, 35
    need for evidence-based approaches, vii
    being nonjudgmental, 150, 154
    point of view, considerations about, 110–111
    practice over research, 205
    proper attitude toward tasks, 124
    relationship with client, 14, 15, 41, 113–114
    as respectful cultural anthropologists, 49
    rigor and imagination of, 37
    sensitivity, 155
    understanding everyone's premises, motives, language, and positions, 49
    using their existing skill sets, 30–31, 66–67, 116
practitioner's judgment, 150, 160–161
precontemplative phase in stage of change model, 46
predicting relapses, 135, 137–138, 146
prediction tasks, 130–131
preparation phase stage of change model, 46
preserve, 123, 174
presuppositions, 119
    embedded in questions related to outcomes, 120
    use of pre-suppositional language, 63–64, 92
Price, J., 144
primary caregivers
    determining who is, 47
    empowering, 20, 45, 47
    engaging, 20
    as principal agents of change, 46

priming, 101
prioritizing, 22
probation officers (POs)
    acknowledging improvement, 141, 177
    ahead of family, 167
    in-home treatment versus, 139
    role at termination, 177
    teen's fear of the court, 141–142
problem definition, summary of basic skills, 78
problem-generated systems, 21
    validation and, 49
problem maintaining behavior. *See* interactional patterns
problem patterns, 19, 20, 24, 112, 152. *See also* interactional patterns
problems
    conceptualizing in relational terms, 16
    deconstructing in hopeful way, 74
    defining interactionally, 64
    difficulties turning into, 16
    domino effect, 110
    exploring unsuccessful attempts to solve, 70
    fluctuations in, 13
    humans as meaning makers, 151
    information about attempts not tried, 104–105
    mapping effects of
    multiple, 65
    new problems, 177–178
    overthinking or oversimplifying, 68, 172–173
    paradoxical tasks for, 131
    persistence of, 64–65
    problem-free periods, analyzing, 13
    problem identification basic skills, 78
    problem-saturated vicious cycle, 11
    solution-generated, 17
    as spirals of interaction, 1
    from systems perspective, 42
    think in opposites, 131–132
    tracking how clients frame problems, 103–104
    two criteria for, 64
    understanding the big picture, 47
    utilizing family's theories about, 106–107
    as vicious cycles, 1
    viewing them in behavioral terms, 65–66
    view of, 111
    youth being validated, 49
problem-saturated story, 11, 73, 112
    blaming, 113–114
Problem Severity Scale, 206, 209–210, 211, 212–213, *212, 214, 215,* 218–219, 221–223, *222, 224, 226,* 227–228, 229, 230–231, 232
procedures, 116
    definition, 14
    guidelines for developing, 152–153
psychotherapy
    as deficit-based approach, 112
    evidence-based common factors, 4–5
    integration, vii
    outcomes analyzed, 14
    stage model, 206

questions
    changing frames with, 120–123
    choice, 122

questions (*Cont.*)
  cognitive behavioral approach, 120
  comparison, 122
  connection, 122
  coping-type, 76–77
  difference, 122
  exception-type, 62, 75, 122
  exception-type, skills for, 75
  exploring, 122
  feasibility, 122
  functions of, 119
  goal setting and defining, 90–91
  helpfulness, 122
  indicator, 122
  as indirect method of suggesting new behavior, 122
  to initiate a self-evaluative process, 122–123
  interactional exceptions follow-up, 73
  as an intervention procedure, 119, 124
  leading to change, 119
  to learn status of problem, 74
  mere measurement effect, 119
  ownership, 122
  planning, 122
  power of, 119–123
  practitioner's response to clients' answers, 123
  pre-suppositional language in, 63–64
  "process," 71
  to reinforce or change behavior and interaction, 121–122
  relationship, 123
  scaling, 123
  sensitivity and skills, 174
  tracking habitual interactions and exceptions, 71, 74–77
  use of, 26
  use by supervisor, 172

Rains, L. A., 208
Randall, J., 187
rationales
  client acceptance of, 14
  developing effective treatment, 151
  framing and reframing procedures, 25
  as motivation for client action, 83
  practice procedures, 20
  task frames, 100–101
  for tasks offered, 125
  treatment frames and, 98–99
  validating the client, 117
reactance, 132
reactivity, 132
readiness, 115
reality, 11
  behavioral confirmation, 95–96
  "beneficial," 63
  deconstructing problems, 73–74
  first-order change and, 17
  multiple usable versions, 12–13
  positive reframing, 55
  role of language, 63–64
  socially constructed, 18
reframing, 95. *See also* deframing; framing
  effective, 100
  escalations in response to change, 146
  essential elements, 107–108
  as intervention procedure, 26
  key phases, 25
  positive reframing, 54–56
  practitioner adjusts to client responses, 102
  practitioner understandings, 151
  priming for spontaneity, 102
  for second-order change, 17
  three-step sequence, 31–32
  as trial balloon, 100
relapse
  after end of in-home treatment, 139–140, 141
  agency teams, 199
  anxiety as response to change, 135
  celebrating change to prevent, 115
  improvement ignored leading to, 135
  predicting, 135, 137–138, 146
  predicting and developing a prevention plan, 145–146
  prescribing a, 145–146
  strategies to build resilience, 26
relationship
  changes or shifts, 110
  practitioner-client, 14, 15, 110
relationship building, 113
relationship questions, 123
removal of child from the home, 141
  challenges, 187
research, 37
  additional studies on I-FAST, 231–232
  at-risk youth, I-FAST and MST compared, 223–231
  efficacy of I-FAST from 2004 to 2012, 219–223
  organization of chapters, 36
  original efficacy study, 207–219
  rationale for the research program, 205–207
resilience
  assumptions about, 22
  in face of challenges, 52
resilience building, 20
  conceptualizing, 134
  implementing, 137–139
  key phases, 26
  strategizing, 134–136
  tips for, 144–147
responsiveness
  assessing, 134
  guidelines for observing and responding to procedures, 153
  tracking change, 137
  types of responses to change, 134–136
  utilizing practitioner response to supervisor ideas, 161–162
restraints from change, 132, 137, 168
Rogers, C. R., 50
Rowland, M. D., 187

safety issues
  authorities' involvement, 89–90
  goals and, 88–89
  physical abuse, 88
  physical discipline, 93
safety plans, 69

Safranske, E. P., 160
Sanders, M. R., 148, 149
scaling questions, 123
    amplifying incremental changes, 144
    small steps to achieving goals, 121
Schoenwald, S. K., 187
school behavior problems, 135
    research on, 231–232
school phobic boy, 107, 137
second-order change, 17. *See also* first-order change
    goal setting and, 84
    interruption of habitual interactional patterns, 112
    positive framing and, 55
    reframing, 100
    strengths-based position, 112
    summarized, 19
Segal, I., 70
self-determination, goal setting and, 82–83
self-esteem, questions to change frame, 120
self-evaluative process, list of questions, 122–123
sense of purpose, developing a common, 83
sensitivity, 155
    with questions, 174
sequences of interaction, 51. *See also* interactional patterns
    systems perspective, 63
session break, 184
Sexton, T. S., 17
sexual molestation example, 58
Shiang, J., 28
single parent, teammate for, 144
skills
    evaluating practitioner's, 163
    expanding practitioner's, 162–163
    I-FAST treatment skills, 150–153, 163
Snyder, C. R., 84
social constructivism, 11–12. *See also* constructivism
    basic tenets, 11–12
    client view of reality, 12–13
    framing, 12–13
    I-FAST, 4
    parenting patterns, 11
    strengths-based perspective, 13
    summarized, 18
    utility of, 5
social interactions, knowledge of reality, 11
Socratic questioning, 121
soft restraints from change, 132
solution amplifying, 110
solution-focused practitioner
    questions to change frame, 120–121
    scaling questions, 121
solution-focused therapy, 74, 116, 120, 121, 162
solution-generated problems, 17
Soteria project, 81
spirals of interaction, problems and resolutions as, 1
spirals of problem, 1
Sprenkle, D. H., 14, 16
staff morale, 198–199
    models and settings, 162
    supervisor contact, 165
    team day, 181, 199

staff retention, agency, 192–193
stage of change model
    goals aligned with, 86–87
    phases, 46
    readiness, 115
stakeholders, 65
    domino effect, 110
    EB model adoption, 193
Stanton, M. D., 138
Staudinger, U. M., 44
stepparents, 136, 173
strategic involvement, assumptions about, 23
strategies
    definition, 99
    treatment rationales, 99
strategizing, 36
    engaging process, 45–49
    frames, framing, and deframing, 97–107
    goal setting, 84–90
    initiating change, 113–116
    problem defined, 64–65
strategy level. *See* I-FAST, Level II
strength-based language, 63
strength-based supervision, 160
strengths
    amplifying something desired, 7
    assumptions about, 22
    belief in, in systems theory, 11
    clients identifying, 52
    coping questions emphasizing, 77
    definition, 13, 44
    of each individual, 13
    in face of adversity, 52
    framing and, 97
    identifying interactions, 64
    tasks and, 126
strengths-based perspective, 13
    assumptions of, 44–45
    following up on interventions, 176
    initiating change, 112–113
    philosophical foundation, 13
    success with presenting problems, 44
    training in agencies, 33
structural family therapy, 127
supervising
    collaborative communication, 151
    listening to supervisees, 160
    training for supervisors, 200–201
    utilizing practitioner response to supervisor ideas, 161–162
supervision
    24/7 line of sight, 69
    case consultation, 164–165
    clinical supervisors, 201
    collaborative, 160
    flexibility in, 159
    identifying interactions, 171–172
    implementing, 164–186
    live, 182–185
    organization of chapters, 36
    as parallel process, 159
    practitioner adherence to model, 159
    strategizing, 162–164
    strengths-based, 160

supervision (*Cont.*)
    struggles with colleagues, 168
    supervisor/practitioner relationship, 160
    sustainability of empowerment model, 33
    sustained, 23
    team, 198
    team day, 181
    unit of analysis and getting unstuck, 172–173
    video use in, 180–181
    weekly consultation suggestions, 165–168
supervisors
    empowering, 197
    training, 197–198
supportive structure, 14
sustainability
    agency/model fit, 190–191
    consultant-supervisor relationship, 33
    of EB approaches in agency settings, 187
    of effective treatments, 189–190
    long-term, 191–193
    sustaining outcomes, 193–195
    three levels, 190, 202
    training and implementation, 191–193
sustained supervision, 23
systems
    definition, 5
    definition in I-FAST model, 21
    goals and functioning, 6
    integrative, use of term, 21
    multiple embedded, 17–18
    problem-generated, 21
systems approach, 1
systems collaboration, 17–18
    aligning goals, 88
    engaging (two-step) process, 59
systems-contextual perspective, 190
systems theory, 5–7
    change is constant, 10–11, 63
    described, 16
    engaging and, 42
    family as a system, 16
    I-FAST, 4
    initiating change, 109–110
    interactional patterns, 16
    interconnectedness and wholeness, 9–10
    practical implications, 9
    summarized, 18
    tracking interactions, 62–63
    utility of, 5
    vicious cycles, 7–8
    virtuous cycles, 8–9
Szapocznik, J., 57

tantrums, 63, 131
task frames, 100–101
tasks, 124–133
    between-session tasks, 128–129
    for changing identifying exceptions, 124
    for changing interactional patterns, 124
    common errors related to, 175–176
    complexity and goal attainment, 80
    devising, 125, 131, 174–176
    devising, steps involved, 174–175
    "enactments," 31
    as experiments, 167
    following-up on, skill sets, 126
    formula first session task, 130
    framing, 100–101
    framing so they will be accepted, 125
    in-session tasks, 72–73, 126–126
    keep track of current successes, 130
    making the task the client's, not the practitioner's, 126
    making use of whatever response the client gives, 126
    out-of-session tasks, 126
    paradoxical, 131
    practitioners' existing skill sets, 31
    prediction, 130–131
    proper attitude toward, 124
    skills for offering, 124–125
    strengths and, 126
    supervising practitioner use of, 174–176
    tracking responses to, 72–73, 125–126
    types of, 126–127
    use of, 26
teaching
    flexibility, 163
    I-FAST model, 159
    processing the interview, 184
    in supervision context, 159, 186
    videos for, 180
team day, 181
    live supervision, 182
    multiple goals, 198–199
team supervision, 198
teamwork and supervision models, 160
terminating
    common problems, 177–178
    conceptualizing, 139–140
    key phases, 26
    practice procedures, 20
    practitioner disengagement difficulties, 177–178
    strategizing, 140–141
    summary, 143–144
termination
    defining successful, 140
    developmentally appropriate behaviors after, 142
    as goal achievement, 140–141
    issues for home-based treatment, 141–143
    medications and psychiatrists, 142
    practitioner disengaging from, 142–143
    problems in supervision, 177–178
therapeutic alliance, 15–16
    change not occurring after, 58
    contextual model, 15
    definition, four elements of, 15
    elements in evidence-based approaches, 15–16
    goals of, 4
    as process of engagement, 41
    supervising, 169–170
therapeutic approaches analyzed, 14
therapeutic bond, establishing, 59
therapeutic contract, 85
therapeutic rationale, 19
therapeutic relationship, developing interventions and, 113–114
therapy, use of term, 21–22

think in opposites, 131
   positioning in relation to positions of others, 132
Third World episode of care models, 80–81
Todd, T. C., 138
tracking
   building resilience and terminating (phases), 26
   how clients frame problems, 103–104
   interactional exceptions, 73–77
   sustained supervision, 23
tracking change, 137
tracking interactions, 61–62
   assessing interactional patterns by interview, 70–71
   essential elements of, 77–78
   key phases, 24–25
   practice procedures, 20
   skills for, 70–77
   specific problem orientation, 64–65
   summary of basic skills, 77
   systems theory and, 62–63
   tracking interactional exceptions as focused skill, 73–77
   tracking interactional patterns, 70
tracking intervention, 70–78
tracking power, 57
   by observing decisions made and conflicts resolved, 57–58
"trainer of trainers" model, 197, 200
training, in agency setting, 191
   costs, 191–192
   hidden (uncompensated) costs, 192
   how other professionals receive the model, 193
   issues, 197–198, 200
   new staff, 200
   phases, 200–201
   staff productivity, 192
   staff retention, 192–193
   strategically designed packages for, 200–201
   strengths-based, 33
transform, client's statement to new frame, 123, 174
treatment
   active client involvement related to outcome, 50
   agency settings, 194–194
   assessing where the case is in the process, 166
   behavioral experiments or trial balloons, 36
   bona fide approach, 205–206
   changing who participates, 176–177
   clear directions for, 82
   clinical choices, 29–30
   continuity of care, 194–195
   decisions and key choices, 28–30
   experimental nature of, 134
   flexibility, 36
   focus on common sense of purpose, 83
   focus on something specific, 67
   goal setting for, 82, 85–86
   how to make therapeutic choices, 30, 32
   importance of goals, 79, 82
   listing what worked/successes, 146–147
   location for, 48
   need to adjust if no progress, 14
   as parallel to supervision, 159
   path of least resistance, 110
   powerful family members and, 57
   practitioners' existing skill sets, 31, 66–67
   problems, 178–180
   pure form family treatment approaches, 3–4
   in stages, 110
   sustainability, 189–190
   use of term, 21–22
   whom to include, guidelines, 45–46, 67
treatment fidelity, measuring, 208, 218, 220, 225, 230, 232
treatment frames
   flexibility with, 97–98
   rationales and, 98–99
treatment models
   adherence to, 148–149
   allegiance to, 149
treatment problems, 178–180
treatment process
   of change, 23
   outcomes as common factors, 23
treatment rationales, 96, 98–99
   assumptions about, 22
   practice procedures, 19
   strategies and, 99
triangulation. *See* interactional patterns
Turner, J., 160
Tyron, G. S., 85

undiagnosed medical problems, 54
unique outcomes, identifying, 121
unit of analysis, 66
   changing as case unfolds, 68
   clinical choices, 29
   dictated by the manual, 29
   getting unstuck, 172–173
   guidelines for deciding on, 66–68
   pros and cons of small units, 68
   supervising, 172–173
utilization, utilizing how clients respond to problems, 104
utilizing the family's beliefs and theories, 106–107

validation
   allowing time for airing problem, 172
   client receptiveness and, 73
   as crossover intervention, 117
   as directional and empathic, 51
   empathy and, 50–51
   of practitioner concerns, 165
   as practitioner-initiated process, 49
   second-order change, 117
values. *See* client values
vicious cycles, 7–8, 7
   assumptions about, 22
   as a common factor, 17
   concept summarized, 19
   dynamics of, 11
   in family systems, 16
   interactional patterns, 7–8
   linear interventions, 10
   as negative escalating change, 10
   not desirable, 7
   positive feedback loops, 7
   practice procedures, 19
   practitioner approach, 7

vicious cycles (*Cont.*)
   problems as, 1, 8, *8*
   repeated interactions, 7, *8*
video use in supervision, 180–181
   tips for video review, 181
viewing and doing, 5
   concepts or frames of stakeholders, 65
   problems in behavioral terms, 65–66
viewpoint, individual as meta-frame, 13
virtuous cycles, 8–9
   assumptions about, 22
   concept summarized, 19
   definition, 9, *9*
   interactional exceptions, 9, *9*
   positive feedback loops as, 7
   practice procedures, 19
visitors, family as, 115

Wampold, B. E., 14, 15, 98, 148, 149, 205
Ward, D. M., 187

Watkins, C. E., 160
Watzlawick, P., 62
Weakland, J. H., 70, 140
Western medicine, 80–81
Whitaker, C., 45
Winograd, G., 85
Woodhouse, S. S., 51
working alliance, 19
World Health Organization (WHO), 80

youth
   acting-out, 105
   conduct disorder, 127–128
   fear of the court, 141–142
   hostile exchanges with parents, 64, 90–91
   low self-esteem, 106
   power struggle, 106, 154
   safety plan for out-of-control teens, 69
   suicidal, 106
   teen defiance, 73, 87, 123

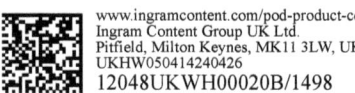
www.ingramcontent.com/pod-product-compliance
Ingram Content Group UK Ltd.
Pitfield, Milton Keynes, MK11 3LW, UK
UKHW050414240426
12048UKWH00020B/1498